MANUAL FOR
VASCULAR MEDICINE
AND
SURGERY

CONTRIBUTORS

George Constantinopoulos, M.D.
Fellow in Vascular Surgery, Department of Surgery,
Hahnemann Medical College & Hospital, Philadelphia, Pennsylvania

Norman Doherty, M.D.
Fellow in Vascular Surgery, Department of Surgery,
Hahnemann Medical College & Hospital, Philadelphia, Pennsylvania

A. Mohsen Kholoussy, M.D., F.R.C.S.
Assistant Professor, Director of Surgical Research,
Department of Surgery, Hahnemann Medical College & Hospital,
Philadelphia, Pennsylvania

Teruo Matsumoto, M.D., Ph.D., F.A.C.S.
Professor and Chairman, Department of Surgery,
Hahnemann Medical College & Hospital, Philadelphia, Pennsylvania

Thomas J. Matulewski, M.D.
Assistant Professor, Department of Surgery,
Hahnemann Medical College & Hospital, Philadelphia, Pennsylvania

David Naide, M.D.
Associate Professor of Medicine, Chief, Division of Vascular Disease,
Department of Medicine, Hahnemann Medical College & Hospital,
Philadelphia, Pennsylvania

Stanley Spitzer, M.D.
Professor of Medicine,
Hahnemann Medical College & Hospital, Philadelphia, Pennsylvania

MANUAL FOR
VASCULAR
MEDICINE
AND
SURGERY

Teruo Matsumoto, M.D., Ph.D., F.A.C.S.

Professor and Chairman
Department of Surgery
Hahnemann Medical College & Hospital
Philadelphia, Pennsylvania

and

Chairman, Department of Vascular Surgery
Haverford Community Hospital
Havertown, Pennsylvania

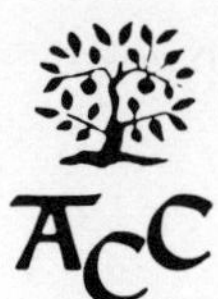

APPLETON–CENTURY–CROFTS/Norwalk, Connecticut

Prentice-Hall International, Inc., London
Prentice-Hall of Australia, Pty. Ltd., Sydney
Prentice-Hall of India Private Limited, New Delhi
Prentice-Hall of Japan, Inc., Tokyo
Prentice-Hall of Southeast Asia (Pte.) Ltd., Singapore
Whitehall Books Ltd., Wellington, New Zealand

Library of Congress Cataloging in Publication Data
Main entry under title:

Manual for Vascular Medicine and Surgery.

Includes index.
1. Blood-vessels—Surgery. I. Matsumoto, Teruo.
[DNLM: 1. Vascular surgery—Handbooks. WG 170 H236]
RD598.5.M36   617′.413   81–17638
ISBN 0–8385–6132–2   A6132–3

Text and cover design: Jean M. Sabato

CONTENTS

PREFACE

A sound understanding of the clinical significance of vascular diseases is essential. Training in the interpretation of new laboratory data is sadly lacking in medical and postgraduate course work.

Rapid development in the sophisticated technology of diagnosis and progress in surgical procedures as well as in formal training in vascular medicine and surgery have resulted in rapid progress in the management of peripheral vascular diseases in which loss of limb or life was not uncommon in years past.

The objective of this book is to combine medical and surgical approaches for the diagnosis and management of peripheral vascular disease. Therefore, this book is designed to supply students, residents, and clinicians with current information regarding pathophysiology, methods of instrumentation, precise surgical indication, and clear techniques. All controversial aspects of management are limited to a simple, well-accepted concept.

The editor wishes to convey his appreciation to Ruby M. Padolina, M.D., our excellent anesthesiologist, and the many physicians in and out of this institution who provided me with numerous complicated cases. ''Medical Views'' was written by David Naide, M.D., and I want to thank him for his understanding in giving me the liberty to exercise editorial prerogative on this part. My special gratitude is extended to Catherine M. Donahue, R.N., my longtime scrub nurse, for her encouragement to complete this book within the deadline. My sincere appreciation is also extended to Joyce Palczewski, R.N., who worked with me for over eight months. The interest, assistance, and support of the publisher is, of course, most greatly acknowledged.

Teruo Matsumoto, M.D., Ph.D
Bryn Mawr, Pennsylvania

PART ONE

Medical Views

CHAPTER ONE

Arteriosclerosis Obliterans

INTRODUCTION

Evaluation of patients with arterial insufficiency, especially of an *atherosclerotic nature,* must reflect the natural history of the disease. In spite of best efforts of treatment, these patients continue to have an unremitting *progression of lipid deposition* with further arterial narrowing even with successful bypass grafts. Many of these patients have other medical problems, including *angina, emphysema,* and *diabetes,* so that a holistic approach must be assumed before the performance of invasive studies and/or arterial reconstructive surgery.

DIAGNOSIS

History

The most common symptom of diminished arterial flow to the extremity is *intermittent claudication.* An important aspect of this symptom is how it affects the patient's activities of daily living, especially if it alters his ability to earn a living. The level of occlusion determines the location of the claudication. In addition, as the process becomes more severe, the patient may develop ischemic nonhealing *ulcerations* of the feet and/or *rest pain.* When either of these conditions is present, it becomes imperative to proceed with further work-up. Ischemic rest pain tends to be worse at night and is aggravated by elevation or a *cold environment.* Impotence is a common complaint in the male patient with pelvic ischemia secondary to disease of the aortic bifurcation. Acute arterial occlusion may produce severe ischemia because of the lack of time to develop adequate collaterals. These patients may manifest neurologic deficits. Patients with ischemic neuritis require prompt attention to prevent it from becoming permanent.

Physical Examination

Bedside evaluation of a patient with arterial insufficiency can be done in a relatively short period of time. From the information obtained by physical examination, the level of an existing arterial occlusion and the *degree of ischemia* can be determined. All of the peripheral pulses should be examined, including pedal pulses, radial and ulnar pulses, and subclavian pulses. Pulses may be graded from 0 to 4 where 0 is absent, 3 is normal, and 4 *represents an aneurysm.* The popliteal arteries should always be examined since an existing popliteal aneurysm will be overlooked if examination is not directed to this area. The popliteal is one of the more difficult pulses to palpate and requires firm bimanual pressure with the fingertips in the popliteal space and *counterpressure with the thumbs* in the front of the knee with the knee joint relaxed. It often takes several seconds of this firm pressure to palpate the popliteal pulse. It is often not immediately palpable possibly because of the relative insensitivity of the fingertips from the firm pressure.

The examiner should carefully auscultate for bruits over the carotids, subclavians, femorals, and popliteals as well as the abdominal aorta and iliacs. A *bruit,* when present, indicates flow turbulence, which might indicate stenosis or aneurysmal dilatation of the vessel.

Delay in *capillary filling time* indicates skin ischemia. First, the skin of the foot should be blanched by digital pressure. On release of pressure, a delay in *reactive hyperemia* indicates poor arterial inflow. One of the most useful bedside maneuvers for evaluating peripheral perfusion takes only 1 minute. This involves elevating the feet for one full minute and observing for abnormal pallor on elevation. The degree of pallor may be graded with 0 representing no pallor in 60 seconds and 3 representing pallor in less than 30 seconds. The feet normally retain a mild pink color even after a full minute of elevation. The feet are then quickly placed in the dependent position, which should produce blushing or color return to the feet within 5 seconds and venous filling of the veins on the dorsum of the foot within 15 seconds, provided that the arterial inflow is normal. However, if the patient has varicosities or venous insufficiency, there may be retrograde venous flow producing rapid venous filling of the feet, which, of course, would invalidate this test as a measure of arterial flow. A severely ischemic foot will develop rubor, a red-blue intense discoloration, on prolonged dependency (1 to 2 minutes).

The Allen test can be used to confirm patency of the radial and ulnar

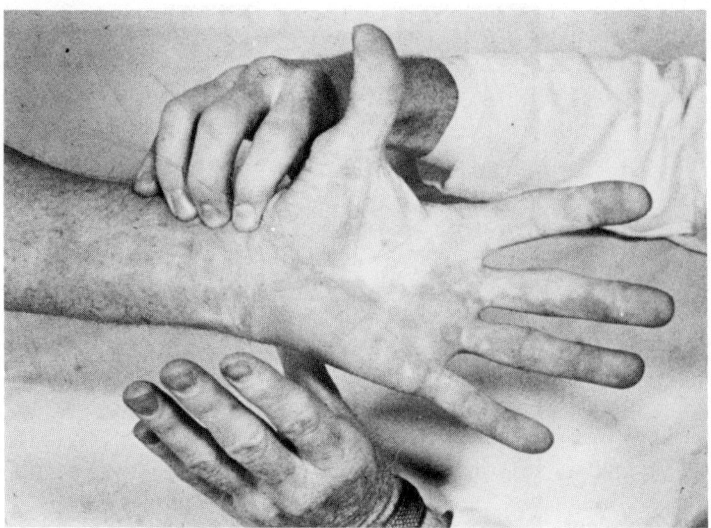

Figure 1-1. Positive Allen test.

arteries in the upper extremity (Fig. 1-1). It is performed by elevating the arm, applying firm pressure over the radial and ulnar arteries to occlude the flow, and having the patient open and close his fist three or four times. This will produce blanching. The hand can then be placed in a dependent position, and the radial or ulnar artery is selectively released. The hand is observed for return of flow down the side on which the arterial inflow was released. The extremities should be checked for temperature changes; in particular, the left and right extremities should be compared for differences in temperature. The skin of the hands or feet should be carefully examined for trophic changes secondary to the ischemia. The skin of a foot with chronic lack of circulation is rather thin and atrophic, perhaps with development of calluses at pressure points of the soles. The nails often show irregular and rather slow growth, and there is frequently a decrease or absence of hair growth on the toes, especially in the presence of severe ischemia. The presence of hair growth on the toes of a foot with chronic ischemia implies adequate arterial flow for healing of an ischemic lesion.

Oscillometric readings can be helpful. The cuff of an oscillometer or, if not available, the cuff of any sphygmomanometer is placed around the ankle, calf, thigh, upper extremity above the wrist, or forearm. The cuff is inflated between systolic and diastolic pressures. Movement of the needle with the aneroid-type sphygmomanometer or bouncing of the mercury with the mercury-type sphygmomanometer represents a semiquantitative measure of arterial flow.

There are two interesting observations that can be made in patients with ischemia: (1) Should a patient have a distal superficial femoral or popliteal occlu-

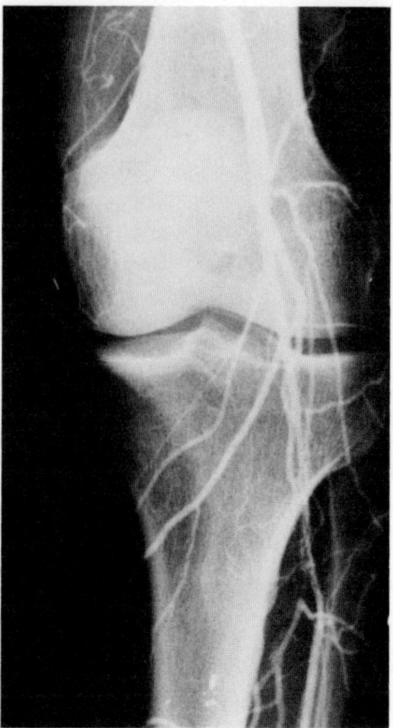

Figure 1-2. The genicular collaterals.

sion, the knee area is often found to be much *warmer* than the other parts of the limb. At times, this is thought to represent an inflammatory process in the knee. However, the explanation is that with this type of popliteal occlusion there is shunting of blood through the collaterals, which, in this case, are the genicular arteries located superficially (Fig. 1-2). The shunting leads to added warmth in the skin about the knee. (2) Patients who have severe ischemia and rest pain may present with significant lower-extremity edema as well as rubor in the involved limb. We have found the reason for this is that the rest pain is aggravated by elevating the legs or by lying flat in bed. Apparently, these patients often sleep in a chair or with the ischemic limb hanging in a dependent position, over the side of the bed. This constant day-and-night dependency leads to significant edema.

Physical examination of the arterial system can usually be completed within 5 minutes. Should abnormalities be found or if the physical examination does not agree with the history, then further studies are indicated.

Noninvasive Evaluation

Many institutions now have a noninvasive laboratory for evaluation of peripheral vascular disease. Valuable information can be obtained with the *Dop-*

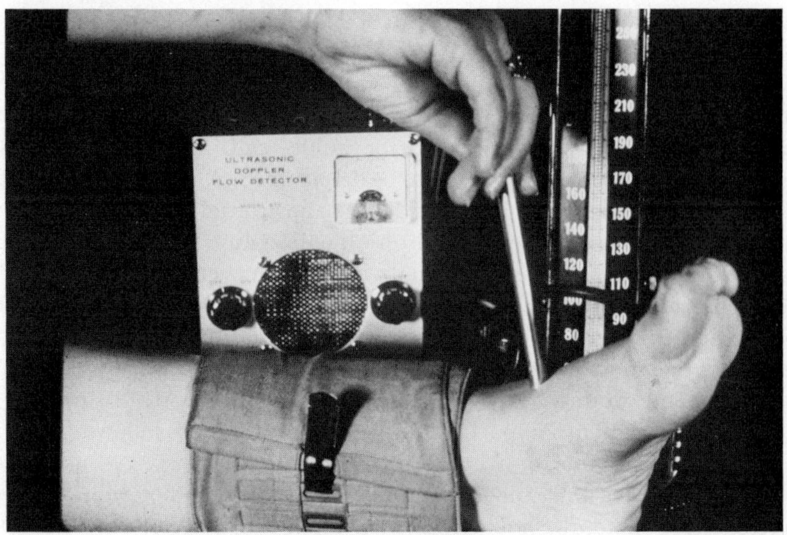

Figure 1-3. Doppler pressure measurement.

pler ultrasound blood flow detector and an ordinary blood pressure cuff (Fig. 1-3). The Doppler instrument is able to detect blood flow in small vessels such as the pedal arteries, even in the absence of a pulsatile flow. A blood pressure cuff is inflated around the ankle, calf, or thigh until the flow sound disappears or until the flow sound reappears as the pressure cuff is released. This procedure detects the blood pressure at the level of the cuff. Blood flow is not significantly lowered until an artery is 70 to 80 percent stenotic. Beyond 80 percent stenosis, flow is rapidly reduced (Fig. 1-4). Although information about blood flow is more important

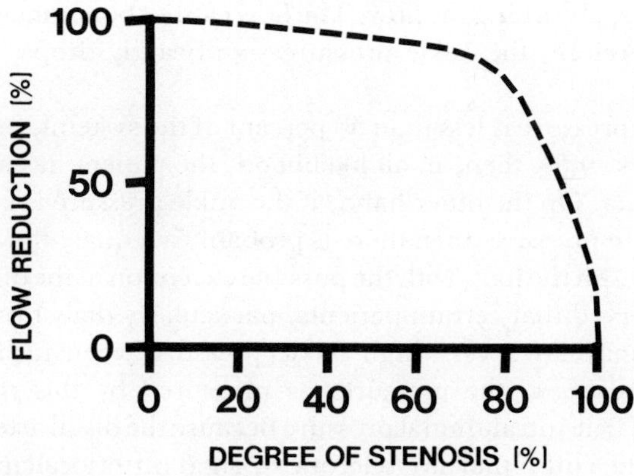

Figure 1-4. Arterial stenosis and flow reduction.

than information about blood pressure, blood flow cannot be precisely measured by noninvasive means.

Increased resistance such as occlusion of all three popliteal trifurcation vessels increases the popliteal artery pressure, but the flow remains very low. Pressures can thus be determined at the ankle, calf, and thigh level. Arm pressure (systemic pressure) should also be determined. A significant drop-off in pressure at any level is presumptive evidence of an arterial stenosis or an arterial occlusion proximal to the level of the drop-off in pressure. In addition, the quality of the flow sound can be helpful in that a biphasic or even triphasic type of flow sound represents normal peripheral flow with no proximal obstruction. However, if the flow sound is heard distal to an arterial occlusion, the second or third part of the flow sound is dampened, and a broader-based, lower-pitched, or flat type of flow sound is heard. Measurement of ankle blood pressure with the Doppler can be useful in comparing one leg with the other, in following up a patient over a period of time, or in evaluating the results of arterial reconstruction.

Measurement of ankle blood pressure with the Doppler before and after exercise can be very helpful. Should a patient present with a history of typical intermittent claudication and with physical examination showing the presence of all peripheral pulses, reassessment of ankle blood pressure after exercise is very important. The patient can be exercised by the treadmill or by jogging in place for 30 to 60 seconds. Under normal circumstances, ankle blood pressure changes little, if at all, after exercise. However, should there be proximal arterial stenosis such as a narrowed segment in the abdominal aorta or iliac arteries, the ankle blood pressure, which may have been minimally reduced before exercise, usually markedly drops immediately following exercise and gradually returns to the baseline reading within a few minutes. This confirms a diagnosis of proximal arterial stenosis. Also, in this situation, pedal pulses will disappear, and oscillations will drop. The explanation is that adequate flow at rest renders palpable pedal pulses and good ankle blood pressure, but with exercise the vascular bed in the muscle dilates, absorbing the flow. The flow cannot be augmented because of the stenosis; therefore, the ankle pressure significantly drops, and the pedal pulse disappears.

If the ankle pressure is less than 50 percent of the systemic or arm pressure (ischemic index < 0.5), then, in all likelihood, the patient has a rather severe degree of ischemia. On the other hand, if the ankle pressure is greater than 50 percent of the arm pressure, then there is probably adequate flow for healing of an ischemic lesion on the foot, with the possible exception of the diabetic patient. Lastly, it is observed that certain patients, particularly diabetics with sclerotic distal arteries, may have very high ankle pressure when measured by this method. In these cases, the pressure, as measured by this method, is not representative of true intraluminal pressure because the distal arteries cannot be compressed by the cuff if they are sclerotic or rigid (arteriocalcinosis).

Instrumentation for studying venous disease will not be discussed at this time. A *pulse volume recorder* (PVR) may also be used by itself and in conjunction with the Doppler. Pulse *waveforms* can be recorded graphically and analyzed. Other types of plethysmography include the mercury strain gauge type and pneumatic types. These have been used but are more complex and less useful in the clinical evaluation of patients.

The response of skin temperature in the toes or fingers to exposure to cold or heat of the trunk may give information about the extent of vasospasm and the extent of peripheral perfusion. These texts are usually done at constant room temperature (20°C). Patients with vasospasm will take a longer time to begin warming up and will do so more slowly; eventually, however, they reach a reasonably normal temperature level. If there is arterial occlusive disease, body heating is much slower and never reaches a normal level.

Isotopic measurements of blood flow are performed by injecting radioisotope into the calf muscle and measuring the disappearance rate. The better the arterial blood flow to the limb, the more rapid the disappearance of the isotope. This procedure has been useful more on a research than on a clinical basis; in fact, it has not been used clinically to any great extent. However, another isotope study that also fits into the noninvasive category is an *isotope angiogram* in which radioisotope technetium (Tc 99) is injected into an arm vein. Scanning can then be performed in indicated areas such as the abdominal aorta or iliac area. Crude but sometimes helpful displays that give some information about the extent of arterial occlusive disease can be obtained. In addition, the isotope angiogram has proved helpful in the determination of the patency of bypass grafts in which there may be a question of graft occlusion.

Arteriography

In general, arteriography is not indicated unless arterial reconstructive surgery is contemplated. The patient's symptoms dictate the need to proceed with arterial reconstructive surgery, and the patient must be agreeable to the surgical approach. Arteriography alone is not necessary to map out the extent or level of arterial occlusion unless this information is used in the management of the patient.

For a lower-extremity problem, the usual procedure is the introduction of a catheter through a needle into an appropriate artery, usually the common femoral artery. This is the *Seldinger technique.* If there is no femoral pulse, catheter introduction may be done through the axillary artery. On rare occasions, neither of these sites is suitable, and resort to a translumbar aortogram is indicated. If there is a good femoral pulse and there is no question of stenosis proximal to the common femoral artery, a less extensive study may be performed by a needle puncture femoral arteriogram. In either case, it is important to obtain films of the distal leg for evaluation of the runoff. In addition to mapping out the appropriate arterial system, it is important to assess the inflow proximal to the area where arterial reconstruction is contemplated, and it is even more important to examine carefully the *runoff* below the contemplated lower end of the graft anastomosis. Should the runoff be inadequate to maintain a good flow through the graft, the chance of maintaining graft patency is significantly reduced.

TREATMENT

Medical Management

Treatment of patients with atherosclerotic occlusive disease should reflect assumption of a progressive disease. However, of all patients with arterial occlusive disease, only about 10 percent require or have arterial reconstructive surgery. The remaining 90 percent of patients must be managed medically. The aims of treatment include (1) avoiding breakdown of skin, (2) attempting to promote development of collaterals to relieve pain, (3) treating areas of skin breakdown when they develop, and (4) treating underlying medical conditions that might affect the peripheral circulation, including diabetes, hypertension, and obesity.

Prophylactic foot care remains the cornerstone of avoiding skin breakdown that may lead to amputation. Many amputations start out with faulty trimming of the toenails. Therefore, patients must be carefully instructed on toenail care as well as daily inspection and cleansing of the feet, especially between the toes. In the case of poor vision or unsteady hands, the toenails should be trimmed by a podiatrist, not by the patient. Ingrown toenails, corns, and calluses should be promptly treated by a podiatrist, who should be aware of the patient's arterial insufficiency. Patients should be carefully instructed on avoiding unnecessary mechanical or thermal injury to the feet. Tight shoes that may create a blister should be avoided. Patients must avoid unnecessary exposure to cold, which has a vasoconstrictive effect. It is strongly recommended that people who smoke give up this habit. Patients who *cease* smoking have a lower incidence of amputation. Blood lipids are checked, and if they are abnormal, appropriate diet is recommended. If there is elevation of the pre β-lipoprotein (triglycerides), the patient is placed on a low-carbohydrate diet. Should there be elevation of the beta lipoprotein (cholesterol), the proper diet is one of low fat. The return of blood lipids to normal does not necessarily reflect a slowing of the progression of atherosclerosis. In any case, significant elevation of blood lipids should be treated. The best stimulus for the development of collaterals is lower-extremity exercise. Patients are encouraged to walk frequently. Other forms of exercise, including jogging, bicycling, and swimming, are helpful if the patient is able to engage in these activities.

There is no convincing evidence that vasodilator drugs are of any great value to patients with chronic arterial occlusive disease. To patients with vasospastic problems, these drugs may have some value. When skin breakdown develops, it can be treated with room temperature or lukewarm compresses (never hot) and, on occasions, very meticulous débridement. It is important to emphasize that extensive débridement of an ischemic lesion should never be done because more often than not a larger lesion results. Analgesics should be administered to patients with ischemic lesions, especially those with rest pain. This pain is often more noticeable at night, and for many patients bedtime is the only time an analgesic for relief of rest pain is necessary. Patients with rest pain often obtain relief at night by a 5-inch elevation of the head end of the bed, allowing the benefit of gravity to direct blood flow to the lower extremities. The heel and malleoli of a peripheral ischemia patient who is in bed for any prolonged period are especially prone to breakdown from pressure against the sheet or mattress. Therefore, these areas should be properly padded, or the leg itself should be minimally elevated so that the heel and malleoli do not touch the sheet. Compound tincture of benzoin applied prophylactically to the heel may help prevent breakdown. It is very discouraging to find that a patient hospitalized for a nonvascular problem such as hernia repair, myocardial infarction, or hip surgery complains of discomfort in the heel about 1 week after admission and that on examination a black ulcerating area is discovered over the heel. *These pressure sores are usually preventable.*

Indications for Arterial Reconstruction

The aim of arterial reconstructive surgery is to preserve the limb and to maintain or provide an improved level of function in the extremity. Arterial reconstruction does not increase life expectancy but makes life more comfortable. There are three main indications for proceeding with surgical intervention for peripheral ischemia. These are: (1) nonhealing *ischemic ulceration* or break in the skin on the foot. If an ischemic lesion develops and the existing blood supply appears inadequate to achieve healing in a reasonable period of time, arteriography with a view toward bypass surgery is indicated. Delay until the ischemic ulcer is large should be avoided because such ulceration may precipitate loss of a limb due to extensive irreversible tissue necrosis. Indeed, one should attempt to ascertain that the limb is salvageable before proceeding with arterial surgery. (2) A second important indication for surgery is *disabling claudication*. What is disabling for one person may not be disabling for another. If the claudication interferes with the patient's earning a livelihood or with the patient's enjoying activities of daily living, bypass surgery is considered in light of the patient's ability to tolerate the proposed surgery from a general medical standpoint. For example, a 50-year-old whose two-block claudication prevents him from pursuing his or her usual employment is a candidate for arterial reconstruction. A 70-year-old with two-block claudication who does very little walking is not a candidate. (3) The third indication for surgical intervention in the treatment of peripheral ischemia is *rest pain*. When the peripheral tissues are severely ischemic such that ischemic rest pain is present, even the slightest trauma is likely to lead to skin breakdown with threat of loss of limb. A patient in this situation frequently has constant pain and is unable to sleep at night. Therefore, bypass surgery should be considered for such a patient. Arteriography should be undertaken only when arterial surgery is indicated and the patient is willing to undergo the proposed surgery. For instance, a patient presenting with a good femoral pulse such that a femoropopliteal bypass graft is indicated to revascularize the foot is a more likely candidate for surgery than a similar patient who requires an aortobifemoral bypass graft. A holistic approach in the evaluation of patients is necessary before the performance of surgery. There is no point in relieving one-block intermittent calf claudication in a patient who is likely to develop angina secondary to coronary insufficiency or dyspnea secondary to emphysema. Years ago *diabetics* were not considered as candidates for bypass surgery because of distal small vessel disease. Today, arteriography is undertaken whether or not the patient has diabetes, and a decision as to the feasibility of bypass surgery is made, depending on the findings. Information to be obtained by arteriography includes (1) the site of occlusion, (2) the status of the inflow vessels proximal to the primary occlusion, and (3) the runoff or outflow tract distal to the level of occlusion. Should the distal runoff prove insufficient to maintain adequate flow through the bypass graft, arterial reconstruction is not indicated.

Nonoperative Treatment of Atherosclerotic Obstruction

As a bridge between medical treatment and surgical intervention in the management of patients with arterial occlusive disease, percutaneous transluminal arterial dilatation is now available. The original impetus for this work came from Charles Dotter, who first reported a percutaneous approach to the dilation of arteries by forcing progressively larger catheters over a spring guide wire down the femoral artery. More recently, this procedure has been refined and further developed by Gruntzig. The procedure is known as *percutaneous transluminal angioplasty* (PTA) or balloon catheter dilatation. It involves passing a very thin catheter via a percutaneous approach through a stenotic area in an artery. The balloon is then inflated to a point where it will compress the athermanous material. The action of the balloon is analogous to an individual's stepping on to deep powdered snow and thereby compressing the snow (Fig. 1–5). The Dotter procedure never gained wide acceptance. However, the Gruntzig procedure, which seems less likely to produce distal emboli, has recently been performed in various centers. While initial results of selected cases such as a localized, non-calcified stenosis appear promising, long-term assessment cannot be made for a number of years.

Types of Arterial Reconstruction and Graft Material

Arterial reconstructive surgery has been performed only for the last 25 years. It is interesting that a 1950 textbook on peripheral vascular disease makes no men-

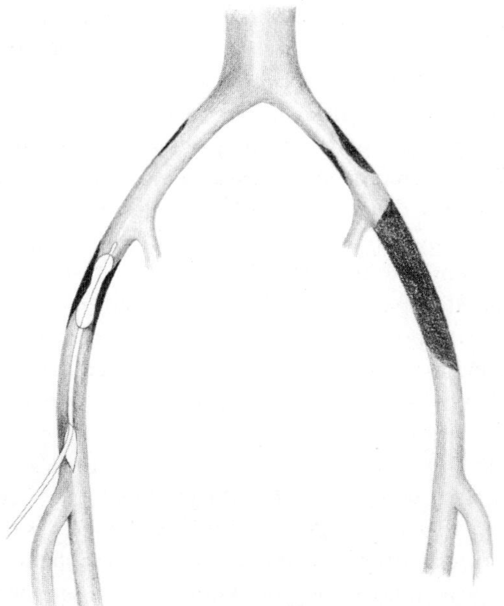

Figure 1-5. Intraluminal balloon angioplasty.

tion of bypass surgery or other reconstructive procedures. The only operations for arterial insufficiency performed at that time were sympathectomy and amputation.

Again, it is emphasized that proper indications based on symptomatology, physical findings, and noninvasive studies should be present before proceeding with arterial reconstruction. In addition, the patient must be agreeable to the procedure and must be able to tolerate the proposed surgery from a medical standpoint. From a morbidity standpoint, arterial reconstructive surgery can be divided into two categories. (1) Those procedures, such as an aortofemoral bypass, that produce relief of obstruction above the *inguinal* ligament are considered major surgery. (2) A bypass procedure in the leg of a patient with no significant proximal lesion and in whom the primary site of occlusion is below the inguinal ligament is just as time consuming and even more meticulous than an aortofemoral bypass. However, a femoropopliteal bypass procedure carries with it a lower morbidity rate. Even patients in their eighties will usually tolerate a femoropopliteal bypass graft, especially if it is done under regional anesthesia, whereas the same patients would have an increased morbidity and greater risk of mortality with an aortofemoral bypass.

If the site of occlusion is in the infrarenal abdominal aorta or in the iliac artery, the procedure of choice is aortofemoral or aortoiliac bypass, which is usually performed with prosthetic Dacron grafts. If there is significant bilateral involvement, the graft is Y-shaped, bifurcating to both iliac arteries or both common femoral arteries. Because this represents a major intra-abdominal procedure, the reconstruction of these lesions carries a higher risk.

An interesting group of patients with premature atherosclerosis developing in the aortoiliac segment has been observed. This syndrome is more common in females. Frequently, the distal vessels are either less involved or not involved at all. The narrowing may extend into the femoral area. These patients are best managed with aortobifemoral bypass grafts.

Femoropopliteal bypasses may be constructed above or below the knee joint. Runoff below the popliteal artery with patency of all three popliteal trifurcation vessels (anterior tibial, posterior tibial, peroneal) is considered excellent runoff. If two of these vessels are open, the runoff is considered to be fair. If one vessel is open, the runoff is considered to be poor. The presence of further stenosis in any of the three runoff vessels may modify the above classification. If there is significant narrowing at or below the popliteal artery, reconstruction of a more widely patent vessel in the leg at calf level or below is that of femoral-to-tibial bypass or peroneal artery bypass. The reversed saphenous vein is the ideal conduit for this bypass. If the saphenous vein is not present or if it is found to be unsuitable as a graft, synthetic grafts or an arm vein of adequate length is used. Various synthetic graft materials such as Dacron and Dacron-Velour have been used in the past. In recent years, several new materials have been employed. These include: (1) expanded, reinforced polytetrafluoroethylene (PTFE) (Goretex®; Impra®) grafts. At this time, they show promise of an improved patency rate. One advantage of these grafts is that if they thrombose, the clot is not very adherent, and thrombectomy can be performed even several weeks after thrombosis. However, long-term conclusions cannot be drawn. (2) Glutaraldehyde-*tanned human umbilical cord vein.* These umbilical cord veins are surrounded by a Dacron mesh for additional support. Again, more widespread use over a longer period of time is necessary before any conclusions can be drawn about the efficacy of this graft material. In summary, the present state of the art requires the statement that the ideal material for bypass graft below the common femoral artery is still the reversed saphenous vein.

Several other procedures are worthy of note. Some vascular surgeons advocate *endarterectomy* for relatively short segmental occlusions. While this procedure may bring about excellent initial results, development of reaccumulation of atheromatous material in the previously endarterectomized segment is not uncommon. Thus, while a few vascular surgeons might still choose to perform this procedure, it is not indicated as an isolated procedure except at the carotid bifurcation area, in the profunda femoris artery, or, on rare occasions, in the larger vessels such as the abdominal aorta or iliac arteries.

Profundaplasty is another procedure that at times is very useful. The proximal portion of the profunda femoris artery should always be examined whenever a bypass graft is anastomosed to the common femoral region. If any significant stenosis is present, an endarterectomy with or without a vein patch is often indicated. A limb will not survive if both the superficial femoral and the profunda arteries are occluded. Profundaplasty has been referred to as a limb salvage procedure where no other type of bypass is feasible and the patient has a superficial femoral artery occlusion. In this case, the profunda may act as a significant large collateral vessel, and if a proximal stenosis can be relieved, there may be a significant increase in flow to the ischemic foot.

Another group of procedures that should be in the armamentarium of all vascular surgeons are the *extra-anatomic bypass grafts*. If a patient has an aortoiliac occlusion with significant signs or symptoms that necessitate some procedure to increase flow but is too ill to undergo aortofemoral bypass, a synthetic graft from the axillary artery to the common femoral artery may be implanted. This graft is implanted subcutaneously so that neither the thoracic or abdominal cavity is entered. If necessary, this surgery can be performed under local anesthesia. If there is significant involvement on the opposite side, a cross-femoral limb can be added to the graft, making this an axillobifemoral bypass graft. It seems that this procedure has the advantage over two separate axillofemoral grafts inasmuch as it increases the flow through the primary axillofemoral graft, thus ensuring a higher likelihood of long-term patency. If a patient has unilateral iliac occlusion with no stenosis on the opposite iliac artery or in the abdominal aorta and is deemed unsuitable for major abdominal surgery, a cross-over femoral bypass alone is indicated. There are conflicting data in the literature as to long-term patency of extra-anatomic bypass grafts. Some of the most optimistic reports suggest a 70 to 80 percent 5-year patency rate. However, many centers performing extensive vascular surgery do not share this optimistic view.

A rare cause of popliteal artery occlusion is *adventitial cystic degeneration* of the popliteal artery. It is most commonly seen in children and young adults and probably represents a congenital anomaly. The usual treatment involves bypass with a short segment of reversed saphenous vein.

A few other points are worthy of mention in reference to the management of patients who have arterial reconstruction. Conservative measures in the treatment of patients with arterial insufficiency are important. It is of the utmost importance that the patient avoid pressure on the heels and malleoli when lying in bed, as even light pressure will blanch out what little blood perfuses the ischemic foot. A foam-rubber heel protector should be applied, or the leg itself should rest on a soft surface so that the heel and malleoli hang free and do not touch the sheets. As a general rule, there is no clear indication for anticoagulation therapy after bypass surgery unless the patient has a history of or demonstrates evidence of *hypercoagulability*. While mini-dose or prophylactic heparin is sometimes recommended to prevent thrombophlebitis and pulmonary emboli, anticoagulants can cause hematomas by increasing leakage from the vascular anastomoses. Anticoagulant drugs should therefore be avoided unless specifically indicated. Low-molecular-weight dextran has been recommended as a rheologic agent to promote better flow in microvasculature by preventing sludging or agglutination of red cells. This occurs by virtue of the increased electronegative charge on the red blood cells and platelets induced by the dextran. Prophylactic antibiotics are prescribed immediately preoperatively and for a few days postoperatively. Early ambulation is practiced, but patients should avoid bending any joint that has a vascular anastomosis in close proximity.

Complications of Arterial Surgery

Other than thrombosis of the graft, infection remains the most feared problem that can develop after bypass surgery. Infection of the vascular bed around the prosthetic graft is difficult to eradicate. This is less likely to be a problem with a vein graft. It is usually necessary to remove the prosthetic graft and to attempt to run the bypass through another area. If an aortofemoral graft or limb must be removed, an axillofemoral or cross-femoral graft may be inserted, provided that the distal limb is implanted well below the infected area.

When infection is present in the groin area, as from a wound infection from previous bypass surgery, the graft must often be removed, and a new graft cannot be implanted in the same area. This problem has tested the ingenuity of vascular surgeons. One method often used involves the creation of a tunnel from the pelvis through the obturator foramen to connect a graft from the retroperitoneal area to the superficial femoral artery. This graft will pass through a clean field, away from the groin infection. Although this procedure is not commonly performed, it should be part of the armamentarium of vascular surgeons.

Another late complication of aortofemoral bypass surgery is an aortoenteric fistula. This may occur over a period of months or even years. The upper anastomotic suture line may develop a false aneurysm that slowly erodes into the intestines, usually the third portion of the duodenum. These patients may present with sudden massive upper gastrointestinal bleeding, or there may be slow leakage of blood into the duodenum. The usual managment is insertion of extra-anatomic bypass grafts and resection of the original aortic prosthesis.

Lumbar Sympathectomy

Although the first sympathectomy was performed in 1889, its first application in the treatment of peripheral vascular disease did not occur until 1925. Until the advent of arterial reconstructive surgery, sympathectomy was the only surgical procedure available to help improve peripheral flow. Several things are known about sympathectomy. After surgical lumbar sympathectomy, 15 to 40 percent of extremity flow passes through arteriovenous shunts and is therefore not nutritive. Although sympathectomy increases peripheral flow, more of this flow is to skin and bone rather than to muscle. The enchancement of flow associated with sympathectomy is reduced in the face of proximal arterial occlusive disease and even more so by distal small vessel disease. Another observation is the variation of response among different patients to lumbar sympathectomy. Most observers feel that the duration of benefit from lumbar sympathectomy is significant and long lasting as opposed to the duration of the relatively short-lived benefit of upper-extremity sympathectomy.

Lumbar sympathectomy may be considered in a situation in which arterial reconstruction is either not feasible from a technical standpoint or not appropriate because it is felt to be too major a procedure for a patient to tolerate. Sympathectomy is indicated more for patients with nonhealing skin lesions, especially when there is excess moisture on the feet. Sympathectomy should not be considered for relief of intermittent claudication. Sympathetic interruption also may be helpful in treating causalgic pain or ischemia neuritis. Some observers feel that sympathectomy will help with development and/or dilatation of collateral circulation, which in itself may be of benefit and may help maintain the patency of a proximal bypass graft. While the mechanism of this effect seems logical, concrete evidence is lacking. A lumbar sympathectomy may be performed along with an aortofemoral bypass or other abdominal arterial reconstruction, particularly if there is evidence of distal ischemia of the skin.

Amputation

Amputation should not be considered a destructive but rather a reconstructive operation to provide the patient with a well-healed stump that, with the help of a prosthetic device, will permit him to resume his normal life activities. Amputation is indicated when there is *irreversible necrosis* of tissue such that there is little or no hope of limb salvage. The urgency of proceeding with amputation is determined by the extent of tissue damage, the degree of pain present, and the degree of systemic toxicity and/or sepsis. If neurologic signs up to the knee level are present, it is doubtful that successful amputation below this level can be achieved. If there is extensive muscle necrosis, *myoglobinuria,* which can lead to deterioration of renal function, can be present. If this is the case, effort should be rapidly directed to amputation. With acute ischemia, extension of tissue breakdown may be rapid, abruptly necessitating amputation. The presence of chronic ischemia forces the possibility of an amputation, particularly if there is progressive gangrene with infection and severe rest pain. Diabetic patients with arteriosclerosis obliterans have a four-times-greater incidence of amputation than those patients without diabetes.

If the extent of tissue necrosis is minor and bypass surgery may result in limb salvage, arteriography is indicated. However, an arteriogram is not necessary to determine the appropriate level of amputation. Noninvasive studies as well as the clinical examination usually guide the surgeon as to the appropriate level of amputation. As a general rule, the purpose of arterial reconstruction is not to enable a more distal leg amputation. However, if successful arterial surgery might result in preservation of a limb or amputation of only a toe, it is a worthwhile consideration.

The level of amputation should be the most distal location capable of adequate healing, as determined by blood supply. A successful amputation should eliminate all necrotic or gangrenous tissue and should provide relief of pain. The remaining stump should be capable of accepting a prosthesis.

A partial foot amputation is certainly preferred. If gangrene extends to the distal portion of the foot, a transmetatarsal amputation may succeed if there is adequate blood supply at this level. If not, the next proximal level appropriate for amputation is below the knee. On rare occasions, a Syme's amputation just above the ankle joint may be considered. However, the prosthesis for a Syme's amputation does not function any better than the prosthesis for a below-the-knee amputation. If the prospect for healing at a below-the-knee level is poor, an above-the-knee amputation is indicated.

There are various means by which a preoperative determination as to the proper level of amputation can be made. By examining the skin, measuring pressures at ankle, calf, and thigh levels with a Doppler, and reviewing previously performed arteriograms, an adequate determination as to the prospect of healing of a below-the-knee amputation can usually be made. If during a below-the-knee amputation the tissues do not look healthy and there is very little bleeding, the surgeon should stop and immediately proceed to an above-the-knee amputation.

While performing the amputation, the surgeon should have in mind the future functional capabilities of the patient and the type of prosthesis that will be fitted to the stump. Rigid dressings are sometimes helpful in reducing the amount of postoperative edema of the amputation stump. Immediate measurement and fitting for a *prosthesis* are indicated, especially in relatively younger patients and when the tissues of the amputation stump appear to be viable with good vascularity. This situation arises more often with amputations performed for trauma rather than ischemic disease. The advantage of immediate fitting is the saving of 6 to 8 weeks' time of preprosthetic training during which time the patient can use his own prosthesis. The disadvantage is that physicians are not able to carefully examine the stump in the immediate postamputation period. If there is a problem with healing or infection, it may not be obvious for a period of time, and the stump may become necrotic.

Because of venous stasis, there is a higher incidence of pulmonary emboli in patients undergoing amputation. It is therefore important to consider early ambulation and, at times, the use of prophylactic or mini-dose heparin (5000 units subcutaneously every 8 to 12 hours). It is also important to have the patient start physical therapy early, to wrap the stump with Ace bandages to lessen postoperative edema, and to avoid flexion contractures of the knee and/or hip joints. If the patient is doing well, a temporary prosthesis (pylon) may be fitted within a week of amputation so that the patient may quickly assume an upright position and develop a feel for use of his prosthesis. After discharge from the hospital, the patient should be placed in the hands of a physical therapist trained in rehabilitation and prosthetics. The prosthesis may be obtained through in-patient or out-patient rehabilitation.

BIBLIOGRAPHY

Abbott WM: Preparation of veins for arterial bypass grafting in Rutherford RB (ed): *Vascular Surgery*. Philadelphia, Saunders, 6, 1977, pp 359–385.

Baue Arthur: Obturator bypass for lower extremity ischemia, in Rutherford RB (ed): *Vascular Surgery*. Philadelphia, Saunders, 1977, pp. 549–554.

Briel DK, Brenner, BJ, Alpert, J, et al: Crossover femero-femoral grafts followed up five years or more. *Arch Surg* 110:1294, 1975.

Chucken F: Medical management of chronic occlusive arterial disease. *Angiology* 28: 760–769, 1977.

Collens WS, Wilensky ND: *Peripheral Vascular Diseases,* Springfield, Ill., Charles C Thomas, 1953, pp 297–302.

Dardick H, et al: Human umbilical cord—a new source for vascular prosthesis. *JAMA* 236: 2859–2862, 1976.

DeLaurentis DA, Friedman P, Wolferth, CC, et al: Atherosclerosis and the hypoplastic aortoiliac system. *Surgery* 83:27–37, 1978.

DeLaurentis DA, Wolferth CC Jr, Wolf FM, et al: Mucinous adverted cysts of the popliteal artery in an eleven year old girl. *Surgery* 74:456, 1973.

Dotter CT, Judkins MP: Transluminal treatment of arteriosclerosis obstruction. *Circulation,* 30:654, 1964.

Fairbairn JP, Juergens JL, Spittell, JA (eds): *Peripheral Vascular Diseases,* ed 4, Philadelphia, Saunders, 1972, pp 4–44.

Gruntzig A, Mahler F, Jumpe D, et al: Die Erfahrung mit der perkutaneu Rekanalisation chronischer arterieller Verschulusse Bach Dotter. *Schweiz Med Wochenschr,* 106: 422–44, 1976.

Lieberman JS: Newer diagnostic methods in peripheral vascular disease. *Cardiovasc Med* 2:729–743, 1977.

Linton, RH: Indications and comparative results of reconstructive arterial surgery, in Haimovici H (ed): *Surgical Management of Vascular Diseases.* Philadelphia, Lippincott, 1972, pp 95–105.

Mannick JA, et al: The late results of axillo-femoral grafts. *Surgery* 68:1038, 1970.

Moore WS: Extremity amputation for vascular disease, in Rutherford, RB (ed): *Vascular Surgery.* Philadelphia, Saunders, 1977, pp 1305–1343.

Peabody CN, Kaunel WB, McNamara PM: Intermittent claudication: surgical significance. *Arch Surg* 109, 693–697, 1974.

Raines JK, Darling, C, Buth J, et al: Vascular laboratory criteria for the management of peripheral vascular disease of the lower extremities. *Surgery* 71:21–29, 1976.

Schata IJ: Medical management of chronic occlusive disease of the extremities, In Peripheral vascular disease. Gifford RW (ed), *Cardiovasc Clin* Philadelphia, Davis 1971, pp 93–102.

Siegel, ME, Wagner HH, Jr: Radioactive tracers in peripheral vascular disease. *Semin Nucl Med* 6, 1976. 253–278.

Veith FJ, Moss CM, Fell SC, et al: Comparison of expanded PTFE and vein grafts in lower extremity reconstruction. *J Cardiovasc Surg* 19, 341–344, 1978.

CHAPTER TWO

Arterial Aneurysms

ABDOMINAL AORTIC ANEURYSM

A true aneurysm must be differentiated from a false or pseudoaneurysm that may develop after arterial injury or at the site of an arterial anastomosis (Fig. 2-1). Of all aneurysms found in clinical practice, abdominal aortic aneurysms are the most common. Many remain undiagnosed unless they become symptomatic or are found on routine physical examination, x-ray, or ultrasound studies performed for other reasons. Almost all abdominal aneurysms are believed to be atherosclerotic in nature. While atherosclerotic plaques may be present, the atheromatous process may lead to degeneration and breakdown of the elastic fibers, allowing the aneurysm to occur and enlarge. Fortunately for the surgeon, it is rare (1.5 percent incidence) to find an abdominal aneurysm that extends above the level of the renal arteries. If the aneurysm is above the renal arteries, it is more difficult to remove from a technical standpoint, and the operative morbidity and mortality are higher because of the necessity of crossclamping the aorta above the level of the renal arteries.

Abdominal aortic aneurysms may be asymptomatic or may produce anterior abdominal, flank, or back pain. Erosion of the vertebra by the enlarging aneurysm does occur, but it is rare. Laminated thrombus is frequently present within the lumen of the aneurysm, and fragments of the thrombus may break loose, causing distal embolization. On occasion, a patient with an aneurysm

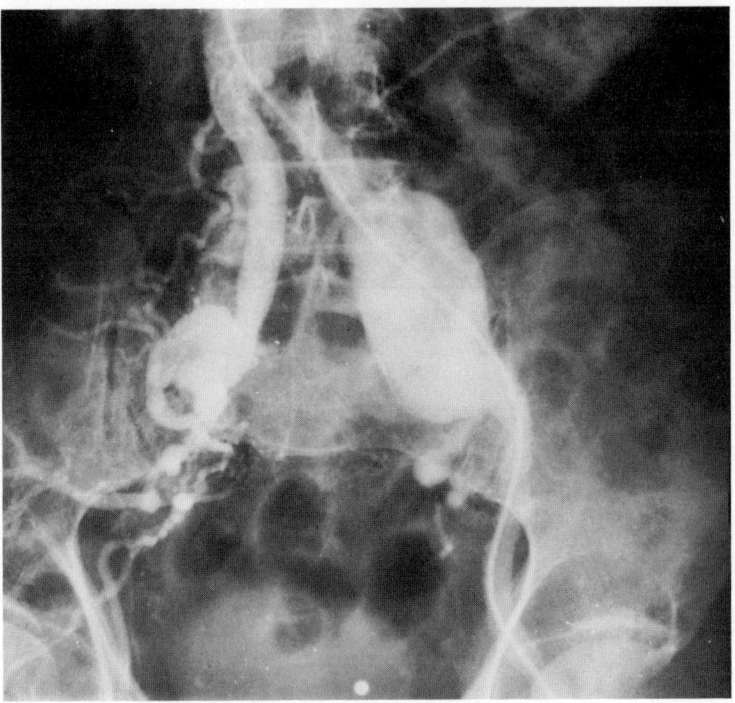

Figure 2-1. Anastomotic aneurysms.

may present with symptoms of peripheral atheroemboli. Abdominal aneurysms may eventually thrombose, causing the patient to present with aortoiliac occlusion. The diagnosis of abdominal aneurysm can frequently be made on physical examination of a pulsatile, expansile mass with or without a bruit. Since the aortic bifurcation is usually located at about the *level of the umbilicus,* the aneurysm is usually palpated above the umbilicus, usually near the midline. One differential diagnosis of abdominal aneurysm on physical examination is a tortuous aorta. This is usually located more to the left of the midline. A very thin patient may have an easily palpable normal aorta. A tumor such as a pancreatic carcinoma may be palpable and pulsatile if it is located anterior to the aorta. It may be confused with an abdominal aneurysm on physical examination. In recent years, abdominal B-mode ultrasound scans and computerized tomography of the abdomen have helped not only with determining the presence of an abdominal aortic aneurysm but also with delineating the presence and size of a thrombus within the lumen of the aneurysm. A plain x-ray may help diagnose an abdominal aneurysm if there is calcification in the anterior and posterior walls, as seen on a lateral film of the abdomen. Aortography is not routinely necessary if the diagnosis of abdominal aneurysm is established. In fact, the dye study may be misleading if the aneurysm is filled with laminated thrombus, so that the channel of blood flow is the size of the normal aorta. However, in some patients, especially if there is additional arterial occlusive disease, an aortogram may be helpful. Aortography will also help ascertain the patency of the superior mesenteric artery since the inferior mesenteric artery is usually sacrificed with aneurysm removal. The presence of an enlarged marginal artery of Drummond is a sign of prior occlusion of the superior mesenteric or inferior mesenteric artery. Occasionally, patients present with generalized or multiple fisiform dilatation of the aortoiliac and perhaps femoral vessels, which appears to represent an entity different from that of the typical abdominal aortic aneurysm. These patients are felt to have an ectasia or generalized weakness of the elastic layer of the arteries, and surgery is usually indicated only if there are areas of extreme dilatation.

With improved surgical techniques and lowered operative mortality, the indications for removal of an abdominal aneurysm have increased. Studies have shown that aneurysms less than 4 to 5 cm in diameter have a low incidence of rupture over a 5-year period. However, larger aneurysms have a marked increased incidence of rupture during a 5-year period, especially when they are greater than 6 to 7 cm. Since current operative mortality rates for unruptured aneurysms are in the range of 1.5 to 4 percent, it is recommended that if a patient is in good general health, all abdominal aneurysms, regardless of size, should be resected and replaced with an aortoaorto, aortoiliac, or aortofemoral bypass graft. However, if the patient is felt to be a poor risk for aneurysm resection, if the aneurysm is less than 5 cm, and if there are no symptoms referable to the aneurysm, it seems reasonable to watch the patient and obtain serial ultrasound studies to determine if there is a progressive increase in size of the aneurysm. This may force the issue of surgical resection of the aneurysm.

The operative mortality rate for ruptured abdominal aneurysm is in the range of 50 percent. The diagnosis should be suspected in older male patients with shock and especially in those patients with abdominal or back pain and a falling hematocrit. If the leak is slow, there may be time to condition the patient for the operating room.

EXTREMITY ANEURYSMS

Ninety percent of all peripheral artery aneurysms occur in either the femoral or popliteal artery segments (Fig. 2-2). Less commonly, aneurysms occur in the carotid, subclavian, brachial, or iliac artery. A patient with one peripheral injury aneurysm stands a 75 percent chance of having multiple peripheral aneurysms. The most common cause of these aneurysms is atherosclerosis. Traumatic, mycotic aneurysms and those occurring at the anastomosis of an im-

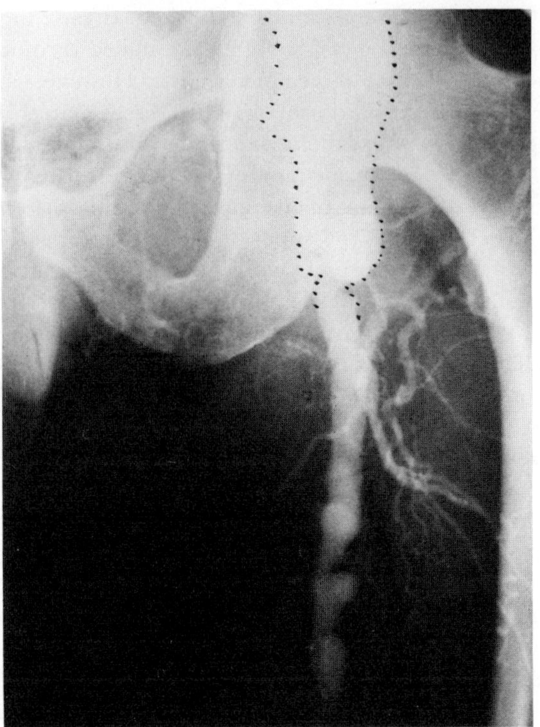

Figure 2-2. Femoral artery aneurysm.

planted bypass graft are less common. The presenting complaint may be that of a pulsating mass or pain. *Popliteal aneurysms* occasionally cause pressure and obstruction in the popliteal vein, leading to thrombophlebitis. Any patient presenting with distal microemboli should be carefully examined for evidence of peripheral artery aneurysms. Any patient with a peripheral artery aneurysm should be carefully evaluated for other aneurysms and for other evidence of atherosclerosis, such as coronary artery or cerebrovascular disease. Peripheral arterial aneurysms (1) may thrombose, leading to sudden severe peripheral ischemia, (2) may cause peripheral embolization as fragments of laminated clot break loose from the aneurysm and embolize distally, and (3) may cause problems with venous compression as the aneurysm expands. When a femoral or popliteal aneurysm clots, there is often extensive thrombosis at and below the aneurysm, leading to severe peripheral ischemia and frequent loss of the limb. Once this occurs, it is often difficult to perform arterial reconstructive surgery because of the extensive propagation of the clot. By the same token, once embolization of fragments of clot from an aneurysm occurs, it is impossible to retract these or to open the occluded distal small arteries. In order to prevent these various complications of peripheral arterial aneurysms, all peripheral artery aneurysms should be resected when found.

VISCERAL ANEURYSMS

Visceral aneurysms are rare but can occur in the splenic, hepatic, or renal arteries and, less often, in the branches of the celiac or mesenteric arteries. Splenic aneurysms are more common in females, with a 4 to 1 ratio. These tend to be asymptomatic unless they rupture. They are often accidentally discovered during angiography for other reasons or on plain x-rays if calcification is present in the aneurysm. Rupture of visceral aneurysms is infrequent, and it is probably reasonable to follow these patients rather than resect the aneurysm unless it is shown to be enlarging or the patient contemplates pregnancy. The incidence of rupture is much higher during the third trimester of pregnancy.

THORACIC ANEURYSMS

While the etiology of thoracic aneurysms may be syphilitic, traumatic, or mycotic, by far the most common cause at the present time is *atherosclerosis*. X-rays in several planes as well as ultrasound may help in the diagnosis. The indications for surgery must be individualized since the operative morbidity and mortality rates are much greater with abdominal aneurysms. The most serious complications of surgery are related to spinal cord and/or visceral ischemia, which may occur during resection of a thoracic aneurysm. Various techniques have been utilized to attempt to preserve blood flow to these vital areas during the surgical procedure.

DISSECTING ANEURYSMS

The prerequisite for the development of the usual dissecting aneurysm appears to be *cystic medial necrosis* of the aortic arch. There is a question as to whether this represents a true pathologic state or a part of the physiologic aging process. In selected patients, rupture of the vasa vasorum may occur, resulting in an intramural hematoma.

After the initial rupture through the intima and various degrees of thickness of the media, a cleavage plane (a new channel) develops within the media of the aorta. After this initial event, the clinical picture varies depending on (1) the extent of dissection of the hematoma, (2) obliteration of the aortic branches by the hematoma, (3) self-decompression of the hematoma by its reentering the aortic lumen, and (4) external rupture of the dissecting aneurysm into the pericardial sac, pleural space, or mediastinum, which usually leads to fatal hemorrhage. This occurs most commonly in the *ascending aorta* and to a lesser degree in the proximal descending aorta. It occurs infrequently in the abdominal aorta or transverse arch. The frequency of intimal tear in the ascending aorta may be related to fixation and greater stress in this area. When it occurs, a dissecting aneurysm may extend proximally as far as the aortic valve, leading to aortic insufficiency, and may extend distally as far as the inguinal ligament. A dissecting aneurysm usually involves one-third to two-thirds of the diameter of the aorta, and any branch of the aorta may be involved.

The older DeBakey classification lists three types of dissecting aneurysms. Type I involved the entire thoracic aorta; type II was limited to the ascending aorta; and type III began distal to the left subclavian artery. The more popular present classification labels as type I those dissecting aneurysms that involve the ascending aorta and/or aortic arch, while type II dissecting aneurysms are limited to the thoracic aorta distal to the left subclavian artery with no involvement of the ascending aorta. This later classification is more useful from a therapeutic point of view since type I dissecting aneurysms require fairly prompt surgical intervention while type II dissecting aneurysms can be medically treated for a few weeks before surgery is considered.

Dissecting aneurysms occur more commonly in men and usually in patients between the ages of 40 to 70 years old. A history of hypertension is often present. The typical complaint is sudden onset of severe, tearing, or ripping type of chest pain starting in the thorax and occasionally extending into the abdomen over several hours' time, perhaps lessening in the chest at that time. Occasionally, there is no pain. The patient may have sudden syncope and/or collapse from cardiac tamponade or hemorrhage into the pleural space or mediastinum. If any branches of the aorta are sheared off, symptoms referable to the ischemic extremity and/or organ may be present. There may be neurologic symptoms if the cerebral or lumbar vessels are involved. There may be sudden congestive heart failure from retrograde dissection into the aortic ring producing aortic insufficiency. The clinical picture can be quite variable, and one must think of the possibility of dissecting aneurysms in order to make the diagnosis as frequently as possible. One clue to dissecting aneurysm (or other left mediastinal mass) *is prominence of the left jugular vein* due to compression of the venous return through the left innominate vein. The electrocardiogram should help rule out acute myocardial infarction. The chest x-ray may be helpful in establishing the diagnosis by revealing a widened mediastinal silhouette. If the diagnosis is suspected and the patient is reasonably stable, aortography may be helpful in establishing the diagnosis as well as the site of origin and extent of the dissection. In addition, one may be able to ascertain which, if any, branches of the aorta have been involved. Other causes of dissecting aneurysms include Marfan's syndrome and torsal trauma. Sudden acceleration may lead to a tear of the thoracic aorta and a chronic dissection.

Without treatment, the mortality is extremely high both acutely and over the first few weeks. Even if a reentry should occur, there is still the possibility of external rupture, which is the most common cause of death in patients with dissecting aneurysms. With improved surgical technique in the last 10 to 15 years, mortality rates have been improved somewhat. However, the greatest advance in the management of patients with dissecting aneurysms has been the advent of so-called medical treatment as first advocated by Wheat et al. Their approach was to attempt to alter the forces that are likely to cause the dissection to continue or extend. The objective was to decrease myocardial contractility and mean arterial pressure by reducing the rate of ventricular fiber shortening. The current regimen includes the use of trimethaphan (Arfonad), reserpine, or nitroprusside as antihypertensive agents. The aim is to lower systolic blood pressure to 100 to 120 mm Hg or to minimum pressure for organ perfusion. In addition, these agents help to deplete catecholamines and reduce myocardial contractility. Propranolol may also be helpful for these patients. With this regimen, Wheat has reported a high one-year survival rate. However, other authors are not as optimistic, and the ideal approach for patients with dissecting aneurysms is still not absolutely clear. The current recommendation for type I dissections (these involve the ascending aorta) is to quickly stabilize the patient and then treat surgically. For the type II lesion, which starts distal to the left subclavian, the medical regimen should be used for 4 to 5 weeks, after which a decision can be made as to surgery. However, earlier surgery is indicated for impending rupture of compromise of the arterial flow in various organs.

BIBLIOGRAPHY

Buda JA, et al: The results of treatment of popliteal artery aneurysms: a follow-up study of 86 aneurysms. *J. Cardiovasc Surg* 15:615, 1974.

Siegel ME, Wagner HH, Jr: Radioactive tracers in peripheral vascular disease. *Semin Nucl Med* 6, 1976.

Szilagyi, DE, Smith RS, DeRusso FJ, et al: Contribution of abdominal aortic aneuryurectomy to prolongation of life. *Annals of Surgery.* 164:678–699, 1966.

Weaver DH, Fleming RJ, Barnes WA: Aneurysm of the hepatic artery. Value of arteriography in the surgical management. *Surgery* 64:891, 1968.

Wheat MW Jr, Harris PD, Malm JR, et al: Acute dissecting aneurysms of the aorta, treatment and results in 64 patients. *J Thorac Cardiovasc Surg* 58:344–350, 1969.

Wheeler WE, Beachley MC, Ranniger K: Angiography and ultrasonography—a comparative study of abdominal aortic aneurysms. *Am J Roentgenol* 126: 95–100, 1976.

CHAPTER THREE

Other Arterial Diseases

TAKAYASU'S DISEASE

This entity, also known as occlusive thromboaortopathy (OTAP) is a chronic inflammatory arteriopathy of unknown etiology that involves the aortic arch and its main branches and also may involve the pulmonary, renal, celiac, or superior mesenteric arteries. Females are involved more often than males, and while there is a higher incidence in Orientals, the disease effects all races. The usual onset is between ages 10 and 30, and onset is rare past 40. Pathologically, there is an inflammatory process with diffuse thickening, destruction of muscular and elastic tissue, and infiltration with lymphocytes and plasma cells and occasionally giant cells. As the lesions evolve, there is eventual scarring and thickening and an increased incidence of hypertension and aortic dissection.

Some people classify the disease in two phases. The early, *prepulseless phase* is noted for systemic symptoms such as malaise, fever, joint symptoms, and anorexia; during this phase, the inflammatory process occurs. There may be a very high erythrocyte sedimentation rate and elevated levels of gamma globulin. In the late or *pulseless phase,* the scarring produces occlusion of the main branches of the aortic arch with resultant symptoms of decreased arterial flow to the brain or upper extremities predominantly. There also may be involvement of the pulmonary artery.

During the early or inflammatory phase, corticosteroids have produced remarkable remissions in some patients, which result in much less later arterial fibrosis and therefore fewer symptoms of ischemia. Patients who are in the late or pulseless phase are occasionally amenable to improvement by arterial reconstruction and bypass surgery. A more recent classification divides patients into four groups in an effort to develop a method of prognosis. Group I includes patients with narrowing or occlusion of two or more branches of the aortic arch without complications, and these patients have the best prognosis. Group II-a patients have the same symptoms as group I patients, which are mild to moderate, and have one of the following complications: retinopathy, secondary hypertension, aortic regurgitation, aortic or arterial aneurysms. Group II-b patients have the same symptoms as group II-a patients except that they have severe involvement. Group III patients have two or more of the above complications and of course have the poorest prognosis.

THORACIC OUTLET SYNDROME

This entity involves pressure on the *brachial plexus* or less commonly on the subclavian artery or vein with resultant symptoms on the involved side in the shoulder or upper extremity. Symptoms tend to be aggravated by various positions of the arm and head, especially on elevation of the arm. There are usually *neurologic symptoms* and *vascular signs*. The thoracic outlet is considered to be outlined by the anterior portion of the first rib, the clavicle and the scalenus anticus muscle. The subclavian artery and vein and the brachial plexus transverse this area as they leave the neck and head toward the shoulder. The three structures travel together except that the subclavian vein passes anterior to the scalenus anticus muscle. There are various areas of potential musculoskeletal narrowing that can apply pressure to the subclavian artery or vein or brachial plexus. However, the most common site of compression is between the clavicle and anterior portion of the first rib. The next most common site is beneath the pectoralis minor muscle. By far the most frequent symptoms are those of brachial plexus compression and are located in back of the neck in the shoulder or down the arm into the hand. *Pain,* if present, tends to be a dull ache, position related, diffuse, and poorly localized. There may be numbness and paresthesias that may be constant or activity related. *Weakness* related to arm elevation (claudication due to arterial compression) may be present. If there is arterial compression, the patient may have Raynaud's phenomenon, distal hand ischemia from emboli, or major arterial insufficiency of the upper extremity. The most common differential diagnosis is that of (1) *carpal tunnel* syndrome and (2) *cervical disc* syndrome. Less common differentials include shoulder problem, neurologic disease, angina pectoris, and ulnar neuropathy.

The actual compression may occur as a result of (1) a fibrous band, (2) congenital bony narrowing, (3) tightness or spasm of muscles leading to outlet narrowing, (4) trauma resulting in muscle spasm and/or hematoma, or a (5) congenital cervical rib. The physical diagnosis may help establish the presence of a thoracic outlet syndrome by demonstrating neurologic deficit in the upper extremity or finding evidence of arterial compression such as a decrease or absent radial pulse and/or development of a subclavian bruit during abduction of the arm with the head turned in the direction of the involvement (*Adson maneuver*). It should be pointed out that it is not uncommon to create a subclavian bruit in normal individuals, especially younger people, by performing the Adson maneuver. This maneuver is therefore not considered positive unless there is a marked decrease or disappearance on the involved side of the radial pulse in a symptomatic patient. It should also be mentioned that many patients with significant nerve compression in the thoracic outlet may have no arterial component to their problem and thus might have a negative Adson maneuver or arteriogram. If there is arterial narrowing, there may be poststenotic aneurysmal dilatation with the possibility of thrombus formation in this area and resultant distal emboli to the hand. If there is venous compression, which is uncommon, there may be cyanosis and/or venous distention in the extremity.

The most difficult differentials are those of cervical root irritation, thoracic outlet syndrome, and carpal tunnel syndrome. The *Tinel test* (paresthesias in the median nerve distribution in the hand on tapping on the median nerve at the wrist) may help to rule out a carpal tunnel syndrome. A *nerve conduction* study of the median nerve above and below the wrist is usually diagnostic of carpal tunnel and should be done if there is any question. Other electromyographic studies may be unable to differentiate cervical root irritation from thoracic outlet nerve compression.

Before considering surgery, one would like to be fairly certain of the diagnosis, and the patient should have significant symptoms compatible with the diagnosis. The outlet maneuvers should be positive. Other problems that might mimic the diagnosis should be ruled out. If the symptoms are severe enough to warrant consideration of surgical correction, arteriography of the appropriate subclavian artery with the arm in various positions may help confirm the presence of pressure in the location of the thoracic outlet. Cervical spine film should be examined to rule out cervical ribs as well as degenerative changes in the cervical vertebra.

Once the diagnosis is established, shoulder-girdle exercise should be tried to attempt to increase the tone of the muscles in the shoulder area. Generally, these exercises are of little value. Surgery is indicated if there are moderately severe symptoms, history suggestive of distal embolization, or evidence of poststenotic dilatation. One of the better methods involves removal of the *first rib* to create surgical decompression of the brachial plexus. One must decompress the space between the highest rib and the clavicle. Also, any congenital bands that may be present, as well as cervical ribs, should be removed. Other surgical techniques involve removing the middle third of the clavicle or sectioning of the scalenus anticus muscle. Statistically, surgery will cure 50 percent of patients and give a good result in another 20 percent.

ACUTE ARTERIAL OCCLUSION

The majority of cases of sudden ischemia are due to arterial emboli. The most common source (94 percent) of arterial emboli are: (1) atrial fibrillation, (2) rheumatic valvular heart disease, (3) recent myocardial infarction, (4) ventricular aneurysm, (5) cardiomyopathy, or (6) tumor of the heart. In addition, small fragments of thrombus and/or platelet cholesterol material may break loose from abdominal or peripheral aneurysms and embolize distally. Emboli tend to lodge at areas of branching or tampering of the arteries. The majority of emboli end up producing ischemia in the extremities, although visceral emboli occur and perhaps 20 percent of all emboli that leave the heart enter the cerebral circulation. Patients with chronic atherosclerotic occlusive disease may eventually have thrombosis at an area of severe stenosis. However, in this situation, the patient will tend to have developed collateral circulation. Therefore, acute ischemia is unlikely to occur. A much less common cause of acute arterial occlusion is *arterial injury* either blunt or penetrating. *Drug abusers* attempting to give themselves intravenous drugs may accidentally inject the drug into an artery, which can produce severe peripheral vasoconstriction and at times digital gangrene.

The diagnosis is usually clear when a patient presents with a sudden onset of a *cold, pulseless, painful extremity.* If ischemia is severe, there may be paresthesias and paralysis. In a patient with acute ischemia and the presence of a neurologic deficit secondary to the sudden ischemia, it is necessary to restore flow as soon as possible. Should the neurologic deficit remain present more than 24 hours, it may become a permanent neurologic problem in spite of restoration of normal arterial flow. Therefore, an immediate embolectomy should be attempted in this type of patient. The use of the Doppler may help in localizing the location of the arterial block. Arteriograms are not always necessary as part of the preoperative evaluation. The degree of ischemia secondary to an embolus will depend on the degree of preexisting arterial occlusive disease, the extent of the emboli, and the location and availability of collateral flow.

From a therapeutic standpoint, the advent of the *Fogarty catheter* has made embolectomy a much simpler procedure. The earlier it is performed, the better the chances of success. However, embolectomies have been successful even as late as 10 to 14 days after the onset of symptoms. If the lower extremity has suffered severe ischemia for more than a few hours and the ischemia is then relieved by embolectomy that restores normal arterial flow, occasionally one will see the development of an anterior tibial *compartment syndrome*. It may produce marked swelling in the anterior compartment, which is limited by fascial planes. This can lead to damage to peripheral nerves and even to arterial occlusion secondary to the great pressure applied to the soft tissues. If one suspects that this may develop, at times, a prophylactic fasciotomy is indicated. The procedure can usually be performed under local or epidural anesthesia. It is often helpful to have an epidural block started prior to the embolectomy, which will help to relieve secondary vasospasm. Postoperatively, moderate heparinization may be undertaken to prevent recurrent emboli. When the patient's condition will tolerate it, a search should be made for the source of embolus. Ultrasound studies and occasionally dye studies are indicated to attempt to determine the presence of thrombus in the heart. If the possibility of recurrent emboli exists, then the patient may be kept on oral anticoagulation for a period of time. More recently, some physicians have advocated the use of fibrinolytic therapy with streptokinase to attempt to dissolve arterial emboli. This method works well on fresh thrombus but not on emboli that may have formed more than 1–2 weeks before.

VASOSPASTIC DISORDERS

Raynaud's Phenomenon

The most common vasospastic disorder is *Raynaud's phenomenon*. This condition may be defined as an increased or unusual sensitivity to cold or emotional factors resulting in arterial and arteriolar vasoconstriction with resultant pallor, cyanosis, and hyperactive and reactive hyperemia on rewarming. It produces symptoms of coldness, pain, numbness, and paresthesias in the hands and fingers. Symptoms tend to come and go quickly with changes in ambient temperature. People speak of the *blue, white, and red* color changes of Raynaud's phenomenon. If there is moderate vasoconstriction, a small amount of blood, which is relatively stagnant and results in cyanosis or a blue color, passes through the digits. If the vasospasm is severe so that there is almost no flow, then the *digits are a dead white color*. After rewarming, there is a reactive hyperemia, which gives the fingers a red appearance.

Raynaud's disease was originally described over 100 years ago by Maurice Raynaud as bilateral symmetrical gangrene. Since this is not what we usually see today, we choose to speak of the entity as Raynaud's phenomenon, calling it primary if there is no obvious underlying cause and secondary if the condition occurs as part of another disease process. Primary Raynaud's phenomenon tends to be bilateral, symmetrical, and intermittent, with only localized necrosis, and symptoms should have been present for 2 years without evidence of underlying problems.

Secondary Raynaud's phenomenon may occur in association with collagen vascular disease (such as SLE, scleroderma, or polyarteritis), thoracic outlet syndrome, Buerger's disease, myxedema, or any vascular process that involves the upper extremity. It also may be secondary to certain occupations such as those of pianist, typist, and people who work with pneumatic drills. Raynaud's phenomenon is much more common in females, usually starts in the second, third, or fourth decade, and tends to involve fingers asymmetrically and the thumbs rarely. The degree of severity is quite variable, and the secondary type is more likely to have fingertip necrosis than primary Raynaud's phenomenon.

The pathophysiology is not well understood. Some observers have felt there was an abnormality in sympathetic nerve function. Most people feel that the arteriolar wall displays an unusual reaction to cold exposure. Symptoms are most often precipitated by cold exposure, but this does not necessarily have to be an unusually cold temperature, as some people develop symptoms even in a warm room when their body is hit by cool air from an air conditioner. Physical examination is usually not very rewarding unless the patient is seen during or immediately after cold exposure. Raynaud's phenomenon will develop when the body is chilled even if the hands are kept warm. Careful attention should be given in the physical examination to ruling out large vessel disease as well as thoracic outlet syndrome.

The usual laboratory work-up for this entity includes a sedimentation rate, platelet count to rule out thrombocytosis, serum protein electrophoresis to look for evidence of abnormal proteins, including cryoglobulins or cold agglutinins, and ANA and DNA antibody determination. Of course, all of these studies will be negative in primary Raynaud's phenomenon without underlying disease. The prognosis in a patient with primary Raynaud's phenomenon when followed for a 10-year period is that about one-third to one-half will have little or no change, one-third will gradually show improvement and eventual disappearance of symptoms, and the remainder may gradually become worse. The diagnosis of the secondary type of Raynaud's phenomenon is that of the underlying disease process.

Cervical sympathectomy is not usually indicated unless there is significant tissue breakdown and threat of loss of digits. When cervical sympathectomy is performed, one expects only a short-term benefit, as it is not uncommon to be able to demonstrate evidence of return of sympathetic function within 6 to 12 months after upper-extremity sympathectomy. Various drugs have been advocated in an effort to deplete catacholamines at the neuroarterial junction. Intra-arterial *reserpine* has been used with reported improvement. However, in our patients, we have not found this to be very helpful. Other oral drugs that have been tried include guanethidine, 10 to 30 mg daily; phenoxybenzamine, 10 to 30 mg daily; prazosin MCI, 1 mg b.i.d.; and alpha methyldopa and tolazoline. Again, final reports of benefit from these drugs are awaited Inderal tends to aggravate this syndrome.

Acrocyanosis

Another vasospastic disorder similar but more mild than Raynaud's phenomenon is acrocyanosis. This usually presents as a painless but more *persistent* coldness and cyanosis of the distal parts of the upper and/or lower extremities. Although symptoms are worse on cold exposure, they may be present even in a warm environment, and unlike Raynaud's phenomenon, the continuous cutaneous arteriolar spasm tends to be much more long lived even after returning to a warm room. Patients with acrocyanosis do not develop ischemic changes or tissue breakdown and have no underlying disease.

Livedo Reticularis

Another vasospastic disorder is characterized by focal and prominent mottling and blotchy or reticular, reddish-blue discoloration of the skin of the extremities. The physiology of this entity is not too dissimilar from that of acrocyanosis. Here there is spasm of certain cutaneous arterioles, apparently in a random distribution with secondary dilatation of the associated capillaries and venules. This condition is primarily of cosmetic and of very little medical concern. Although usually primary, this condition may occasionally be secondary to connective tissue disease. Chronic ulcerations have been reported to occur on occasion. There is no specific treatment other than avoidance of cold.

Ergot Intoxication

Ergot preparation can induce intense *vasospasm,* which is supposed to be its mechanism of action for relief of migraine headaches. When excess amounts of ergot preparations are taken for relief of migraine headaches in a patient who is unusually sensitive to the drug, severe, symptomatic peripheral vasoconstriction can occur not only in the arterioles but even in the small and medium-size arteries. Patients will usually not progress to gangrene from the vasospasm alone unless the vasoconstriction is so severe and so prolonged that thrombosis occurs. Epidemics of ergot poisoning have occurred in Europe as a result of humans ingesting ergotized *grain* or grain products. Ergot intoxication is rare from orally ingesting ergotaine or related alkaloids but can occur after rectal suppository or injections of ergotamine preparations for migraine headaches. Should a patient present with unusual vasoconstriction, particularly if it affects multiple extremities, one should think of the possibility of ergot intoxication and question the patient about migraine headaches and/or the use of ergot preparations. It is important to point out from a therapeutic standpoint that the ergot preparations act distally on the neuroarterial junction, the vasoconstricting effect will not be interrupted by any type of sympathetic ganglion block, and there are no drugs to counteract the constricting effect distally. Symptomatic treatment is indicated until the effects of the drug wear off.

VASCULAR CONDITIONS RELATED TO ENVIRONMENTAL TEMPERATURE

Pernio Syndromes

Pernio syndromes are those in which the peripheral blood vessels react to cold. It is possible that patients who develop the syndrome have some inherited predisposition. The skin temperature tends to be maintained at a lower than normal level and to warm up more slowly than normal.

Acute pernio (acute chilblains) occurs in people who go out into the snow or cold especially in wet weather without adequate protection for their feet and legs. They tend to develop a reddish-blue dermatitis associated with intense itching and burning in the affected areas, usually on the lower extremities. These lesions gradually subside over a 2-week period. The lesions tend to be bilateral and symmetrical. *Chronic* pernio (chronic chilblains) represents the clinical situation of chronic cutaneous erythematous, ulcerative, and hemorrhagic lesions that often leave residual scarring and fibrosis. This develops in patients who have repeated episodes of cold exposure. The lesions are more active in the cooler months and may subside during the warm weather.

Trench Foot

Trench foot occurs when there are changes in the peripheral circulation and tissues caused by exposure to environmental temperatures about 32° F or somewhat higher. This may be aggravated by moisture, dampness, or immobility and requires prolonged exposure.

Immersion Foot

Immersion foot is a similar condition that occurs after prolonged immersion of the feet in cool or cold water. Dependency and immobility again are aggravating factors. Pathologically, there is fibrosis and thickening of the smaller arteries as well as an inflammatory reaction in the venous system. There is usually little or no organic occlusion.

Frostbite

Frostbite is defined as a condition in which actual freezing of tissues occurs as a result of cold exposure. There is a discrepancy as to whether the damage in this ''slow freeze'' type of frostbite occurs as a result of actual freezing of skin and tissues or as a result of changes that occur in blood vessels. Initially, there is intense *vasoconstriction* producing severe ischemia, and when the situation is severe, there may be thrombosis of smaller arteries and eventual tissue death. Aggravating factors for frostbite include: dampness, wind, immobility, orthostatic edema, and underlying arterial occlusive disease. Although most frostbite occurs from outdoor exposure to the cold, on rare occasions we have seen frostbite develop when a patient has packed his hand or foot in ice for pain relief from an injury. Frostbite can be prevented by adequate prophylactic measures.

The treatment of mild frostbite is *rapid rewarming*. This is best done by placing the frostbitten part against a warm area of the body. The exposed part should never be exposed to warmth greater than body temperature because of the possibility of burning and harming the ischemic tissues. With severe frostbite, the same rapid rewarming and the avoidance of trauma and infection are indicated. If tissue damage is present, antibiotics are indicated. Vasodilators, anticoagulants, and steroids have been tried but are not of proven value. If seen early, a frostbitten extremity may be thawed quickly by placing the exposed tissue in a warm bath of 40° to 42° C for 15 to 20 minutes but not longer.

ERYTHERMALGIA (ERYTHROMELALGIA)

This syndrome is one of *painful red areas* of skin on the extremities. Although not a common problem, it is seen on occasion. The majority of cases are primary with no underlying etiology. Secondary erythermalgia can occur in association with myeloproliferative disorders, hypertension, diabetes, venous insufficiency, and collagen vascular disease. The primary features of this entity are increased temperature of the skin and associated hyperemia, with the development of pain when the extremity is above a certain temperature, usually 32° to 36°C. The etiology is not one of pure vasodilatation. Symptoms are aggravated by dependency and relieved by elevation or by direct pressure on the skin. The usual complaints are of burning distress, usually in the hands and feet, worse on walking or after lying down at night. Symptoms are also aggravated by warmth and are more intense in the summer. Relief is often obtained by exposure to cool air or water. To make this diagnosis, one should establish that the pain is associated with increased skin temperature. There are no serious complications of this disorder. From a therapeutic standpoint, some patients obtain marked relief with *acetylsalicylic acid.*

VASCULITIS AND SMALL VESSEL DISEASE

There are a number of diseases that have as a common part of their picture an inflammatory and sometimes proliferative process involving small arteries. The causes, pathology, and signs and symptoms are quite variable and often nonspecific. The inflammatory change may be looked upon as the end result of trauma, infection, radiation, thermal injury, autoimmune mechanism, allergens, toxins, or ischemia. The pathology tends to be nonspecific with edema, fibrin deposition, and leukocyte infiltration. At times, it is helpful to attempt to establish a tissue diagnosis by biopsy of the vascular lesions, especially if specific therapeutic measures (for example, high-dose steroid therapy or immunosuppressive therapy) may be indicated. We will discuss some of these arteritidies at this point. In some of these entities, the etiology is felt to be a hypersensitivity reaction secondary to either autoantibodies, drugs, or viruses. If foreign antigen is injected into a host, antibody appears that soon forms an antigen-antibody complex. These are removed from the circulation and deposited in blood vessels and glomeruli, producing clinical syndromes. These complexes also bind complement, leading to a decreased serum complement level. In addition, there is an attraction to polymorphonuclear cells, which release enzymes causing tissue necrosis.

Polyarteritis Nodosa

This disease is characterized by inflammation and necrosis of small and medium-sized arteries in almost any organ of the body. The lesions involve all three coats of the arterial wall and are present in different stages (acute, chronic, or healing) throughout the body. From a clinical standpoint, these patients tend to have fever, anorexia, weight loss, arthralgias, skin rashes, petechiae or nodules, peripheral neuropathies, bronchitis or asthma, myalgias, increased incidence of duodenal ulcer, congestive heart failure, and occasional renal involvement. There is a suggestion that treatment with corticosteriods increases long-term survival. The two factors most important in prognosis are hypertension and renal disease.

Allergic or Hypersensitivity Angiitis

Allergic or hypersensitivity angiitis is similar to polyarteritis except for lack of involvement of medium-size arteries and the fact that all lesions are in the same stage at any one time, which suggests a single precipitating event such as a drug reaction as the etiology. A variant of this is *Henoch-Schonlein* syndrome of allergic vasculitis in which the predominant features are those of purpura, arthritis, and abdominal pain.

Scleroderma (Progressive Systemic Sclerosis)

Scleroderma has characteristic intimal proliferation in arteries of the lung, kidney, and skin, as well as other organs. Raynaud's phenomenon is often a common occurrence in scleroderma. As the disease progresses, there is a marked change in the skin and subcutaneous tissues, with tightening and stiffening of the skin, especially of the hands, face, and chest. Gangrene of the ends of the fingers may occur. The sclerosis of the skin and subcutaneous tissues eventually may spread to other areas of the body. *Telangiectasias* are common in the advanced stages, and there is resorption of the distal phalanges starting at the distal ends of the bones and progressing proximally. There may be subcutaneous calcification. Also, in the advanced stages, patients tend to have pulmonary fibrosis and esophageal stenosis. Arthralgias are also common. The prognosis is variable, but the course tends to be downhill. Various drugs, including antimetabolites, have been tried, but there is no good evidence of benefit at this time.

Systemic Lupus Erythematosus (SLE)

SLE was first described over 100 years ago and is now characterized by the finding of antinuclear antibodies, anti-DNA, low levels of serum complement, and/or finding of LE cells in the blood. The disease appears to be a complex autoimmune disease in which the patient's own cells somehow become antigenic. Vascular lesions may occur in the pleura, pericardium, peritoneum, and serosa of the joints. In the kidney, there is thickening of the basement membrane of the glomerular capillaries producing the typical "wire loop" lesion. The clinical picture depends on the organs involved. Patients tend to have systemic symptoms, including fever, butterfly rash over the cheeks, polyserositis, muscle and joint pains, lymphadenopathy, nephritis, convulsions, and GI symptoms. They may develop skin infarcts (small vessel disease), painful ulcers, or venous or arterial thrombosis. Raynaud's phenomenon is common. Livedo reticularis may occur. Life expectancy may be weeks to 10 years, and occasional spontaneous remissions occur. Large doses of corticosteroids are indicated for severe acute attacks. The use of immunosuppressive agents may be indicated in some patients.

Temporal Arteritis

Temporal arteritis tends to occur in elderly patients and is characterized by an inflammatory process with giant cells and occasionally granulomas of the aorta and its major branches. The temporal artery, producing pain in the involved vessel in the scalp, is the vessel most commonly involved. Other vessels, including the subclavian, profunda, and visceral arteries, may be involved. The disease is often associated with polymyalgia rheumatica. Headaches and other vague symptoms may occur, but signs of cerebrovascular insufficiency are less common. A dreaded complication is transient or permanent *blindness* related to central retinal artery occlusion, ischemic optic neuritis, or retrobulbar neuritis. The process may start as a "flulike" syndrome with malaise, anorexia, weight loss, low-grade fever, and myalgia. There is usually a mild anemia, moderate leukocytosis, and characteristicly, a very high sedimentation rate, often over 100 mm in 1 hour. If the sedimentation rate is not significantly elevated, the diagnosis is very questionable. If there is any question of the diagnosis, temporal artery biopsy is indicated, making sure to obtain a long enough section of artery to avoid "skip" areas. If there is any likelihood of the diagnosis, the patient should be immediately started on corticosteroid therapy, which usually leads to rapid symptomatic improvement and tends to prevent the development of blindness. Treatment may be necessary for weeks to months, after which one tries to taper the steroids. The disease then tends to run a self-limited course, lasting from 3 months to 3 years. It is a rare cause of aortic dissection.

THROMBOANGIITIS OBLITERANS (BUERGER'S DISEASE)

Buerger's disease is an entity with involvement of small and medium-size arteries and veins in the upper and lower extremities, associated with heavy tobacco intake. The venous element is seen clinically as a *migratory thrombophlebitis.* The arterial component leads to peripheral ischemic problems, usually with skin breakdown and possible gangrene. Ischemic lesions may develop in the hands as well as in the feet. Pathologically, this disease is distinctly different from atherosclerosis. There is an inflammatory and proliferative process involving all three coats of the vessel wall with eventual occlusion. There is absence of calcification or lipid deposition in the arteries. The usual onset is between the ages of 25 and 40 years old, and 90 percent of the cases occur in men. The disease has been found in many ethnic groups throughout the world, and no race or color is immune from the disease. Life expectancy is normal. Although many cases diagnosed as Buerger's disease in the past may in reality have been premature atherosclerosis developing in young people, most vascular specialists agree that there is a definite group of patients who fit the criteria of Buerger's disease today. There appears to be a definite relationship to something in tobacco, and if patients with this problem will discontinue smoking, there usually will be no further progression of the disease. The treatment consists of good skin care, *avoidance of smoking,* and occasionally lumbar sympathectomy. Bypass surgery is usually not feasible because of the distal nature of the arterial problem. The remainder of the management program is similar to that for any arterial occlusive disease other than the application of arterial bypass procedures.

ARTERIOVENOUS FISTULA

An arteriovenous fistula may be acquired or congenital, large or small, and affect the circulatory system to a great or small degree, depending on the size of the fistula. Arterial flow tends to decrease distal to a fistula. On occasion, if there is a large arteriovenous fistula, the peripheral arterial flow may be diminished to the point where the distal tissues are ischemic and the possibility of developing gangrene exists. The flow through an arteriovenous communication tends to increase progressively with time. The bypassing of the capillaries by the arteriovenous communication leads to a marked increased venous pressure both proximal and distal to the fistula. If the arteriovenous connection is present in an extremity prior to the closing of the epiphyses, that limb will tend to grow longer than the opposite limb. In any case, the involved limb becomes warm, swollen, and somewhat cyanotic with evidence of venous distention. A continous trill of bruit is frequently felt or heard over the arteriovenous fistula. There is increased oxygen content of venous blood beyond an arteriovenous fistula. Branham's sign is diagnostic of an arteriovenous fistula. With temporary occlusion by pressure over a large fistula, there is prompt slowing of the pulse. Branham's sign is positive only when there is a large flow rate through the fistula compared with the normal cardiac output. With a large arteriovenous fistula, the hemodynamics are as follows. Because of the increased stroke volume, there may be cardiac enlargement and increased cardiac output as a result of the circulatory demands of the fistula. Also, there is an increased pulse pressure, increased blood volume, and decreased peripheral resistance, which may eventually lead to high-output *cardiac failure*. Venous insufficiency and associated ulceration (the so-called ''hot ulcer'') may develop.

The majority of arteriovenous fistulas are *congenital* in origin; they are frequently small initially and gradually enlarge. Frequently, they are too diffuse to be completely excised, although surgical treatment may occasionally be indicated. Recurrence is common. An *acquired* arteriovenous fistula can occur from any wound, particularly a penetrating wound in which there was arterial injury. To make the diagnosis of arteriovenous fistula, one must have a high index of suspicion. Should the diagnosis of traumatic arteriovenous fistula be established, the fistula is usually allowed to mature for approximately 6 months and is then excised. Some physicians are treating fistulas by embolizing material to thrombose the fistula. An aortocaval fistula may develop as a complication of surgery for herniated intervertebral disc in which the instrument for removal of the disc may injure the aorta or iliac artery and vena cava. It may also develop from a ruptured abdominal aortic aneurysm or from a tumor. If this lesion develops, it will steadily increase in size and require surgical treatment.

Causes of acquired arteriovenous malformations other than penetrating injuries include crushing together of the artery and vein to soft tissues compressed against underlying bone, mass ligature on a vascular pedicle at surgery, mycotic aneurysms eroding into a vein, neoplasms with eroding into vessels, and intracaval rupture of an abdominal aortic aneurysm. Arteriovenous malformations can also occur in the viscera, liver, and lungs. Large hepatic or pelvic arteriovenous fistulas can produce signs and symptoms similar to interatrial septal defect. Bacterial endarteritis is a rare complication of an arteriovenous fistula.

POSTTRAUMATIC REFLEX
SYMPATHETIC DYSTROPHY

This condition produces a burning type of pain (causalgia) following trauma. There may or may not be direct injury to a nerve trunk. This syndrome occurs in the extremities and has been seen in the left upper extremity after myocardial infarction (shoulder-hand syndrome). At times, the trauma may be so minor that the patient does not recollect it. If symptoms are of long standing, bone atrophy may occur in the region or distal to it; this localized osteoporosis is known as Sudeck's atrophy. Immobility and reflex response to pain are aggravating factors.

The pain tends to be diffuse and not directly related to the area of previous injury. Trigger areas may exacerbate the pain, and hyperesthesia and paresthesias are frequently present. The extremity is often held motionless and flexed and may be cold and swollen. Frequently, there is excess perspiration. The syndrome is one of neural dysfunction with secondary vascular changes. The vasoconstriction, swelling, hyperhydrosis, and osseous changes are attributed to autonomic dysfunction.

Treatment should be started as soon as possible and should consist of a warm environment and encouraging the patient to use the painful limb as much as possible. An active physical therapy program, including warm baths, massage, and passive and active exercises, is of utmost importance. Analgesics should be used sparingly, and the patient should be given an optimistic outlook. If these measures fail, a series of sympathetic ganglion blocks are often helpful in producing temporary and frequently permanent relief. If all else fails, then cervical or lumbar *sympathectomy* can be carried out.

BIBLIOGRAPHY

Herman BE: Buerger's syndrome. *Angiology* 26: 713–716, 1975.

Holling HE: Reflex sympathetic dystrophy, in Holling HE (ed): *Peripheral Vascular Diseases,* Philadelphia, Lippincott, 1972, pp 196–198.

Ishikaw Kaichiro: Natural history and classification of occlusive thromboaortopathy (Takayaser's disease). *Circulation* 57: 27–35, 1978.

Porter JM, Snider RL, Bardona EJ: The diagnosis and treatment of Raynaud's phenomenon. *Surgery* 77:11, 1975.

Roos DB: Experience with first rib resection for thoracic outlet syndrome. *Am Surg* 173–429, 1971.

CHAPTER FOUR

Cerebrovascular Insufficiency

INTRODUCTION

For the most part, cerebrovascular insufficiency is related to atherosclerotic involvement of the vessels supplying blood to the brain. Lipid deposition and plaque formation are more severe in certain segments of the cerebral circulation. These sites inlude: (1) the origins of the common carotid and extracranial vertebral arteries, (2) the internal carotid artery at its takeoff from the common carotid bifurcation, (3) several intracranial portions of the internal carotid artery where there is angulation, (4) the middle cerebral arteries, (5) the basilar arteries, and (6) the intracranial vertebral arteries. Arteriography is more helpful in localizing lesions in the extracranial vessels than it is in localizing intracranial arterial lesions.

Occlusive cerebrovascular disease is frequently caused by gradually enlarging *atherosclerotic plaque* with eventual intimal ulceration and thrombosis of the involved vessel, leading to a decreased flow of blood to the brain with resultant symptoms. Often, there is diffuse involvement such that multiple vessels supplying blood to the brain are narrowed. The *extensive collateral network* through the *circle of Willis* might prevent symptoms in some situations even though one or even two major vessels are involved. In a rather unusual situation, a patient can have arteriographically proven occlusion of both internal carotid arteries and both vertebral arteries with only minimal cerebrovascular symptoms because of extensive collateral circulation. When the flow to a specific area of the brain becomes significantly compromised, the patient presents with symptoms related to involvement of the particular *anatomic area* supplied by the ischemic part of the brain. If the compromise of circulation is *vasospastic,* the patient might have a transient ischemic attack (TIA) with temporary interruption of neurologic function. If the final event is one of thrombosis with infarction of the involved area of brain, the patient develops a completed stroke with resultant neurologic deficit.

Another mechanism producing cerebrovascular insufficiency is that of *microembolization* of lipid and/or platelet material that breaks loose from an ulcerating atherosclerotic plaque in the common carotid bifurcation area. These microemboli can settle in any part of the brain. If this mechanism does, in fact, produce a TIA, it remains unclear as to why these microemboli travel to the same vessels each time the patient has a TIA since most TIA patients have repeated episodes of the same neurologic deficit. While it is clear that microemboli from ulcerating plaques, which can sometimes be seen in the retinal arteries on funduscopic examination, do occasionally arise, the percentage of cerebrovascular symptomatology based on this phenomenon has not been determined.

Sudden cerebrovascular symptoms might present as a result of embolization of thrombi from the *heart,* as in the case of an endomural thrombus from the atrium or heart valves of a patient with atrial fibrillation, rheumatic heart disease, or after acute myocardial infarction. Another cause of cerebrovascular accidents is *cerebral hemorrhage,* which occurs from a ruptured atherosclerotic vessel, hypertension, congenital aneurysms, or blood dyscrasias. The hemorrhagic blood destroys and replaces brain tissue, leading to symptomatology.

While most cases of cerebral thrombosis are a result of atherosclerosis with or without embolic phenomenon, other causes should be mentioned even though they are relatively uncommon. These include encephalitis, thromboangiitis obliterans, collagen vascular disease, including polyarteritis nodosa and SLE, polycythemia vera, and mechanical obstruction by tumor.

Patients with occlusion of the main trunk of the *anterior cerebral artery* might present with hemiplegia, mild sensory deficit primarily affecting the lower extremity, and mental confusion. Symptoms of occlusion of the main trunk of the *middle cerebral artery* include coma, contralateral flaccid hemiplegia, hemianesthesia, hemianopsia, as well as profound motor and sensory aphasia if the dominant side is involved. Occlusion of the main trunk of the *posterior cerebral artery* might cause collateral hemiplegia (usually transient), contralateral hemianesthesia, contralateral homonymous hemianopsia, sensory aphasia if the dominant side is involved, and, less often, ipsilateral cerebellar signs, contralateral rigidity, and tremors. Occlusion of the main trunk of the *posterior inferior cerebellar artery* may produce ipsilateral facial analgesia, ipsilateral Horner's syndrome, ipsilateral ataxia, contralateral analgesia, and ipsilateral weakness of the vocal cord or the tongue. Occlusion of the *superior cerebellar artery* might cause ipsilateral ataxia, contralateral hemianalgesia, and contralateral hemianesthesia. Occlusion of the main trunk of the *basilar artery* might cause headache, dizziness, coma, flaccid quadriplegia, areflexia, complete anesthesia, pinpoint pupils, and hyperpyrexia.

COMPLETED STROKE

Once a patient develops a fixed neurologic deficit (stroke, cerebrovascular accident, CVA), primary management is supportive. A CAT scan can be performed to rule out tumor and hemorrhage. While a few surgeons have tried emergency cerebral arteriography and carotid artery surgery for an acute stroke, the results have been poor, and such measures are not generally recommended. Certain disease states predispose a patient to a stroke; when possible, such underlying problems should be treated. Patients with significant *hypertension* should be placed on a low-sodium diet, and antihypertensive therapy should be instituted to maintain diastolic pressure under 90 mm Hg. *Diabetic* patients should be treated with appropriate diet and insulin therapy to keep the blood sugars at a reasonable level. Likewise, *hyperlipemia* should be treated with appropriate diet and medication to maintain lipids at a normal level. *Polycythemia vera* should be treated to lower the possibility of sludging. Anticoagulant therapy to prevent strokes will be discussed under management of TIAs.

TRANSIENT ISCHEMIC ATTACK (TIA)

The most important aspect of cerebrovascular disease is the *transient ischemic attack*. Once a completed neurologic deficit (stroke) has developed, nothing can be done to reverse the process, and the only hope for the patient is moderate return of function aided by rehabilitation. A TIA provides the physician with a *warning* prior to a completed cerebrovascular accident. TIAs tend to occur in patients who have a borderline or a critical amount of flow to an area of the brain. This may be the result of one or more extracranial arterial stenoses or occlusions and may be combined with intracranial occlusive problems. The balance of flow may be tipped to a transient state by vasospasm, sludging, or a temporary drop in cardiac output or systemic blood pressure. The clinical manifestations are those of (1) transient visual or speech disturbances with or without transient numbness and (2) paresthesias, weakness, or paralysis affecting the face and/or extremities. This temporary neurologic deficit tends to last from a few minutes to a few hours. Symptoms that last longer than 24 hours are empirically referred to as a *completed stroke*. Once a patient shows clinical symptoms of cerebrovascular disease such as recurrent TIAs, *arteriography* to determine the presence of a lesion that might be amenable to arterial reconstructive surgery is recommended. However, in some situations in which the patient might have only vague neurologic symptoms or perhaps an asymptomatic carotid bruit or in a single carotid system TIA patient with a negative neurovascular examination, noninvasive studies *prior* to arteriography are indicated.

NONINVASIVE WORK–UP
FOR CEREBROVASCULAR DISEASE

Many new studies are being evaluated for the noninvasive work-up for carotid artery disease. Atherosclerosis of the neck vessels is a relatively common disorder. While symptoms might occur when only *minimal* disease is present, severe disease might be present *without* symptoms. Noninvasive studies should be performed with consideration not only to those patients who have surgically treatable lesions but also to patients who will benefit from having this lesion treated prophylactically, lowering the likelihood of a future stroke. For patients with clear, recurrent carotid system TIAs, these studies are not necessary, and arteriography is indicated. Noninvasive studies cannot differentiate severe stenosis from occlusion and cannot detect intracranial involvement. Noninvasive studies may be of some value for the single carotid system TIA patient with a negative neurovascular examination. The greatest risk for stroke exists in the *first year* and especially in the *first 2 months* following a transient ischemic attack. Thus, if a patient has been asymptomatic for 1 year after a TIA, observation of this patient rather than work-up is indicated.

Many noninvasive techniques are currently available and may be categorized into two major groups. The first group consists of those techniques that *directly* assess the carotid bifurcation. They include (1) carotid phonoangiography (CPA), (2) audio-frequency analysis of bruits, (3) Doppler ultrasonic imaging of the carotid artery and its bifurcation, and (4) real-time ultrasound imaging of the carotid artery. The second group of techniques assesses the hemodynamics of the carotid system distal to the bifurcation and thus *indirectly* provides information about the morphology of the carotid system. These techniques include: (1) ophthalmodynamometry (indirect measurement of retinal artery pressure), (2) thermography, (3) oculoplethysmography (OPG), and (4) directional Doppler flow studies. The latter studies, which are more commonly performed for evaluation of TIAs, will be discussed.

Two techniques of *oculoplethysmography (OPG)* have been developed. One of these, developed by Kartchner, involves the application of suction through a *fluid system* to the sclera of the eyeballs for recording of the flow in the internal carotid artery. A sensor is applied to the ear lobe for simultaneous monitoring of the external carotid circulation. Delay in the arrival time of the pulse waves suggests a proximal stenosis or occlusion. The other type of OPG is based on *air vacuum* suction applied to the sclera of both eyeballs. As the intraocular pressure increases, the circulation in the choroidal and retinal arteries slows down and finally ceases. At this point, the intraocular pressure equals the pressure in the ophthalmic artery and can be accurately measured in mm Hg.

Directional Doppler study (supraorbital Doppler examination) involves placement of the Doppler probe over the supraorbital artery to determine whether flow is coming out of or toward the orbit. This can be determined *directly* by use of a directional Doppler study or *indirectly* by simultaneous listening to the supraorbital Doppler flow sound and compression of the branches of the external carotid artery. The latter indirect method is less satisfactory than the directional Doppler method. If the supraorbital flow sound suddenly disappears on external carotid compression or if the directional Doppler indicates flow back toward the orbit, significant internal carotid stenosis or occlusion with reversal of flow in the supraorbital artery, which then fills via the external carotid branches, exists.

A new technique, that of digital subtraction angiography, is currently being developed and may be useful in the future.

In summary, advanced technology can now evaluate carotid artery disease in a noninvasive manner. What remains to be determined by the physician is whether the symptoms with which the patient presents and the atherosclerosis present in the cerebral arteries are merely coincidental, unrelated findings, or *causally* related.

INDICATIONS FOR CAROTID SURGERY

Carotid reconstruction should not be considered unless the symptomatology can be ascribed to the lesion. When a patient has recurrent carotid system TIAs, angiography is indicated. The brachiocephalic and intracranial vessels should be visualized. Dye may be injected (1) through catheterization of the aortic arch and its branches, (2) by percutaneous puncture of the common carotid artery, or (3) by retrograde countercurrent injection of the brachial arteries. Films of the intracranial circulation are necessary to both identify associated vascular lesions and rule out intracranial mass lesions appearing as cerebrovascular disease. If arteriography reveals a stenosis of greater than 70 percent (Fig. 4–1) or an ulcerating plaque, regardless of the degree of stenosis in the carotid bifurcation, carotid endarterectomy, occasionally with a vein patch, is indicated.

During the period of clamping of the carotid artery, many surgeons prefer to use a temporary shunt to maintain adequate perfusion of the brain. Others prefer to monitor intraoperatively internal carotid artery stump pressure, jugular venous oxygen, and the electroencephalogram and to use a shunt only if necessary. A *vein patch graft* is often applied at the site of closure of the arteriotomy. While this type of surgery is not major, there is a small risk of stroke produced by the procedure. It is noteworthy that in recent years the incidence of intraoperative stroke has decreased as operative monitoring and techniques have improved.

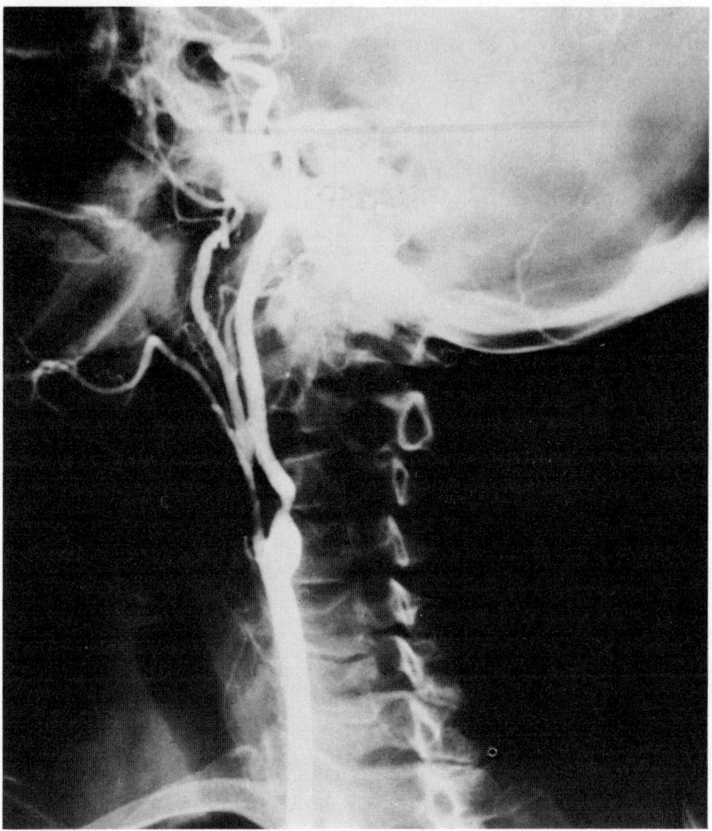

Figure 4-1. Carotid arteriogram.

A bypass for stenosis at the origin of the common carotid artery or stenosis of the vertebral artery involves a major thoracotomy and is not commonly performed. However, various types of *bypasses,* including carotid to subclavian, subclavian to carotid, and subclavian to subclavian, can be performed in the neck area with use of Dacron or Goretex materials.

Mention should be made of the *subclavian steal syndrome,* which involves marked stenosis or occlusion at the origin of the subclavian artery such that flow to the involved arm is via retrograde flow down the vertebral artery on that side, as shown by serial arteriography (Fig. 4-1). This entity might be discovered as an incidental finding on an arch study. Patients with subclavian steal syndrome might develop signs of cerebral ischemia on attempted use of the involved arm. Not infrequently, however, patients with arteriographically proven subclavian steal syndrome have lesions in other arteries, such as the opposite vertebral artery or one or both carotid arteries. Subclavian steal syndrome can be surgically treated by carotid-to-subclavian or subclavian-to-subclavian bypass.

OTHER TYPES OF REVASCULARIZATION

Some surgeons have recently attempted intracranial bypass grafts from branches of the external carotid artery to the middle cerebral artery. At present, evaluation of this procedure is not possible, as it is too new. Where there is marked narrowing of multiple branches of the aortic arch, *multilimb bypass grafts* from the aortic arch to the various segments of the subclavian and carotid systems are placed distal to the occlusion or stenoses. However, since these procedures involve a much greater morbidity rate, it would seem that the so-called extra-anatomic approaches of carotid to subclavian, subclavian to carotid, and subclavian to subclavian would be a more practical solution.

MEDICAL MANAGEMENT
OF A TRANSIENT ISCHEMIC ATTACK

As previously mentioned, any associated risk factor such as hypertension, diabetes, and hyperlipidemia should be controlled. There is no evidence that increased cerebral blood flow to an ischemic brain can be produced by any of the commonly available *cerebral vasodilator drugs*. There is some question as to whether or not drugs with rheologic properties, such as low-molecular-weight dextran, may improve microvascular perfusion. This has not been proven. Dextran acts by increasing the electronegative charge of the red blood cells, thereby lessening sludging or agglutination.

The use of *anticoagulants* for TIA patients remains controversial. There is suggestive evidence that oral anticoagulation with warfarin will decrease the risk of stroke in patients with carotid or well-defined vertebral-basilar TIAs, but this appears to be true primarily in the first few months after the onset of symptoms. There is an increased risk of intracranial hemorrhage in patients on coumadin.

At the present time, antiplatelet drugs, including aspirin, dipyridamole (Persantine), and sulfinpyrazone (Anturane), are being used extensively in patients with cerebrovascular disease. However, there is still no *sufficient* evidence that antiplatelet drugs prevent stroke in a TIA patient or lead to decreased mortality from this problem.

BIBLIOGRAPHY

Asari S, Kinugasa K, Fujesawa H, et al: Extracranial-intracranial bypass in experimental cerebral infarction in dogs. *Stroke* 9:461–464, 1978.

Editorial: Non-invasive techniques for diagnosis of carotid artery disease. *Stroke* 9:427–429, 1978.

Gee W, Mehigan JJ, Wylie EJ: Measurement of collateral cerebral hemispheric blood pressure by ocular pneumoplethysmography. *Am J Surg* 130:121–127, 1975.

Kartchner MK, McRae LP: Non-invasive evaluation and management of the asymptomatic carotid bruit. *Surgery* 82:840–847, 1977.

McDowell FH, Millikan C: Summary of 11th Princeton conference on cerebrovascular diseases (March 1978). *Stroke* 9:429–439, 1978.

Morssy J: Atherosclerosis and its complications in intracranial and extracranial cerebral arteries in Haimovici H (ed): *The Surgical Management of Vascular Diseases.* Philadelphia, Lippincott, 1970, pp 215–220.

CHAPTER FIVE

Venous Disease

The majority of venous problems encountered in medical practice occur in the legs, and most of the following remarks refer to the lower extremities. Phlebitis occurring in other areas will be discussed briefly at the end of this section.

ANATOMY–PHYSIOLOGY

Certain basic facts should be kept in mind when evaluating and treating a patient with problems of the venous system. Blood in the leg veins is fighting gravity. The primary force propelling blood back to the heart is supplied by contraction of the lower-extremity muscles. Thus, it is easy to understand that when a person is sitting or standing motionless without muscle contractions in the legs, there will be a significant increase in peripheral venous pressure. Other factors propelling blood back toward the heart include: (1) a small residual intravascular pressure left over from the heart after blood traverses the arterial system and capillary bed; (2) pressure applied to a vein by an adjoining artery as it pulsates; and (3) negative intrathoracic pressure, which occurs with inspiration, drawing blood up to the heart. The average pressure at the venous end of a capillary at heart level is 12 mm Hg. Eighty-five percent of venous return from the lower extremity is via the deep system.

    In addition, certain anatomic considerations are important. The veins of

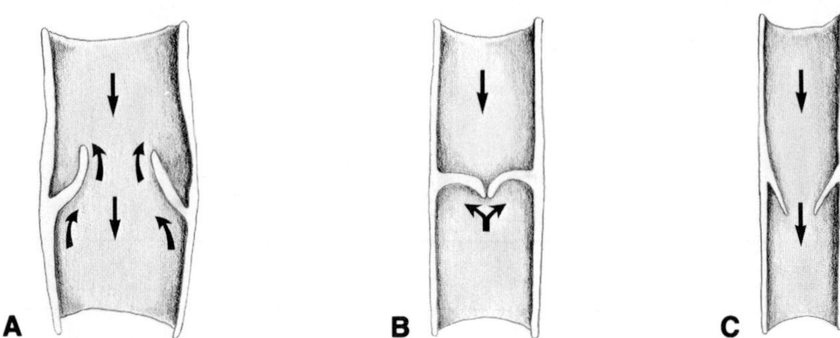

Figure 5-1. Competent (A, B) and incompetent (C) venous valves.

the lower extremities have valves that prevent backflow if the leaflets are competent (Fig. 5-1). Above the groin, the number of valves is very small, with one or no valve present in the iliac area and usually no valve in the inferior vena cava.

In the communicating veins (perforating veins), the flow is normally from superficial to deep, with valves present to prevent backflow from deep to superficial areas. Valves may be incompetent on a congenital basis or may become incompetent as a result of thrombus formation from thrombophlebitis. It is of interest that if there is significant deep venous obstruction such that over a period of time collateral venous pathways develop, the collaterals usually have no valve.

The deep veins of the foot include the deep plantar venous arch and the medial and lateral plantar veins. At the calf level, there are normally three paired sets of veins, including the anterior tibial, posterior tibial, and peroneal veins. It must be stressed that there is considerable anatomic variation from patient to patient, especially in the calf area. The three sets of veins at the calf level usually merge to form a single or paired popliteal vein, which then continues as the femoral vein (primary deep vein of the thigh), where it continues to the inguinal ligament. The primary superficial vein in the lower extremity is the long (greater) saphenous vein, which starts at the medial malleolus and progresses upward along the medial leg and thigh to form the saphenofemoral junction at the groin. The other significant superficial vein is the short saphenous vein, which starts behind the lateral malleolus, runs upward along the lateral border of the Achilles tendon, and then pierces the deep fascia halfway up the leg to run into the groove between the bellies of the gastrocnemius muscle. Usually, it then joins the popliteal vein. In addition, there are many intramuscular veins of the leg, especially in the calf area. These veins are compressed and emptied with calf muscle contraction, provided that the venous pump, which is most helpful in emptying blood that would otherwise pool in the veins of the leg, is intact.

Persons with normal venous circulation will develop edema if their legs are dependent for a long enough period of time. This is due to constant high hydrostatic pressure. If one moves sufficiently during the day and has a period of rest at night with the body parallel to the ground, elevated venous pressure does not develop. However, if one takes a long plane ride, especially if it involves being up day and night and the following day when the legs are not elevated at all, or if soldiers are made to stand at attention for 8 hours without moving, development of edema of the ankles in spite of a normal venous system is not uncommon.

VARICOSE VEINS

The usual cause of varicosities is incompetence in communicating veins, usually of a congenital basis. Over a period of time, increased pressure in the superficial system, as a result of the incompetent communicators, leads to gradual dilatation of the superficial vein, which, in turn, becomes tortuous and develops incompetence in its own valves (Fig. 5–2). Dilated superficial veins may also develop as collaterals if there is significant deep venous obstruction. It should be noted that varicose veins are primarily of cosmetic concern and less commonly cause significant peripheral edema or stasis ulceration.

Varicosities are usually self-evident. The location of communicating vein incompetence can often be ascertained by appropriate tourniquet testing. This involves elevating the leg to empty the veins, applying a high-thigh tourniquet,

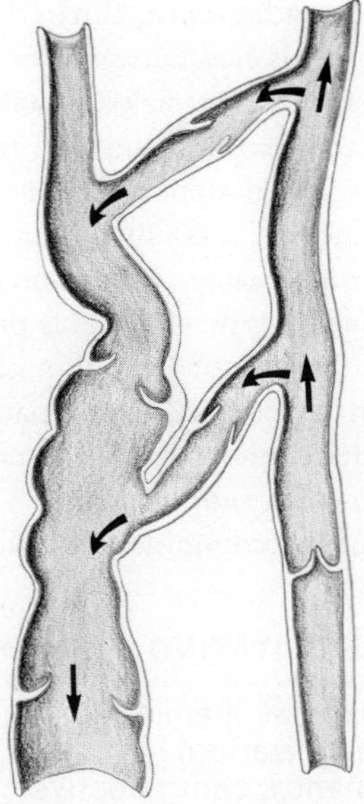

Figure 5–2. Varicose veins.

and then having the patient stand up. This maneuver is repeated with the tourniquet at *progressively lower levels* to determine at what tourniquet level rapid filling of the varicosity is prevented. In addition, the patient can be exercised with a high-thigh tourniquet to test for patency of the deep venous system. With exercise and a proximal tourniquet, the superficial veins should empty moderately if the deep system is open.

As for the management of varicosities, if they are small in size and number, they may be left alone and perhaps treated with proper elastic support and leg elevation. If there are large numbers of veins or veins of great size or if the patient is overly concerned from a cosmetic standpoint, then varicose vein surgery consisting of ligation and stripping is indicated. Prior to this type of surgery, it is important to determine where the leaking communicating veins are located and also to ascertain the presence of a patent deep venous system. This can be done with the tourniquet testing as mentioned before or by Doppler ultrasound study. If there is any question, then a venogram should be performed.

THROMBOPHLEBITIS

The exact etiology of thrombophlebitis is not known, but several factors may play a part (Table 5–1). The first factor is mechanical or chemical injury. If there is direct injury to a vein from trauma or an irritating substance given intravenously, this may lead to endothelial damage within the wall of the vein, which may then lead to platelet adherence, fibrin deposition, and thrombosis. The body normally has many balances between thrombosis and fibrinolysis. A second and most important factor is stasis or slowing of blood flow. When the rate of venous flow in the limb becomes sluggish, there is a greater propensity toward deep vein thrombosis. Dependency and/or lack of the muscle pump are aggravating factors. This may be seen in patients at bedrest, such as with hospitalization for acute myocardial infarction, pneumonia, etc, or in postoperative patients. The same type of stasis is produced when a limb is immobilized by a cast or splint after fractures or other musculoskeletal injuries. We have also seen stasis lead to thromboembolism in patients cramped into an overcrowded plane for an extended trip or who fall asleep in an awkward position, such as with the leg draped over the end of a sofa. The third factor that may be related to the development of thrombophlebitis is hypercoagulability, but it is

TABLE 5–1. FACTORS PRECIPITATING THROMBOPHLEBITIS

1. Endothelial injury (mechanical-chemical)
2. Stasis (dependency-immobilization)
3. Hypercoaguability (pregnancy, contraceptives, malignancy, etc)

difficult to measure in the laboratory. There may be antithrombin III deficiency (familial) or shortened platelet survival time.

During the postoperative or postpartum period, there is an increased generation of thromboplastin, creating a potential hypercoagulable state with a resultant increased incidence of deep vein thrombosis. Likewise, in patients with overt or occult malignancy, there is also increased circulating thromboplastin, which may explain the increased incidence of thrombophlebitis in patients with neoplasms. In addition, patients on oral contraceptive pills have been shown to have an increased incidence of thromboembolism associated with the hormones present in these drugs.

SUPERFICIAL THROMBOPHLEBITIS

Superficial thrombophlebitis involves inflammation as well as thrombus formation in a superficial vein of the extremities. There is usually pain, redness, heat, and local tenderness as well as a palpable cord (thrombosed vein). Systemic signs such as fever and tachycardia are usually not present. There is usually no peripheral edema, although local swelling may be present in the area of the inflamed vein. The differential diagnoses include cellulitis, lymphangitis, and erythyma nodosum. Superficial phlebitis tends to be rather inflammatory, which makes the thrombus more adherent to the wall of the vein. Therefore, the incidence of pulmonary emboli with superficial thrombophlebitis is low, so that anticoagulants are not routinely necessary. The usual treatment involves leg *elevation,* warm compresses, and anti-inflammatory drugs, most commonly phenylbutazone. The process usually improves within 4 to 7 days. It may take several weeks to completely subside. Should the process not respond to treatment, especially if the phlebitis extends progressively up the leg, then heparinization is advisable to prevent the process from extending into the deep system.

DEEP VEIN THROMBOSIS (DVT)

Deep vein thrombosis represents thrombosis in the deep venous system, usually but not always associated with inflammation (Fig. 5-3). Patients who form thrombi as a result of stasis from bedrest or immobilization may have very little inflammation, and it is this type of thrombophlebitis, perhaps more accurately called deep venous thrombosis, which is more dangerous from the point of view of risk of pulmonary embolism. Patients with deep thrombophlebitis usually present with significant edema of the leg associated with pain and tenderness. There may be a dull ache, worse on dependency. The calf is tender on deep

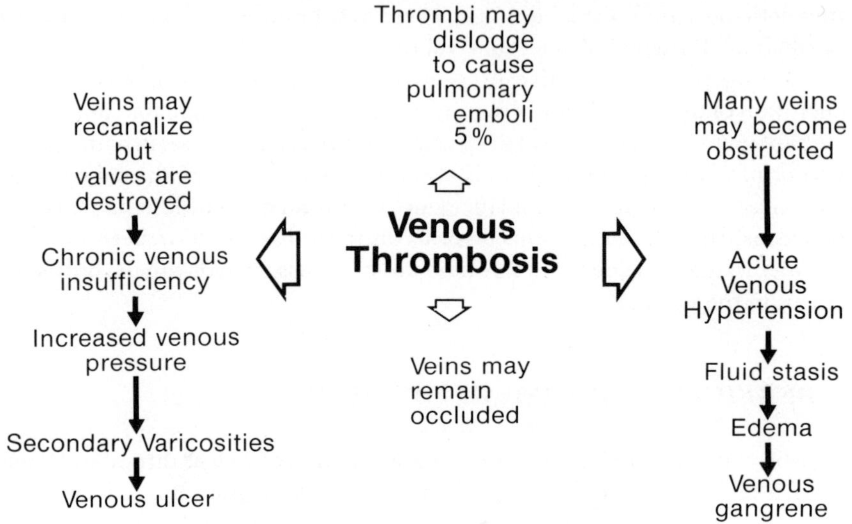

Figure 5–3. Natural history of venous thrombosis.

palpation. There may be pain in the calf on dorsiflexion of the foot (Homans' sign), although it is nonspecific. There are other signs, such as the tibial tap sign and the cuff test (inflating a blood pressure cuff on the calf and comparing the pressures at which pain is produced in the symptomatic and asymptomatic legs). It must be pointed out that all of these tests are nonspecific, are not diagnostic of thrombophlebitis, and may be present in other entities that cause calf pain and tenderness. In addition, other symptoms may include increased warmth, a prominent superficial, collateral venous pattern, and mild systemic signs such as slight fever or tachycardia. The less inflammatory the process, the greater the risk of pulmonary emboli. With proper treatment, the process usually will subside within 1 to 3 weeks.

The clinical diagnosis of acute thrombophlebitis by history and physical examination alone is difficult. Fifty percent of cases of deep thrombophlebitis may be asymptomatic. The differential diagnosis includes Baker's (popliteal) cyst, which may have concomitant thrombophlebitis associated with it, muscle tear (sudden sharp pain in the calf associated with exertion and followed by ecchymoses within several days), cellulitis, lymphangitis, muscle hematoma, sciatica, popliteal artery aneurysm, tension myalgia, lymphedema, and arteriovenous fistula (Table 5–2). It should be pointed out that if thrombophlebitis is present, treatment is necessary to prevent the development of pulmonary emboli and propagation of clots, which occurs in approximately 20 percent of untreated patients. Another interesting observation is that as many as 50 percent of patients referred as chronic recurrent deep vein thrombosis patients have never had the disease.

TABLE 5-2. DIFFERENTIAL OF CALF PAIN.

Thrombophlebitis
Baker's cyst
Muscle tear
Cellulitis
Lymphangitis
Hematoma
Sciatica
Popliteal artery aneurysm
Tension myalgia

EVALUATION

It has been shown that physical examination alone is accurate in only 50 percent of cases of deep thrombophlebitis. This means that half of the patients diagnosed as having thrombophlebitis on clinical grounds do not have thrombophlebitis when further studies are performed. For this reason, other studies are often helpful if the diagnosis remains questionable after history and physical examination. Venography is the standard by which other studies are compared and represents the most accurate means of diagnosing thrombophlebitis, although even this test is not absolute. Because other methods in addition to history and physical examination are frequently necessary and in light of the fact that venography is an invasive procedure, various tests have been developed over the last 10 years to help increase the accuracy of the diagnosis of thrombophlebitis.

Impedance Plethysmography (IMP or IPG)

Impedance plethysmography involves the placement of paired electrodes around the limb through which a minute electrical current is passed from one electrode to the other. Even minute changes in the limb fluid volume will be reflected by an alteration in the electrical resistance. A recording is made so that any variation of the limb fluid volume, such as that which occurs with inspiration and expiration, leads to a change in electrical resistance, which is recorded graphically. A variation of this test is the occlusive IPG where a venous occlusion cuff is placed high on the thigh and changes are sought on release of the cuff rather than on phasic changes with respiration. If deep vein thrombosis is present, the normal variation in limb fluid volume with respiration will be diminished or absent with this test. The accuracy of diagnosis of thrombophlebitis by this method is said to be 40 to 50 percent.

Pulse Volume Recorder (PVR)

The pulse volume recorder test is used to determine the maximum rate of venous outflow from the extremity after venous return has temporarily been obstructed by an occluding blood pressure cuff inflated to below diastolic pressure. As blood pools in the veins distal to the cuff, the limb volume increases, causing a gradual rise in the monitoring cuff pressure. When the occluding cuff is released, limb volume rapidly decreases. However, if there is hemodynamically significant deep venous obstruction, the resistance to flow increases, producing a decreased rate of venous outflow.

Phleborheography (PRG)

Phleborheography involves the application of recording cuffs at five different levels on the extremity and an additional cuff around the thorax to record respirations. These cuffs are connected to a six-channel recorder that simultaneously records the normal respiratory variation of venous pressure. The presence of acute deep venous thrombosis will obliterate these respiratory waves and will also interfere with normal outflow of blood from the extremity in response to rhythmic compression. Proponents of this test claim an accuracy of 80 to 90 percent.

Doppler Ultrasound

The Doppler instrument transmits an ultrasound beam. If the beam strikes moving particles such as red blood cells moving in a vein or artery, the ultrasound beam is altered and reflected back to a small ultrasound receiver in the tip of the probe that is then converted to an audible sound. Venous flow generates a low-pitched sound that does not vary with the cardiac cycle but does show phasic variation with respiration. Occasionally, the venous flow sound may seem pulsatile in tricuspid insufficiency or congestive heart failure or because of a neighboring artery. Venous flow over the femoral, popliteal, and posterior tibial veins can be monitored with the Doppler instrument.

Variations of this venous flow sound with respiration indicate a competent deep venous system from the level of the probe back to the heart. In addition, compression proximal and/or distal to the probe can reveal a clot or venous *valvular* incompetence. With the probe over the posterior tibial vein of a normal deep venous system, calf compression will slow or stop the venous flow sound while release of calf compression will cause a sudden rush of flow at the posterior tibial level. With the Doppler probe over the popliteal vein, calf compression should produce an augmentation of the venous sound in the absence of thrombosis. If the calf veins are occluded by thrombi, there will be little or no augmentation of the venous flow sound. With the probe over the popliteal vein, thigh compression produces no augmentation of the venous sound in the presence of a competent valve system of the deep veins that prevents backflow. An increase in the venous sound at the popliteal level upon thigh compression indicates valvular incompetence of the deep system in that area. With the probe over the femoral vein, compression of the thigh will produce an augmentation of the venous sound in a normal situation and no augmentation of the venous sound with a Valsalva maneuver or with pelvic compression. In experienced hands, the accuracy of the Doppler study is felt to be 60 to 70 percent.

The preceding tests, including impedance plethysmography, pulse volume recorder, and Doppler ultrasound, are shown to be more accurate in the diagnosis of thrombi of the iliac or femoral veins in which the diagnosis of deep vein thrombosis is not as difficult to establish from physical examination. The tests are less reliable in the case of calf thrombophlebitis whose clinical diagnosis by history and physical is much less accurate. Thus, while these studies add to our clinical acumen, there is still a significant number of patients whose diagnoses still remain in question.

Radioactive Fibrinogen Scanning

I_{125}-labeled fibrinogen is injected intravenously, and the lower extremity is scanned daily for 5 to 7 days. The tagged fibrinogen is incorporated with a thrombus. If thrombi form, the level of radioactivity will increase, which will be picked up by the scanning. A greater than 20 percent increase in radioactivity lasting more than 24 hours is significant.

This test is reliable in the calf area but not in the thigh or pelvic areas, and only if it is given prior to the development of the thrombus. It is helpful in monitoring the development of thrombophlebitis in postoperative patients in whom I_{125} fibrinogen should be given preoperatively, before the thrombus forms. Of those who develop a positive scan, about 20 percent will go on to develop *clinical* deep vein thrombosis. Therefore, those patients who have positive scans should be heparinized.

Radioactive fibrinogen scanning is also useful in the study of various means of prophylaxis in the development of phlebitis in groups of patients undergoing surgery. The goal of these studies has been to determine which patients develop thrombi with or without prophylaxis. Radioactive fibrinogen scanning has been shown to be rather inaccurate in the diagnosis of thrombophlebitis in patients who are given the tagged fibrinogen after the development of thrombophlebitis.

Radioisotope Venography

Radioisotopes can be injected into a vein on the dorsum of the foot, and scans can be taken as the isotope flows up the lower extremity. Some centers inject their lung scans this way, thus obtaining the vein scan as well. A crude type of outline of the venous system is obtained, which may give gross information. The outline is poor below the level of the knee. It is difficult to make a diagnosis of thrombophlebitis with this technique. This procedure may be useful if an allergy to contrast media exists. A flow study that does not identify the thrombus but may tell of the collateral pathways is obtained.

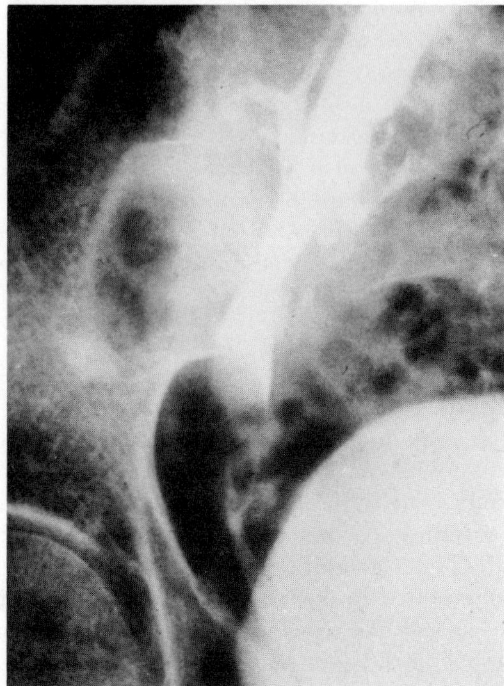

Figure 5–4. Recanalized vein.

Venography

Opacification of the deep venous system with contrast is considered the standard for the diagnosis of deep vein thrombosis. Venography is considered an accurate study, although it is not an absolute tool. Part of the difficulty lies with the fact that there is marked anatomic variation, especially in the calf area. Also, on occasion, the popliteal and/or the superficial femoral veins may be duplicated.

The technique involves injecting contrast into a small vein on the dorsum of the foot and taking x-rays as the dye flows up the leg. Some angiographers prefer to place a tourniquet around the ankle to drive the dye into the deep system, although most angiographers do not feel this is necessary. Any pain associated with the procedure is related to the length of time that the contrast media is in contact with the vein. Abnormalities encountered with this procedure include: (1) sudden cessation of flow in a vein, (2) rounded ghostlike filling defects within the vein with dye flowing around the thrombus (indicating fresh thrombus poorly adhering to the vein), (3) absence of filling of veins normally expected to fill, and (4) an hourglass appearance of a vein, representing a recanalized vein (Fig. 5–4). To obtain good visualization of the iliac veins and vena cava, the contrast media should be injected into the femoral vein. One thing that cannot be determined on the usual venogram is competency of the valves. One can usually see the presence of a valve but cannot tell whether or not the valve leaflets will prevent backflow. Special methods of performing the venogram to determine the competency of valves are available, but these procedures are rather difficult and seldom performed. Doppler ultrasound offers more information about valvular competence than does venography. A venogram is indicated if the clinical and noninvasive evaluation still leave doubt as to the presence of deep vein thrombosis.

TREATMENT

The goals of therapy for thrombophlebitis is to prevent pulmonary emboli and to lessen the degree of permanent damage in the deep venous system, thus reducing the possibility and extent of a postphlebitic syndrome. It should be pointed out that there are an estimated 140,000 fatalities per year in the United States from pulmonary emboli and that 200,000 people are disabled yearly in the United States from a postphlebitic syndrome.

Elevation relieves swelling by producing improved venous return to the heart. Elastic support is usually not necessary while the patient is in bed with legs elevated. However, once the patient begins to ambulate, mild elastic support such as antiembolism stockings may help prevent stasis in the superficial venous system. By compressing the superficial veins, antiembolism stockings produce a greater rate of flow in the deep venous system. In addition to leg elevation, the primary treatment for deep thrombophlebitis consists of intravenous heparin therapy. Warm compresses are of questionable value but may offer symptomatic relief. Thrombectomy with a Fogarty catheter was advocated in the past. Although an initial successful result may be obtained, there is high incidence of rethrombosis; therefore, thrombectomy is seldom indicated except perhaps in the case of massive iliofemoral thrombophlebitis. Ambulation may be started when the patient becomes free of pain, and it should be instituted while the patient is still on heparin. Heparin is usually continued for 7 to 12 days. The patient is usually switched to oral anticoagulants (warfarin) prior to stopping heparin, and the oral anticoagulants are continued for 2 to 3 months.

Should there be a contraindication to heparin therapy such as recent or acute upper gastrointestinal bleeding, low molecular weight dextran therapy should be instituted. This may be beneficial in view of its anti-inflammatory effect and its effect of increased electronegative charge on red blood cells that reduces sludging or agglutination, especially in the microvasculature. While good results in the treatment of deep vein thrombosis with dextran have been reported, it would not be the drug of choice if anticoagulants could be utilized.

Again, the mainstay of treatment for deep vein thrombosis is anticoagulation therapy with heparin. Heparin appears to interfere with many coagulation factors, including thromboplastin and prothrombin, but its main action is in preventing thrombin from reacting with fibrinogen to form fibrin. Heparin is used intravenously either by intermittent intravenous injection every 4 to 6 hours, as originally advocated by the Scandinavians, or as continuous intravenous infusion after an initial bolus injection. With intermittent intravenous heparin therapy, the usual dose is 4000 to 5000 units every 4 hours. Most patients have a good therapeutic response to this regimen. It has the advantages of not requiring an infusion pump and not requiring the patient to be attached to an intravenous line. It is a reasonably safe method provided that the partial thrombin time (PTT) is not "chased." (Attempt to keep the PTT at twice the normal when measured 3½ hours after administration of the dose of heparin.) Many physicians now favor continuous intravenous heparin. It was shown that there is a lower incidence of bleeding complications with continuous intravenous heparin therapy with the PTT kept at 1½–2 times normal compared to intermittent intravenous heparin therapy. Another advantage of continuous heparin therapy is that the PTT may be done at any random hour rather than at a predetermined time, as with intermittent intravenous therapy. The average dose with continuous heparin is 22,000 to 25,000 units per day after an initial bolus of 5,000 to 10,000 units.

Thrombocytopenia (platelet count under 100,000) has been reported to occur during heparin therapy, but it has been seen only infrequently in our experience and does not seem to lead to any problem. The platelet count is found to return to normal levels after heparin is discontinued. The purposes of heparinization are improvement of thrombophlebitis and prevention of thromboembolism. It is questionable whether the PTT must be kept at a specific level for this to occur. Improvement may be seen on venography or even in the clinical setting with less than full heparinization. There may be local factors in the area of the thrombophlebitis leading to increased or decreased sensitivity to heparin that cannot be measured by the usual tests (PTT or LWCT). It is possible that a relatively simple heparin assay that is better for monitoring heparin therapy may become available in the future.

The newest form of treatment for thromboembolism is fibrinolytic therapy with streptokinase or urokinase. Streptokinase became available 15 years ago. However, a newer, more purified form of streptokinase with much less pyrogenicity was introduced for general use in January 1978, and urokinase was also recently placed on the market. At present, these drugs are found useful in situations of massive or life-threatening pulmonary emboli and extensive deep vein thrombosis. When used within 3 days but preferably within 24 hours of the onset of thrombophlebitis or pulmonary embolism, this drug therapy usually produces prompt lysis of the thrombus. This, in turn, allows return of normal deep venous function without damage to the valves in the leg veins and promptly relieves right heart strain associated with massive pulmonary embolism. Streptokinase acts by combining with plasminogen to form an activator that combines with more plasminogen to produce plasmin. Plasmin can hydrolyze fibrin and fibrinogen (Fig. 5–5).

There is a greater possibility of bleeding complications associated with fibrinolytic therapy than with heparin therapy, so the patient must be carefully watched. The patient should have no intramuscular or intra-arterial injection during or within 12 hours of fibrinolytic therapy. A fixed dosage schedule involving a thrombin time or P.T.T. administered prior to therapy and again at 4 and perhaps at 12 hours after initiation of therapy is recommended to test the activation of the fibrinolytic system. Streptokinase, 250,000 IU, is given as an initial loading dose with a maintenance dose of 100,000 IU per hour for 12–24 hours for pulmonary emboli or significant deep vein thrombosis. When necessary, the fibrinolytic state can be reversed by the administration of EACA (epsilon aminocaproic acid). Fibrinolytic therapy should not be used for minor thrombophlebitis. During streptokinase therapy, there may be a reduction in plasma fibrinogen and plasminogen as well as a marked shortening of the euglobulin clot lysis time. Thrombolytic therapy is contraindicated in patients with a bleeding diathesis, in postoperative patients, and in patients in whom a translumbar aortogram was performed within the preceding 10 days. It is also contraindicated in patients with any recent bleeding episode, severe hypertension, or severe liver or kidney disease. There is little question that fibrinolytic therapy leads to lysis of thrombi in the deep veins and in the pulmonary arteries. However, there is a question as to whether there is any lowering in mortality

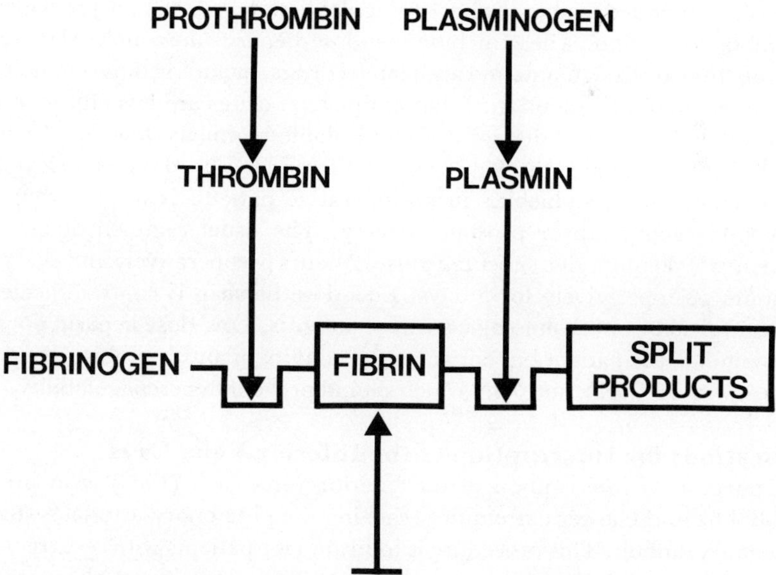

Figure 5–5. Thrombosis and fibrinolysis.

rates or in the incidence of recurrent pulmonary emboli compared with patients treated only with heparin. After streptokinase therapy is completed, the patient should be heparinized until coumadinization can be completed. The patient should then be kept on oral anticoagulants for several months. It is of interest that studies on pulmonary embolism patients have shown greater thrombolysis in the streptokinase-treated group compared to the heparin-treated group after 3 days, but after 10 days of therapy the difference between the two groups became insignificant. It is also interesting to note a greater lytic response in male patients than in female patients.

PROPHYLAXIS OF THROMBOPHLEBITIS

The following groups of patients may be considered as having a higher than usual risk for developing thrombophlebitis: (1) patients at bedrest such as after acute myocardial infarction, congestive heart failure, pneumonia, sepsis, and traction; (2) patients undergoing surgery who are over 40 years of age; (3) patients with leg trauma, especially those with fractures and those with a cast; (4) patients with a history of thrombophlebitis, obesity, or malignancy; and (5) women taking oral contraceptives. To prevent the development of thrombophlebitis, it is recommended that an attempt be made to eliminate stasis by keeping the legs elevated while in bed, exercising the legs frequently, and wearing mild elastic support hose when the legs are dependent. Various drugs have been recommended to alter the hypercoagulable state, which may predispose to thrombus formation. These include low-dose heparin, low-molecular-weight dextran, oral anticoagulants and antiplatelet drugs, including dipyridamole and aspirin. It should be mentioned that antiplatelet drugs are less efficacious for venous than for arterial disease. Of all available regimens, low-dose or minidose heparin has gained the widest acceptance and has been shown to lower the incidence of thrombophlebitis in postoperative patients, except perhaps for those undergoing hip or prostate surgery. The usual regimen of low-dose heparin is 5000 units give subcutaneously 2 hours preoperatively and every 8 or 12 hours postoperatively for 5 days. Low-dose heparin is contraindicated in neurosurgical or ophthalmologic surgical patients. Low-dose heparin does not anticoagulate the patient but enhances the activity of antithrombin III and interferes with X^A, IX^A, and XI^A, which should prevent hypercoagulability.

Indications for Interruption of the Inferior Vena Cava

The purpose of interruption of the inferior vena cava (IVC) is to prevent thrombi from the lower extremities reaching the pulmonary arterial system as pulmonary emboli. This procedure is indicated for patients with recurrent pulmonary emboli while on adequate anticoagulation and for those with pulmonary emboli who cannot be anticoagulated for other reasons such as gastrointestinal bleeding. Less common indications include septic pulmonary emboli and paradoxical emboli with a patent right to left shunt. It should be emphasized that if recurrent pulmonary emboli occur at a time when the patient is not adequately anticoagulated, an increased level of anticoagulant therapy as opposed to inferior vena cava (IVC) interruption is indicated. It is rare for a patient on even a moderate amount of heparin to have a fatal pulmonary embolus. Interrupting the vena cava is effective in preventing further embolization during the initial 6 to 12 months, but after that time contrast studies usually show large collateral pathways so that it is again possible for thrombi to leave the lower extremities and enter the pulmonary circuit. Caval interruption will not prevent (1) recurrent pulmonary emboli with a double cava, (2) thrombi proximal to the interruption of the inferior vena cava, or (3) emboli arising in the upper-extremity, veins or right heart.

The surgical methods of interrupting the IVC are ligation and plication. By comparison, the plication method by either suture plication or by one of the available clips is preferred. The plication method allows passage of some venous flow, thereby lowering peripheral venous pressure (Fig. 5–6). This lower peripheral venous pressure will reduce the incidence of postphlebitic syndrome and peripheral edema. It also reduces the possibility of development of large collateral pathways and thus may protect the patient for a longer period of time

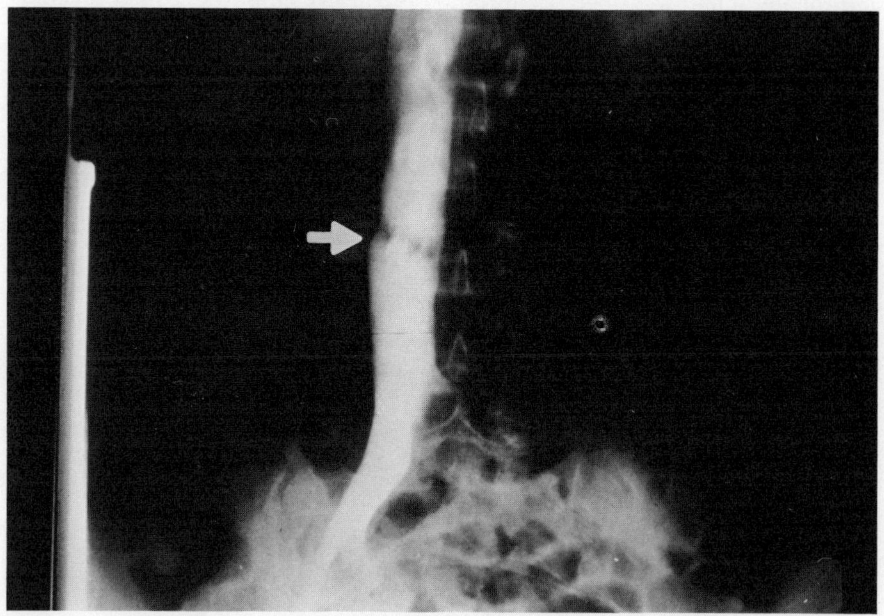

Figure 5–6. Caval plication.

from further pulmonary emboli. It is possible that a certain number of plications become the same as a ligation if the plicated area thromboses, but even if this occurs, the patient is no worse off than if he originally had a ligation. In patients too ill to undergo surgery, the IVC may be interrupted by a filter inserted percutaneously. The Mobin-Uddin umbrella can be inserted via the right jugular vein or the Kimray-Greenfield filter can be passed into the IVC via the femoral vein.

VENOUS GANGRENE (PHLEGMASIAS)

The phlegmasias represent an extension of an iliofemoral thrombophlebitis. With iliofemoral thrombosis, there is significant peripheral edema and increased peripheral venous pressure, but the more distal and collateral venous pathways are patent, and arterial inflow is normal. Should this process worsen so that there is extensive deep venous thrombosis throughout the lower extremities, arterial inflow is reduced because of obstruction in the venous outflow tract. The patient will present with a mildly ischemic leg with perhaps some decrease in peripheral pulses and pallor but no skin breakdown. This condition is referred to as *phlegmasia alba dolens.*

Should the process worsen even further so that even the smallest venules and collateral pathways become thrombosed, arterial inflow becomes severely compromised. The leg may become cadaveric and distally develop frank gangrene. This results from the inability of arterial flow to enter the capillary bed because of severe obstruction in the venous system (Fig. 5–7). In spite of the severe ischemia, the limb is usually not cold because of extensively pooled venous blood. This condition is referred to as *phlegmasia cerulea dolens.* Most cases of phlegmasia cerulea dolens occur in patients with malignancy or in patients who have an occult neoplasm, which later becomes apparent. It is not uncommon for these patients to progress to a point requiring amputation of the limb because of gangrene, which is actually secondary to venous disease. Should a pa-

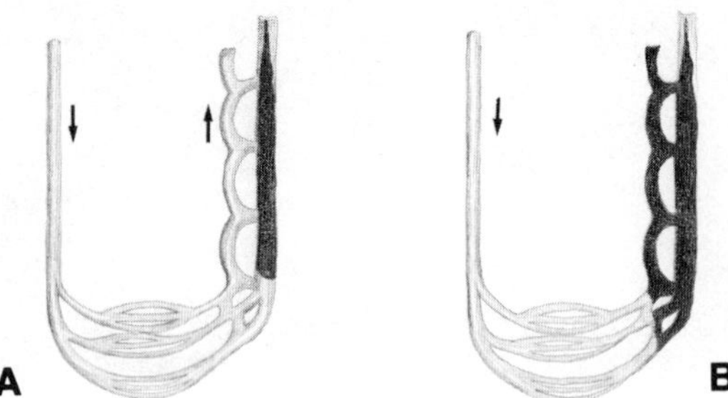

Figure 5–7. Phlegmasia alba dolens (A) and cerulea dolens (B).

tient with phlegmasia cerulea dolens present without evidence of neoplasm, a thorough examination should be instituted since almost all of these patients will eventually develop a neoplasm. From a therapeutic standpoint, treatment consists of large doses of heparin. If the patient is seen within the first few days of onset of this process, administration of streptokinase is recommended in view of the serious nature of this problem, particularly if adequate venous outflow cannot be obtained. Phlegmasia cerulea dolens rarely occurs in the upper extremities.

OTHER TYPES OF THROMBOPHLEBITIS

Upper-Extremity Thrombophlebitis

Superficial thrombophlebitis may be seen in the upper extremity secondary to the presence of an intravenous catheter or to the administration of intravenous medication, which is irritating to the vein. If a large catheter is placed into a vein, thrombosis may occur because of the lack of normal venous flow around the catheter. There is usually an intense local inflammatory reaction, but pulmonary emboli are uncommon. Warm soaks are indicated, and heparin may be helpful, especially if there appears to be propagation of the thrombus.

An uncommon but interesting type of venous thrombosis occurs in the axillary or subclavian area and is referred to as *effort or axillary thrombosis* (Fig. 5–8).

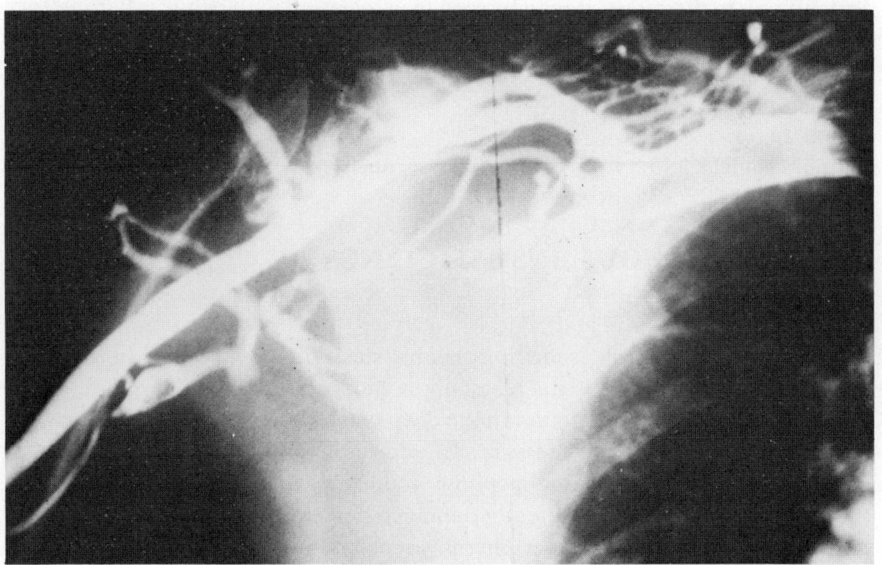

Figure 5–8. Effort thrombosis.

The mechanism here is some unusual or strenuous exertion of the upper extremity leading to a small endothelial tear in the subclavian or axillary vein with platelet or fibrin deposition and thrombosis. These patients present with a swollen, cyanotic, painful arm with dilated superficial veins. It is interesting that as many as 25 percent of patients with subclavian vein intravenous lines have venogram-proven but usually asymptomatic thrombi in the area.

Doppler examination may fail to show flow in the axillary vein. The usual treatment is full heparinization for 10 to 12 days, followed by warfarin for 3 months, during which time recanalization or collateralization develops. With this treatment, patients usually become asymptomatic by the end of 3 months. Attempts at Fogarty-catheter thrombectomy do not usually produce long-lasting patency of the vein, and it is therefore not indicated. We have seen this entity occur after heavy lifting, bowling, and filing objects on high shelves.

Superior Vena Caval Syndrome

Superior vena caval syndrome is usually caused by neoplasms, neoplasm of the lung being the most common. There may be an intraluminal lesion or external compression. Signs and symptoms depend on (1) the location and the degree of obstruction, (2) the chronicity of the condition, and (3) the presence of collaterals, which are demonstrated by infrared photography.

Pelvic Thrombophlebitis

Pelvic thrombophlebitis undoubtedly does occur, but its incidence is uncommon and difficult to diagnose. It may be seen in association with pelvic inflammatory disease. Otherwise, there is no specific sign. The usual type of venography fails to opacify the pelvic veins.

Tumors

Tumors such as leiomyosarcoma are rare causes of venous thrombosis.

CHRONIC VENOUS INSUFFICIENCY

Chronic venous insufficiency is also referred to as *postphlebitic snydrome* and results from any process producing chronic stasis of venous blood in the lower extremities. It is frequently the result of previous episodes of thrombophlebitis, which leave residual obstruction in the deep venous system, which, in turn, increases peripheral venous pressure. In addition, the collateral pathways that develop lack valves to prevent backflow. If the deep venous system recanalizes, the valves are usually permanently damaged and eventually become incompetent. This leads to increased peripheral venous pressure. Chronic venous insufficiency may also result from compression of the deep veins by tumors, extensive hemangiomas, arteriovenous fistulas, or congenital absence of valves in the deep veins.

To once again review the physiology, there are superficial veins, deep veins, and communicating or perforating veins that run from the superficial to the deep venous system. Valves prevent backflow. The peripheral venous pressure drops markedly with walking or lower-extremity exercise, and this is referred to as the *muscle pump*. However, in the presence of valve incompetence of the communicating or deep venous system or obstruction in the deep venous system, the peripheral venous pressure remains high even during exercise. A chronically elevated peripheral venous pressure, even with ambulation, leads to increased capillary pressure with congestion and development of edema in the interstitial tissues.

Thus, in the early stages, patients develop peripheral edema, usually only in the foot or lower leg but not in the toes. These symptoms may intensify with progression of the day. As years pass, the patient may develop brown pigmentation, especially on the medial lower leg, as a result of hemosiderin deposits that lead to dermatitis with irritation and itching and, sometimes, dry scaly skin. If this condition goes untreated, the extent of edema and pigmentation worsen, and induration often associated with fibrosis develops in the subcutaneous tissue. If more years pass without treatment, the patient may again develop a typical stasis ulceration of the medial lower leg (Fig. 5–9), which may be moderately painful and cause a significant degree of disability. It is estimated that at any one time 200,000 people in the United States are unable to work because of stasis ulcerations.

Many of the problems associated with stasis dermatitis and ulceration can be avoided before they develop with proper medical management, which involves elastic support and leg elevation during the day and mild leg elevation at

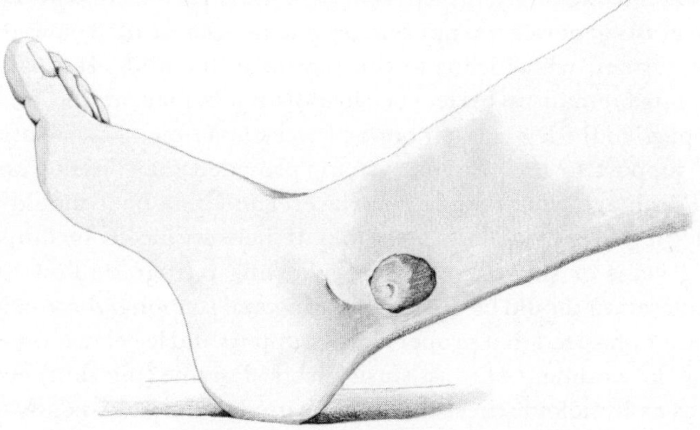

Figure 5-9. Venous ulcer.

night. The pressure applied against the skin by women's support hose is in the neighborhood of 6 to 8 mm Hg. So-called antiembolism stockings, or men's support hose, apply a pressure of about 12 mm Hg. Custom-made, heavier elastic stockings may have a pressure of 20 to 50 mm Hg. The proper type of elastic support for any one patient will vary depending on the basic underlying pathophysiology and clinical situation. Ordinary Ace bandaging of the leg may prove satisfactory in some cases, but a uniform pressure all the way up the leg as the Ace bandage is wrapped around the limb is difficult to obtain.

The appearance of a stasis ulcer is not too much different from other types of leg ulcers. These are generally only moderately painful, or there may be no pain. The etiology can be traced to the location of the ulcer and to the appearance of the surrounding skin and the leg itself. If there is no history of thrombophlebitis or past venous problem and no evidence of surrounding pigmentation, chronic edema, or dilated veins, it is difficult to make a diagnosis of venous stasis ulceration. In fact, if there is no other abnormality in the leg and the ulcer is over the lateral portion of the lower leg, it is unlikely that the ulcer is caused by chronic venous insufficiency.

The most important aspect of the management of a patient with a stasis ulcer is leg elevation. If the patient keeps off his feet for a period of a few weeks and receives good local care to the ulcer with compresses and clean dressings, most stasis ulcers will show significant improvement. At times, especially if the ulcer is not improving, skin grafting is indicated to speed up the healing process. As for the local care of the ulcer, enzymatic debriding ointments may be helpful. If there is a moderate amount of drainage, hydrophilic beads of dextranomer (Debrisan) may be used to help clean up the ulcer surface. Rarely, a chronic, open ulceration may manifest malignant changes.

In an effort to improve peripheral venous flow in patients with deep vein occlusion, surgeons have attempted venous bypass grafts; unfortunately, however, these grafts generally do not remain patent because of the low-flow state in the venous system, which leads to thrombosis of the graft. If a patient with a stasis ulcer must remain on his feet because of his job, for example, an Unna boot may be applied to the leg and left on for 1 week at a time. This is satisfactory in providing support to the venous system, provided there is not an excessive amount of drainage from the ulcer surface. The Unna boot should be applied when the leg is as free of edema as possible. If there are locally incompetent communicating veins or superficial varices allowing retrograde flow to the ulcer area, consideration should be given to ligating and stripping these veins. Again, it should be emphasized that proper elastic support and leg elevation will usually prevent the development of most stasis ulcers. Porcine (pig skin) heterografts, which act as a physiologic dressing, may be used and changed daily to improve healing of leg ulcers.

In the discussion of venous stasis ulcers, it is important to mention other types of leg ulcers of the lower extremities. Those associated with arterial insufficiency are usually initiated by *trauma,* such as a bump, or by the rubbing of a shoe against the skin of the foot where the arterial inflow is inadequate for healing to occur. Thus, the etiology is trauma, and the lack of healing is due to ischemia.

Another common type of ulceration is the *neurotrophic or neuropathic ulcer.* This results from repeated or persistent trauma of which the patient is unaware because of lack of pain sensation secondary to his neuropathy. This may be seen in diabetics or, rarely, in patients with other neurologic problems, including spinal cord injury. The neurotrophic or neuropathic ulcer may also be seen in patients with leprosy. These lesions tend to occur over pressure points and are most commonly seen on the sole of the foot, where they may become quite large before the patient is aware of them. These are not due to lack of arterial flow or to venous insufficiency.

On rare occasions, unusual infections may cause resistant leg ulcerations. Various types of *vasculitis* may lead to ulcerations, which are often difficult to heal because of end-artery (arteriolar) disease. These start as bruiselike lesions. The skin then breaks down, forming very painful ulcers. Satellite lesions may develop. Some observers feel that the so-called hypertensive ulcer that occurs on the legs results from vasculitis. Small skin infarcts that ulcerate may occur as a result of microemboli to the leg from an ulcerating atherosclerotic plaque in a more proximal artery. Other rare leg ulcers include those associated with tumor infiltration, ulcerative colitis, chronic pernio, erythema induratum (tuberculosis), and factitial or self-induced ulcers.

LYMPHEDEMA

The purpose of the lymphatic system in the extremities is to carry away excess tissue fluid that accumulates outside the vessels in the interstitial spaces. The lymphatics do not selectively absorb fluid but admit material forced on their outer surface. Lymph fluid is propelled up the leg by muscle contraction, and backflow is prevented by valves in the lymph vessels. Problems may arise if there is a developmental defect or obstruction of the lymph channels that develops as a result of inflammation, invasion, or compression. These patients have nonpitting edema without pain but with thickening and induration of the skin of the leg, including the toes. There is little or no pigmentation or ulceration.

The most common type of lymphedema seen in clinical practice is *lymphedema precox.* This occurs predominately in females, and symptoms usually start between the ages of 10 and 25 years. Occasionally, it may start later, and this is known as *lymphedema tarda.* The swelling is spontaneous and without obvious cause. The degree of severity of lymphedema will vary depending on whether or not there is aplasia or hypoplasia present in the lymphatic system. Lymphangiography can help determine this, but it is often not necessary. Contraindications to dye studies are iodine sensitivity, lymphangitis, and decreased pulmonary function because the oily dye settles in the lung.

Lymphedema tends to worsen after long periods of activity, during menstruation, and in warm weather. The cause of this is not clear, although a hormonal basis is suspected. The pathophysiology of lymphedema is that there is a congenital underdevelopment of the lymphatic system that is adequate during childhood but becomes inadequate during the rapid growth of adolescence and during adulthood. When lymphedema is not only congenital but also inherited, being found in several blood relatives of a family, it is referred to as *Milroy's disease*.

The *obstructive* type of lymphedema has a fairly clear etiology. It may be caused by (1) direct invasion of lymph nodes by tumor, (2) surgical removal of lymph nodes during cancer surgery, (3) scarring secondary to x-ray therapy, or (4) resection of lymphatic channels during arterial reconstructive surgery. It has been said that painless, progressive swelling of one leg in a male over 60 years of age indicates prostatic carcinoma, until proven otherwise.

In regard to inflammatory problems of the lymphatics, recurrent episodes of cellulitis and lymphangitis may eventually lead to destruction of a sufficient portion of the lymphatics to produce lymphedema. Small breaks in the skin between the toes may be the source of recurrent lymphangitis with eventual lymphedema. This can be prevented by proper treatment of the dermatophytosis, which usually causes cracking of the skin between the toes. *Filariasis* can infect the lymphatic system, but it is seen only in warm climates such as in India, Africa, and the islands of the Pacific.

Medical management of lymphedema can be successful in preventing greatly enlarged lower extremities with connective tissue overgrowth that develops over the course of many years if the process is not treated. The primary objective is to control the amount of edema, and the following measures should be instituted as soon as the diagnosis is established. Diuretics such as hydrochlorothiazide or furosemide taken either daily or every other day will often reduce the amount of swelling that occurs during the course of the day. Leg elevation is important. Most patients will require and benefit from some type of elastic support. A properly measured elastic stocking with a pressure of 35 to 45 mm Hg, a higher pressure than is necessary for venous insufficiency, should be prescribed. Of course, the leg should be free of edema prior to measurement for the elastic stocking. Postmastectomy edema can be controlled in a similar manner. If recurrent lymphangitis is an etiologic factor, measures should be instituted to control dermatophytosis. If lymphangitis cannot otherwise be controlled, then prophylactic antibiotics such as penicillin or erythromycin 250 mg every 6 hours for the first 7 days of each month or intramuscular bicillin once a month are indicated.

In patients in whom lymphedema has been present for many years and in whom enlargement and deformity of the lower extremities has developed, surgical intervention should be considered. Some of the surgical procedures are directed at removing as much of the diseased tissue as possible. Other methods have recently been attempted to induce new pathways for lymphatic drainage, but these have to be considered experimental at this time.

BIBLIOGRAPHY

Bell WR, Tomasulo PA, Alving BM, et al: Thrombocytopenia occurring during the administration of heparin. *Ann Intern Med* 85:155–160, 1976.

Beninson J: Lymphedema: pathophysiology and clinical concepts. *Angiology* 26:661–664, 1975.

Cranley JJ, Canos AJ, Sull WJ, et al: Phleborheographic technique for diagnosing deep venous thrombosis of the lower extremities. *Surg Gynecol Obstet* 141:331–339, 1975.

Fagen G: *Varicose Veins.* Springfield, Ill., Charles C Thomas, 1967.

Flanc C, Kakkar VV, Clarke MB: The detection of venous thrombosis of the legs using I_{125}-labeled fibrinogen. *Br J Surg* 55:742–747, 1968.

Romasy RS, Barnhart MD, Schinagl EF: Application of dextranomer beads (Debrisan [Rx]) in the treatment of exudating skin lesions: results of a cooperative study. *Angiology* 29:675, 1978.

Salzman EW, Deykin D, Shapiro RM, et al: Management of heparin therapy. *New Engl J Med* 292:1046–1050, 1975.

Sautter RD, et al: The limited utility of fibrinogen I_{125} leg scanning. *Arch Intern Med* 139:148–153, 1979.

Seaman AJ, Common HH, Rosch J, et al: Deep vein thrombosis treated with streptokinase heparin. *Angiology* 27:549–556, 1976.

Sigel B, Felix R, Popky GL, et al: Diagnosis of lower limb thrombosis by Doppler ultrasound technique. *Arch Surg* 104:174–179, 1972.

Sy WM, Lao RS, Bay R, et al: (99 [m]Tc) Pertechnetate radionuclide venography. *J Nucl Med* 19:1001–1006, 1978.

Wheeler HB, O'Donnell JA, Anderson FA, et al: Occlusive impedance plethysmography: a diagnostic procedure for venous thrombosis and pulmonary embolism. *Prog Cardiovasc Dis* 17:199–205, 1974.

PART TWO

Surgical Views

CHAPTER SIX

Preoperative Evaluation of the Vascular Surgery Patient

INTRODUCTION

This chapter is intended as a guide to the preoperative medical evaluation of the vascular surgery patient. Emphasis will be placed on the cardiopulmonary preoperative evaluations. However, metabolic and hematologic disorders as well as renal function be evaluated.

The initial history and physical examination are the hallmarks on which diagnoses are made and further diagnostic studies ordered. The present illness should be painstakingly elucidated with accuracy and precision. Past medical history is crucial, including current and past medications, drug allergies, family history, bleeding tendencies, mental disorders, and previous surgery. An orderly sequence in the physical examination is important so that no findings are overlooked.

In order to further aid in the initial assessment of the patient, a number of laboratory tests have been shown in the past to be of help. Recommended initially are complete blood count, urinalysis, SMA–12, chest x-ray, electrocardiogram, prothrombin time, partial thromboplastin time, platelet count and serum creatinine level. Additional studies may be indicated depending upon the patient's surgical and/or associated medical conditions, and these tests will be discussed further.

On the basis of information obtained by history, physical examination, and laboratory tests, the necessity for surgery and the urgency with which it must be performed can be ascertained. This, in turn, will aid in determining the risk of surgery.

Generally, the risk of surgery is divided arbitrarily into three groups: the ''good risk'' patient is one in excellent health and who is going to have surgery on a lesion of local nature that has no systemic effects. There is no disease immediately apparent involving other organ systems. Other than the studies mentioned previously, no further diagnostic tests are indicated, and the patient is ''cleared for surgery.'' The ''poor risk'' patient is one whose surgical lesion has produced severe systemic effects and who may have, in addition, severe disease of one or more vital organ systems. Such diseases will require further investigation prior to surgery and therapeutic measures to improve or correct the condition prior to surgery.

The third category is the ''intermediate risk'' group, which requires future investigation other than routine and may require additional therapy prior to surgery. However, the severity of the surgical condition and/or the assorted medical problem is of a mild to moderate nature, not severely affecting the body's homeostasis.

CARDIOVASCULAR EVALUATION

One of the most widely used techniques for the preoperative assessment of surgical risk, as described by Dripps, is an excellent predictor of perioperative noncardiac complications but not necessarily of perioperative cardiac problems. Recently, Goldman et al presented a multifactoral approach to the estimations of cardiac risk in noncardiac surgical procedures. They identified nine independent correlates of life-threatening and fatal cardiac complications: (1) preoperative third heart sound or jugular venous distention of cardiac origin; (2) myocardial infarction in the preceding 6 months; (3) more than five premature ventricular contractions per minute, documented at any time before the operation; (4) rhythm other than sinus or premature atrial contraction on preoperative electrocardiogram; (5) age over 70 years; (6) intraperitoneal, intrathoracic, or intra-aortic operations; (7) emergency operation; (8) significant valvular aortic stenosis; and (9) poor general medical condition. By application of a risk index, estimation of cardiac risk independent of direct surgical risk can be made. Table 6–1 illustrates the computation of the cardiac risk index as described by Goldman et al. In their experience, if the point score was 0 to 5, life-threatening complications occurred in .7 percent of their patients; 6 to 12 points, 5 percent incidence of life-threatening complications; 13 to 25 points, 11 percent incidence of life-threatening complications; and greater than 26 points, 22 percent incidence of life-threatening complications.

TABLE 6-1. THE GOLDMAN CARDIAC RISK CRITERIA.

Criteria	Points
1. Age over 70 years	5
2. Recent myocardial infarct (last 6 months)	10
3. Aortic stenosis	3
4. S3 gallop	11
5. Nonsinus rhythm	7
6. Ventricular arrhythmias	7
7. General status (COPD, hypokalemia, acidosis, uremia, liver disease)	3
8. Aortic, intrathoracic, and intraperitoneal surgery	4
9. Emergency surgery	4
Total	53

The presence of the above criteria with the assigned score points correlates well with the associated morbidity.

In evaluating the advisability of surgery, one of the first organ systems to be evaluated is the cardiovascular system. The cardiovascular system can be considered in four broad categories: (1) congenital heart disease, (2) rheumatic heart disease, (3) hypertensive cardiovascular disease, and (4) arteriosclerotic heart disease.

Atherosclerosis is present in all age groups. It is found in increasing degree with the advance toward old age. Atherosclerosis may involve the cardiovascular system, yet the patient may be completely symptom-free. However, the history is very important in evaluating the patient with arteriosclerotic heart disease. One should inquire regarding prior myocardial infarction and as to the frequency, severity, initiating events, and method of relief of an angina pectoris attack. Symptoms of congestive heart failure must also be elicited during the interview with the patient. These include easy fatigability, dyspnea, orthopnea, paroxysmal nocturnal dyspnea, and peripheral edema. The physical examination in patients with arteriosclerotic disease can be unrevealing. However, one should carefully auscultate for an atrial gallop or ventricular gallop sound, systolic murmurs, and pulmonary rales.

The chest x-ray is usually normal. However, it can give an estimation of cardiac size, pulmonary congestion, and, hence, information regarding the presence of congestive heart failure.

General anesthesia should not be given to patients 30 years or older without a preoperative electrocardiogram. The electrocardiogram can provide essential information not only for prognosis but also for diagnosis and may suggest the need for preoperative therapy, particularly regarding antiarrhythmic agents.

The electrocardiographic diagnosis of a prior myocardial infarction is well established. However, the electrocardiogram cannot provide a time frame. Surgery performed within 6 months of an acture myocardial infarction is associated with an increased risk; hence, the history must supplement the electrocardiogram.

Various arrhythmias may be present preoperatively. An occasional atrial premature beat does not require therapy. If frequent atrial premature beats are present there is clinical evidence that this arrhythmia is resulting in hemodynamic compromise, quinidine sulfate, 200 mg, every 4 hours is recommended. A rare premature ventricular contraction likewise does not require therapy. If the premature ventricular contractions are occurring more frequently than one every ten beats, are multifocal, are occurring two in a row, or are occurring early in the cycle close to the T-wave, therapy should be instituted. There are a number of antiarrhythmic agents that are effective for premature ventricular contractions. Lidocaine, 100-mg bolus intravenously, and a continuous intravenous infusion of appropriate dose is usually used. Quinidine sulfate, 200 mg, every 4 hours is a suitable oral agent. Procainamide, 375 to 500 mg, every 4 hours is a suitable alternative to quinidine. Paroxysmal ventricular tachycardia is a serious but uncommon condition requiring prompt therapy. Electrical cardioversion or intravenous lidocaine could be used for treatment.

Atrial fibrillation and atrial flutter with rapid ventricular response are best treated with digitalis preparation. Digoxin is preferred. For rapid digitalization, digoxin in a dosage of .5 to .75 mg may be given intravenously with additional doses of .25 mg every 4 hours until the rate slows to 80 to 100 beats per minute. Quinidine or electrical conversion may be tried in an attempt to convert this dysrhythmia to sinus rhythm. Sinus tachycardia is not an arrhythmia. Sinus tachycardia is caused by increased sympathetic tone or decreased vagal tone, frequently secondary to hypoxia, hypovolemia, dehydration, drugs, and infection. Treatment is directed at the cause.

In recent years, there has been great concern regarding the risk of advanced heart block in surgical patients, especially in patients with bifascicular block, particularly right bundle branch block and left axis deviations. Cardiologists at our institution are frequently consulted regarding the question of standby cardiac pacemaker placement in patients with this electrocardiograph abnormality who require surgery. Patients with complete heart block commonly have preceding right bundle branch block and left axis deviation. The incidence of progression to complete heart block is less than 10 percent. The assumption has been that the stress of surgery and anesthetic induction may further predispose these patients to complete heart block. A recent prospective study by Pastore et al indicates that temporary pacemaker insertion is rarely required in patients with chronic right bundle branch block and left axis deviation who require noncardiac surgery.

Patients with advanced second- or third-degree atrioventricular block as well as those with a clear history of Stokes-Adams attacks require pacemaker insertion prior to noncardiac surgery.

The administration of digitalis preparations to patients with coronary artery disease who are scheduled for noncardiac surgery is a subject of considerable controversy. General anesthetics tend to be myocardial depressants. In patients with limited cardiac reserve, it is postulated that digitalis given prior to anesthesia may negate the myocardial depression caused by general anesthesia and enable the heart to increase its output efficiently. Digitalis should, of course, be given to all patients in congestive heart failure. The functional status of the heart is the major determinant of digitalis therapy. In the exhibition of digitalis preparations, one must be aware of recent knowledge in the pharmacodynamics of the drugs. There are several digitalis preparations available; however, digoxin is preferred. Digoxin is excreted principally by the kidney. Dosages should be reduced in those patients with impaired renal function or the elderly who usually have reduced clearance of digoxin. In addition, one must be alert to electrolyte disorders, particulary hypokalemia, which may potentiate digitalis toxicity. Metabolic disturbances such as hypothyroidism and pulmonary disease also will require reduction in the dose of digoxin. Digoxin has a rapid onset of action and a relatively short half life. If the patient has an arrhythmia, such as rapid atrial fibrillation that requires a cardiac glycoside, then the glycoside in the form of digoxin should be given preoperatively. Prophylactic digitalization, however, is not indicated.

Congenital heart disease in the adult is uncommon; however, it does occur, and all murmurs in the patient who is scheduled for surgery should be investigated prior to surgery. Echocardiography has proven to be of great value in this regard, and in selected patients this study will be diagnostic. In patients with pulmonary hypertension, large left-to-right shunts, or right-to-left shunts, noncardiac surgery should not be performed unless the basic surgical lesion is life threatening to the patient. Prophylactic antibiotics are recommended.

All patients with rheumatic heart disease who are to undergo surgery should have bacterial endocarditis prophylaxis according to the American Heart Association's recommendations. New York Heart Association class III and class IV cardiac patients should not undergo noncardiac surgery unless the basic surgical condition will significantly shorten the life of the patient.

When the clinician must prepare a hypertensive patient for a surgical procedure, he needs to evaluate carefully the antihypertensive therapy so that untoward complications will not arise during and following the operation. A main principle of antihypertensive therapy is that patients may require multiple drugs attacking the three major sites of increased peripheral vascular resistance: (1) the central vasomotor sympathetic center, (2) the peripheral sympathetic nervous system, and (3) the arteriolar smooth muscle directly. There is available today a large number of antihypertensive agents, and of some significance to the surgeon and anesthesiologist are the affects of these compounds on vascular responsiveness. Diuretics (natriuretic agents) probably produce their antihypertensive effect by reduction in blood volume, reduction in total body sodium and potassium, as well as reduction of sodium and water content of the arteriolar wall. The thiazides compose a large group of commonly used antihypertensive diuretic agents. In addition, there are other more potent diuretics that can be used to treat hypertension, namely, furosemide and ethacrynic acid. There are also potassium-sparing diuretics that are weak antihypertensives but may be employed in the treatment of hypertension because of their potassium-sparing effect. Spironolactone and Triampterene are such examples.

Several agents act as smooth muscle dilators and hence decrease peripheral vascular resistance and lower blood pressure. Hydralazine and prazosin are such examples. When hydralazine does lower blood pressure, baroreceptor-mediated augmentation of cardiac rate may occur, and, as a result, the use of a ß-adrenergic receptor blocking agent such as propranolol should be used with this drug. Reflex tachycardia is not a problem with prazosin, but it does occur in approximately 5 percent of patients.

Propranolol is a ß-adrenergic receptor blocking drug that can be used alone in the therapy of hypertension. Propranolol causes bradycardia and a decrease in cardiac output.

α-Methyldopa, a false neurotransmitter, is an excellent antihypertensive agent that is usually used with a diuretic in the treatment of mild to moderate hypertension. It can be used intravenously as well as orally.

Adrenergic-inhibiting antihypertensive drugs will not be discussed because they not only reduce peripheral vascular resistance but also cardiac output and interrupt vascular reflexes with resultant postural hypotension.

Before therapy is instituted, one has to categorize the patient: (1) mild hypertensive, diastolic blood pressure 110 mm Hg or less; (2) moderate hypertensive, diastolic blood pressure 110 to 130 mm Hg; and (3) severe hypertension, diastolic blood pressure greater than 130 mm Hg.

The mild hypertensive can usually be controlled with a diuretic agent alone such as furosemide 40 mg daily or hydrochlorothiazide, 50 mg daily. α-Methyldopa, 250 mg, once a day may be added if required. Once the patient's blood pressure is in normal range, 140/90 or less, then surgery may be performed.

For the moderately severe hypertensive, a diuretic plus α-methyldopa should be instituted initially and the dose of α-methyldopa increased up to 2 gm/day before adding an additional agent such as clonidine or propranolol.

The severe hypertensive will require intensive therapy usually with a diuretic, vasodilator, and ß-adrenergic receptor blocking agent, all in combination.

Very often, the mild to moderate hypertensive on bedrest will experience a reduction in blood pressure and not require antihypertensive agents preoperatively. Even if the diastolic blood pressure is 90 to 100 mm Hg, one may wish to withhold antihypertensive therapy until the postoperative period in order to avoid volume depletion and sodium and potassium loss preoperatively. The concentration of sodium and potassium in the extracellular fluid seems to determine responsiveness to vasoconstrictor impulse and administered vasopressor agents; consequently, the long-term use of electrolyte-depleting diuretic carries a serious potential for hypotension during surgery, which needs to be recognized prior to the initiation of surgery.

PULMONARY EVALUATION

The recognition of preoperative decrease in ventilatory reserve may allow useful treatment prior to surgery. In addition, appropriate diagnostic studies may be ordered to help differentiate dyspnea due to decrease in ventilatory reserve or due to cardiac failure or combined compromise of respiration and circulation. Once again, it must be emphasized that a skillful history and systemic physical examination will often allow the physician to distinguish between pulmonary or circulatory causes for respiratory insufficiency. The diagnostic skills of the physician are extended when additional information is obtained from the electrocardiogram and chest x-ray. Every patient who is going to have vascular surgery should have a preoperative chest x-ray, and this film should be carefully reviewed with the radiologist prior to surgery. Mass lesions, infiltrative processes, cavitary lesions, and evidence of pulmonary hypertension preclude elective surgery until further diagnostic and therapeutic measures are performed. If the surgery is an emergency and the life of the patient is threatened by the primary surgical problem, then the information obtained by the above measures has to be taken into consideration in the post- and intraoperative management of the patient. If the history, physical examination, electrocardiogram, or chest x-ray suggests the presence of pulmonary disease, further assessment of pulmonary function should be performed. The recent development of small electronic devices has allowed accurate bedside determinations of forced vital capacity and forced expiratory volume to be performed on the patient. Forced vital capacity (FVC) measures the size of the lung in contact with the environment, the volume expelled by a fully inflated lung. Lung volumes are influenced by degrees of inspiratory and expiratory pressures and by age, height, and sex. Body position is also important. Supine position results in a reduced vital capacity compared to the upright position. Compromise in FVC generally means restriction of lung parenchyma, which can be due to multiple causes. One should be aware of reduction in FVC, particularly if major abdominal or thoracic surgery is to be performed since it is likely that these procedures will result in further reduction in FVC and levels may be reached that will necessitate respiratory support.

Forced expiratory volume (FEV)in 1 second is an assessment of air flow in expiration. Flows are largely dependent on respiratory muscular effort, force of elastic recoil, and the diameter of the airways. The initial forced expiratory effort achieves a peak flow extremely rapidly, normally with the first 100 msec, and is dependent on muscular effort. The flow decreases steadily with decreasing lung volume, is determined by the lung elastic recoil and the patency of the airway, and is largely independent of muscular effort. Reduction in FEV indicates impairment of elastic recoil in the case of emphysema and increased airway resistance in the case of chronic bronchitis or bronchial asthma.

In addition to aiding in the diagnosis of ventilatory insufficiency and planning therapy, these studies are also of value in assessing the risk of surgery. Most patients with FVC, 2.0 liters or greater, and FEV, 1.0 liter/second or greater, will tolerate elective surgery, but the greater the impairment of spirometic measurements, the greater the risk of postoperative ventilatory failure.

Blood gases, of course, are essential in evaluating respiratory homeostasis. These determinations should be made preoperatively in all patients who are to undergo major surgery or in whom there is a suspicion of pulmonary or cardiac pathology.

There are a number of other pulmonary function tests that can be measured, particularly in the pulmonary function laboratory. However, these tests are used to further classify disease status and are not indicated "routinely" in the preoperative evaluation of the vascular surgery patient unless there is a specific indication.

The patient with obstructive pulmonary disease presents a particular problem with regard to the preoperative assessment. Frequently, if not always, these patients are heavy cigarette smokers, and one cannot emphasize too strongly the need to stop cigarette smoking preoperatively. If there is a significant reduction in FVC and FEV, a bronchodilator should be used preoperatively in an attempt to improve pulmonary function. Respiratory failure postoperatively can be a major cause of postoperative mortality. Acute respiratory failure has been defined as a situation in which the arterial PO_2 is below the predicted normal for the patient's age, often assumed to be 50 mm Hg, or the arterial PCO_2 is above 50 mm Hg in the absence of metabolic acidosis. Causes of respiratory insufficiency following surgery may include hypoventilation, diffusion defects, abnormalities in ventilation/perfusion ratios, and shunting, all of which may occur in patients with chronic obstructive pulmonary disease.

The presence of left ventricular dysfunction in the presence of chronic obstructive pulmonary disease is controversial. Kachel concluded that the bulk of the evidence indicates that the clinical symptoms of left-sided failure are unreliable in those with obstructive disease of the airways and that the great majority of patients have normal left ventricular function once other causes are excluded. A small group of patients have some abnormality in left ventricular performance, but this is not clinically significant. Patients with significant left or right ventricular failure should be treated with digitalis and diuretics prior to surgery. Patients with congestive heart failure have more frequent problems with venous rather than arterial thromboembolism, probably related to stasis produced by relatively high volume pressure and bedrest. Hence, an additional pulmonary problem, that of pulmonary embolism, may be prevented by the treatment of congestive heart failure preoperatively and by early ambulation postoperatively.

Of patients undergoing major surgical procedures, 1.2 to 4 percent are reported as having bronchial asthma. Patients with preoperative bronchial asthma may develop bronchospasms during surgery. The postoperative complications can be reduced by careful preoperative medical management.

The mild asymptomatic asthmatic patient may be managed with minimal therapy. A discussion of the problem with the patient and assurance by the physician that the patient's pulmonary status will be closely observed can allay anxiety.

Theophylline, either orally, rectally, or intravenously, may be employed for its bronchodilatory effect. Theophylline at a serum concentration of 10 to 20 mg/ml is an effective and safe drug in controlling the symptoms of bronchial asthma. Relaxation of the bronchiolar and alveolar smooth muscle is a direct action of the drug. If evidence of infection is present, an appropriate antibiotic should be employed. Cultures should be obtained prior to the use of antibiotics. Recently introduced sympathomimetic agents such as terbutaline and metaproterenol are also effective bronchodilators. These drugs, when given orally, are effective for periods of 4 or more hours; 5 mg of terbutaline every 8 hours or 20 mg of metaproterenol every 6 hours are the usual dosages. An aerosolized bronchodilator may be administered by means of hand-held nebulizers; however, the use of the freon-propelled metered dose canisters is discouraged. High-humidity therapy may also be used to alleviate bronchospasm.

Hydration is a very important therapeutic measure. Oral fluids may be sufficient, but parenteral fluids should be used as indicated. Thick and sticky sputum may be difficult to clear from the bronchial lumen. Hydration may aid in the clearing of such mucus. Aerosol therapy with water or saline may also aid in clearing thick or tenacious sputum. It may act as a lubricant permitting separation of the sputum plugs from the bronchial wall.

Successful management of the patient with bronchial asthma requires consideration of the various precipitating factors and, if possible, their control or removal. Infectious agents, allergic factors, pollens, dusts, irritants, such as fumes, smoke, weather, humidity, and emotional factors, may play a role and need to be controlled in the preoperative period, if possible.

EVALUATION OF THE DIABETIC PATIENT

The patient with clinical diabetes mellitus who is about to undergo surgery presents a challenge to the surgeon, internist, and anesthesiologist. All must be consulted prior to the surgery in order to plan the patient's therapy properly. Duration of the surgery, type of anesthetic agents, nature of the surgery (peripheral vascular, abdominal, thoracic), fluid replacement therapy, plus anticipated time the patient will be unable to take oral nutrition must be thoughtfully evaluated in planning the patient's diabetic therapy. In addition, one must recognize that diabetes mellitus is a syndrome involving multiple organ systems. The heart, kidney, brains, nervous system, as well as the eye may be affected in the diabetic patient. Each of these organ systems must be carefully evaluated prior to surgery to determine the extent of any involvement.

All diabetic patients should have a careful fundoscopic examination to reveal evidence of diabetic retinopathy. Microaneurysms, central waxy exudates, round hemorrhages, and hyaline exudates should alert the physician to ocular involvement.

Diabetes mellitus is characterized by hyperglycemia, usually accompanied by glycosuria. The basic defect appears to be a lack of metabolically effective circulating insulin. The elevated blood sugar level is a result of deficient utilization on the part of peripheral tissues and an increased output of glucose by the liver. Excess glucose comes from dietary carbohydrates, liver glycogen, and glucose formed from protein and fat. In the course of metabolism, free fatty acids are released and metabolized in the liver to an end product of acetoacetate, which by hydrogenation is converted to ß-hydroxybutyric acid or by decarboxydation to acetone. The three products are known collectively as ketone bodies. In diabetes, the breakdown of fatty acids is increased, and since the metabolism of the ketone bodies is limited, they accumulate in the bloodstream and are eliminated via the kidneys. Glycosuria itself produces an osmotic diuresis that is enhanced by the presence of ketone bodies and the associated loss of sodium and potassium. Evaluation of the diabetic patient, therefore, includes not only measuring the blood glucose but also electrolytes, pH, serum acetone, PCO_2, and PO_2. These are in addition to a complete blood count, blood urea nitrogen, creatinine, and complete urinalysis.

The anesthetic agents used may have an effect on carbohydrate metabolism, and, in addition, the stress of surgery with release of epinephrine and glucocorticoids will also affect the state of the diabetic patient. Usually, there is an increased breakdown of glycogen to glucose in the liver, resulting in further hyperglycemia.

As a general principle, it is safer to permit minimal elevations in blood sugar and mild glycosuria to avoid the dangers of hypoglycemia, particularly in the elderly or the cardiac patient, in the intraoperative and postoperative periods. The mild diabetic who is not insulin dependent can be managed by diet alone. The diabetic diet should contain 25 to 35 calories per kilogram of ideal weight divided in terms of 40 percent carbohydrate, 40 percent protein, and 20 percent fat. Immediately postoperatively, a blood sugar should be obtained. If the blood sugar is 250 mg or less, insulin should not be given, but continued dietary or parenteral nutrition should be the controlling factor. The patient in whom diabetes is well controlled with oral agents should continue taking those oral agents until the day prior to operation. Once again, immediately after surgery, a blood sugar determination should be made. If the blood sugar is 250 mg or less, insulin should be withheld. If the blood sugar is greater than 250 mg, regular insulin should be given. Usually, if a patient is well controlled preoperatively with oral agents, the patient will not require very large doses of insulin in the postoperative period. It is recommended to obtain blood sugars every 6 hours and to give regular insulin in a dose of 5 to 10 units subcutaneously or intravenously, depending on the level of blood sugar and clinical state of the patient. If the patient has a Foley catheter in place, a possible alternative method of management is to ''cover'' the urine sugars every 6 hours with regular insulin: (1) 1 plus urine sugar, no insulin; (2) 2 plus and 3 plus urine sugar, 5 units of regular insulin; (3) 4 plus urine sugar, 10 units of regular insulin. At the present time, there is an increasing tendency to avoid this method of diabetic management because the renal threshold of glucose may not have been determined for the patient being treated or a high renal threshold for glucose may be present. There is also some question regarding the accuracy of the determination of the urine glucose. In spite of these potential shortcomings, this method is used, and one should be familiar with it.

A variety of programs is available for the management of the insulin-dependent diabetic who is to undergo surgery. Before discussing these programs, it must be emphasized that the anesthetist should be consulted prior to instituting therapy. If diabetic ketoacidosis is present, surgery should be postponed until the condition can be reversed. The patient in frank diabetic coma is no candidate for surgery regardless of the indication. For a minor surgical procedure, one in which the patient will be able to resume oral feedings within 24 hours, the patient can be given his regular dose of insulin, and the daily carbohydrate requirement is divided into four equal doses and given parenterally as 5 to 10 percent dextrose in water every 6 hours. For the more labile diabetic or for patients in whom surgical treatment is of a greater magnitude, the use of a short-acting insulin such as regular insulin is preferred. This program is started as early as 48 hours prior to the operation and may be continued well into the postoperative period. Administration of insulin immediately prior to surgery is not recommended. However, in the recovery room, a blood sugar is immediately obtained along with serum acetone, pH, and PCO_2, and regular insulin is given either intravenously or subcutaneously, depending on the clinical state of the patient. Usually 5 to 10 units of regular insulin is all that is needed, provided severe acidosis or significant ketonemia is not present. Then the blood sugar is obtained every 6 hours, and regular insulin is ordered according to the blood sugar determination. Hypoglycemia should be avoided.

Another regimen that may be employed in patients who are insulin dependent and taking a single injection daily and in whom complicated postoperative course is not anticipated is: on the day of surgery, the patient is given one-half the daily dose of insulin that was previously required, and, at the same time, an intravenous infusion of 50 gm of dextrose in 1000 cc is started before surgery. The remainder of the dose of insulin may be given, or a small dose of short-acting insulin may be given at the completion of surgery. The next day, the usual dose of insulin is given in the morning prior to breakfast or at the time of starting the intravenous infusion. This program can be modified, if necessary, and the patient can be given small doses of regular insulin 5 to 10 units every 6 hours in the postoperative period until further stabilization of the clinical state.

EVALUATION OF HEMOSTASIS

Failure of hemostasis can be a catastrophe for the vascular surgeon. Disruption in normal hemostasis often can be anticipated. Of paramount importance is the patient's history of abnormal bleeding, particularly with regard to bleeding after tonsillectomy, dental extraction, or other surgery. If the patient has not experienced excessive bleeding in association with such stresses, chances are that if a bleeding disorder occurs, it has been acquired and not congenital. In fact, most adults' bleeding problems are acquired, although occasionally a patient with undiagnosed mild hemophilia, Christmas disease, von Willebrand's disease, or another platelet abnormality will suffer bleeding episodes postoperatively. Cessation of blood flow from an injured vessel, the cumulative phenomenon called hemostasis, occurs as a result of many events and the interplay of multiple factors.

After the initial vascular response to injury, early platelet adherence to subendothelial collagen fibril begins to occur. Then platelets begin to adhere to each other. This platelet aggregation is the result of platelet adenosine diphosphate (ADP) interaction. The platelets begin to compact forming a ''platelet plug.'' Subsequently, a complete series of reactions occurs that ultimately leads to the transformation of the soluble protein fibrinogen to the insoluble fibrin clot, constituting the process of coagulation. Failure at any one of the stages may manifest itself as a potential bleeding disorder.

Fibrinolysis is not necessarily part of the hemostatic mechanism, although excessive fibrinolysis may cause failure of hemostasis. The process of clot dissolution is as complex as the clotting system itself.

The initial laboratory evaluation of hemostatic disorders is aimed at detemining whether a platelet or plasma coagulation abnormality is responsible. Four laboratory tests provide this information: (1) prothrombin time, (2) activated partial thromboplastin time, (3) platelet count, and (4) bleeding time. Prothrombin time assesses the function of the extrinsic pathway. It detects deficiencies of coagulation factors VII, X, V, II (prothrombin), and I (fibrinogen). Concentration of these factors has to be less than 30 percent of normal before the prothrombin time becomes abnormal and there is concern about excessive bleeding.

The partial thromboplastin time evaluates the intrinsic pathway of prothrombin conversion to thrombin. Deficiencies of coagulation factors XII, XI, IX, VIII, X, V, II, and I may be detected with this test. As with the prothrombin time, factor levels have to be less than 30 percent of normal before an abnormality shows up in the partial thromboplastin time.

Together, the prothrombin time and the partial thromboplastin time measure all factors except factor XIII. This factor abnormality is fortunately rare, is usually congenital, and manifests itself prior to adult life. Platelet disorders are best evaluated with a platelet count and bleeding time. The bleeding time indicates the effectiveness of platelet thrombus formation. It is prolonged in severe thrombocytopenia and in disorders such as von Willebrand's disease. If a patient's platelet count and bleeding time are normal, a platelet problem can be ruled out.

If a congenital deficiency of a specific factor is suspected, a coagulation laboratory can confirm the diagnosis and determine that factor's concentration. Replacement therapy is called for in congenital factor deficiencies, depending on the severity of the deficiency and the type of surgery that is to be performed.

Acquired coagulation disorders generally fall into six categories: (1) liver disease, (2) vitamin K deficiency, (3) ingestion of oral anticoagulants, (4) disseminated intravascular coagulation, (5) dilution phenomenon, and (6) circulating anticoagulants. The liver synthesizes the vitamin K-dependent factors (II, VII, IX, X) as well as factors V and XI and fibrinogen. Therefore, prothrombin time and partial thromboplastin time will be prolonged in patients with hepatic dysfunction. It usually takes rather severe diseases to affect the coagulation factors, particularly fibrinogen, and the severity of the liver disease should be clinically obvious.

Vitamin K deficiency should be suspected in patients with very poor nutrition and in those who have been receiving antibiotics for a prolonged period.

These chemotherapeutic measures may reduce bacterial flora of the intestine and stop synthesis of vitamin K, leading to deficiency.

Vitamin K is essential for the synthesis of factors II, VII, IX, and X. Both the prothrombin time and the partial thromboplastin time will be prolonged in vitamin K deficiency states. Ingestion of oral anticoagulants such as warfarin sodium should be suspected in patients who are deficient in vitamin K-dependent factors. These drugs interfere with vitamin K synthesis.

Disseminated intravascular coagulation is a most serious condition, diagnosed by a prolongation of the prothrombin time, partial thromboplastin time, and reduced platelet concentration. In addition, there is usually evidence of fibrinogen degradation products because of a stimulation of the fibrinolytic systems. The condition results from the intravascular activation of thrombi, secondary to injury of body tissues, endothelium, platelets, or red cells. There is a compensatory activation of the fibrinolytic system resulting in a depletion of factors V, VIII, I, II, and platelets.

Dilution phenomenon occurs when profuse bleeding is present. Coagulation factors, platelets, and red cells are lost. As blood volume is replaced, it is necessary to replace these factors as well as labile factors V and VIII, usually with fresh plasma or fresh blood, in order to avoid the dilution phenomena.

Circulating anticoagulants are immunoglobulins that inhibit the action of coagulation factors. Usually either the prothrombin time or the partial thromboplastin time will be prolonged. A coagulation laboratory will be able to more precisely determine the exact nature of the circulating anticoagulants.

BIBLIOGRAPHY

Denes P, Dhingra RC, Wu D, et al: H–V interval in patients with bifascicular block. *Am J Card* 101:35:23–29, 1975.

DePasquale NP, Bruno MS: Natural history of combined right bundle branch block and left anterior hemiblock. *Am J Med* 54:279–303, 1973.

Dripps RD, Lamont A, Eckenhoff JE: The role of anesthesia in surgical mortality. *JAMA* 178:261–266, 1961.

Faling LJ, Weiss EB, Chodash S, et al: The preoperative management of patients with bronchial asthmas, in Oakes WW, JH Moyer (eds.): *Pre and Postoperative Management of the Cardiopulmonary Patient.* New York, Grune & Stratton, 1970, pp 108–119.

Fraser JG, Ramachandran PR, Davis HS: Anesthesia and recent myocardial infarction. *JAMA* 199:318–320, 1967.

Goldman L, Caldera DL, Nussbaum SR, et al: Multifactorial index of cardiac risk in non-cardiac surgical procedures. *New Engl J Med* 297:845–850, 1977.

Griffith GC: Surgical risk in atherosclerosis, in Oakes WW, JH Moyer (eds.): *Pre and Postoperative Management of the Cardiopulmonary Patient.* New York, Grune & Stratton, 1970, pp 288–292.

Hillis LD, Cohn PF: Noncardiac surgery in patients with coronary artery disease. *Arch Intern Med* 138:972–975, 1978.

Hurst JW, Logue, RB, Walter PF: The clinical recognition and management of atherosclerotic heart disease, in Hurst JW, Logue RB, Schlant RC, Wetzl (eds.): *The Heart,* New York, McGraw-Hill, Vol. 4, pp 1156–1167.

Jelliffe RW, Brooker G: A nomogram for digoxin therapy. *Am J Med* 57:63–68, 1974.

Kachel RG: Left ventricular function in chronic obstructive pulmonary disease. *Chest* 74:286–290, 1978.

Kaplan EL, Anthony BF, Bisnoa, et al: Prevention of bacterial endocarditis. *Circulation* 56:139A–143A, 1977.

Likoff W: Indications for preoperative digitalization, in Oakes WW, JH Moyer (eds.): *Pre and Postoperative Management of the Cardiopulmonary Patient.* New York, Grune & Stratton, 1970, pp 305–307.

Morris JF: Spirometry in the evaluation of pulmonary function. *West J Med* 125:110–118, 1970.

Moyer JH: Management of hypertension in elective and emergency surgery, in Oakes WW, JH Moyer (eds.): *Pre and Postoperative Management of the Cardiopulmonary Patient.* New York, Grune & Stratton, 1970, pp 293–307.

Pastore JO, Yurchak PM, Janis KM, et al: The risk of advanced heart block in surgical patients with right bundle branch block and left axis deviation. *Circulation* 57:677–680, 1978.

Perlroth MG, Hultgren HN: The cardiac patient and general surgery. *JAMA* 232:1279–1280, 1975.

Petty TL: Office spirometry and the cardiac patient. *Practical Cardiology* 4:41–51, 1978.

Rogers PH, Sherry S: Current status of antithrombotic therapy in cardiovascular disease. *Prog Cardiovasc Dis* 19:235–253, 1976.

Severinghaus EL: The vitamins, in DiPalma JR (ed.): *Pharmacology in Medicine,* New York, McGraw-Hill, p 1021.

Snider GL: Control of bronchospasm in patients with chronic obstructive pulmonary disease. *Chest* 73:927–935, 1978.

Steen PA, Tinker JH, Tarhan S: Myocardial reinfarction after anesthesia and surgery. *JAMA* 239:2566–2570, 1978.

Stein M, Cassara EL: Preoperative pulmonary evaluation and therapy for surgical patients. *JAMA* 211:787–790, 1970.

Tarhan S, Moffitt EA, Taylor WF, et al: Myocardial infarction after general anesthesia. *JAMA* 220:1451–1454, 1972.

CHAPTER SEVEN

Aortoiliac Occlusive Disease

INTRODUCTION

The terminal aorta is the vessel most frequently involved with arteriosclerotic disease. However, because of the large lumen of this vessel, symptoms due to reduction of blood flow occur either with a high degree of stenosis or with a complete occlusion of this vessel. Symptoms may also appear as a result of distal embolization from an ulcerated atheromatous plaque, often located in the distal aorta. The common iliac, hypogastric, and external iliac arteries are also frequently diseased, and according to the anatomic distribution of their lesions, various patterns of symptomatology will be present.

The response of the body to the presence of arterial occlusive disease in the aortoiliac segment is the development of collateral circulation. (1) High occlusion of the infrarenal aorta with involvement of both iliac systems will stimulate the development of collateral pathways in the abdominal wall via the *lower intercostal* and internal mammary arteries to the inferior epigastric and femoral arteries (Fig. 7–1). (2) Another collateral route starts from the superior mesenteric artery and continues via the *marginal* and superior hemorrhoidal artery, supplying the pelvic vasculature. (3) Finally, occlusion at the level of the aortic bifurcation will be compensated via the collateral pathway of the *lumbar* arteries to the circumflex branches of the external iliac and the deep femoral arteries (Fig. 7–2).

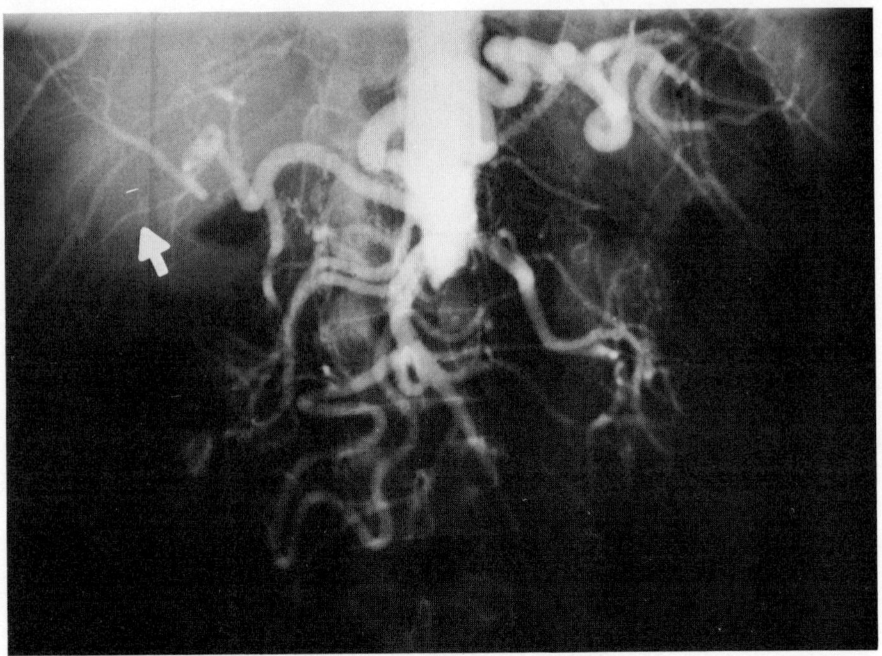

Figure 7-1. Intercostal collaterals.

Unlike patients with femoropopliteal occlusive disease, patients with aortoiliac disease are in a younger age group and have a lower incidence of associated diseases, such as hypertension, coronary artery disease, and diabetes. The operative mortality rate is in the range of 2 to 5 percent. The results of anatomic as well as extra-anatomic reconstructions are excellent with complete disappearance of the symptoms in 40 percent of patients, very good with considerable improvement in 50 percent of patients, and fair to poor in 10 percent of patients who experience no relief.

DIAGNOSIS

History

The majority of patients with aortoiliac disease present with symptoms of inadequate perfusion of the muscles during exercise. The distribution of the occlusive disease will determine which muscle groups will become symptomatic. Unilateral occlusion of the common iliac artery will present with claudication of the buttock, thigh, and calf. If only the external iliac artery is occluded, the gluteal muscles will be adequately perfused, and the symptoms will be referred to the

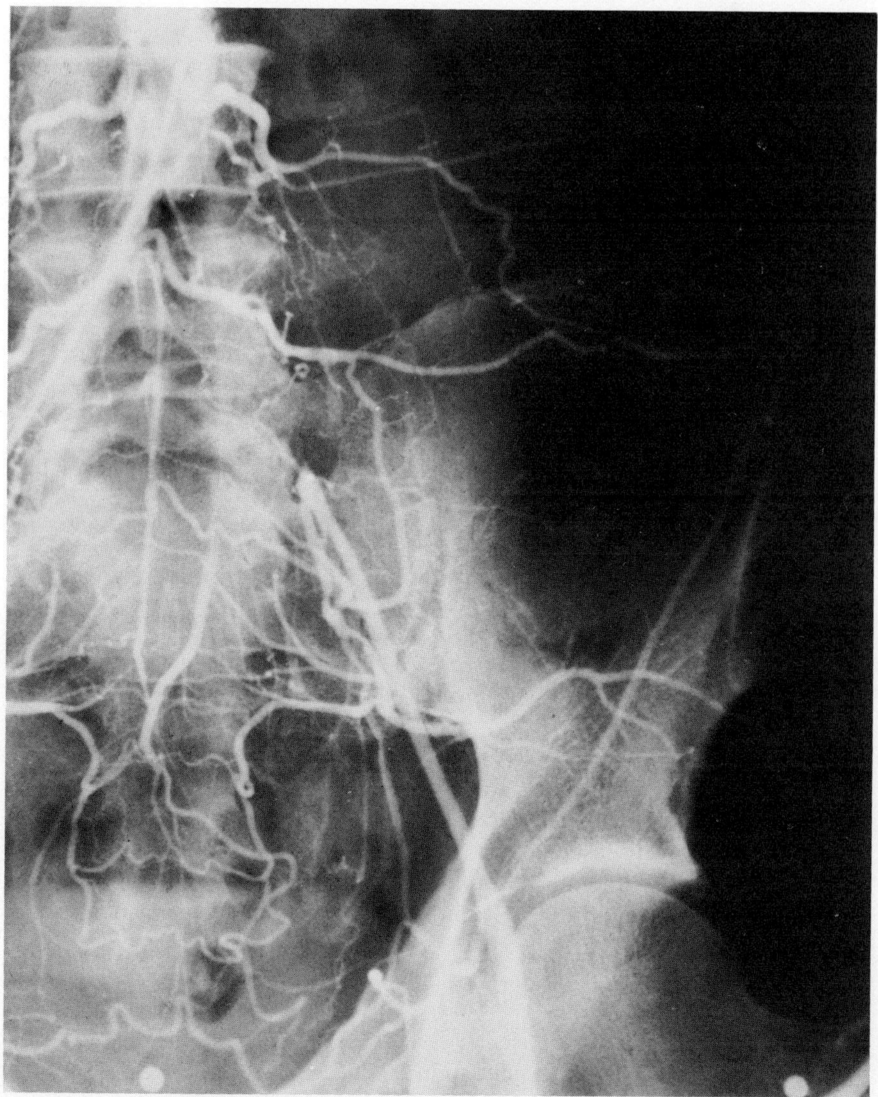

Figure 7-2. Lumbar and visceral collaterals.

thigh and calf. In the male patient, occlusion of the distal aorta or both common iliac arteries will result in *impotence* due to inadequate flow to the hypogastric vasculature. Impotence, bilateral claudication, and absent pulses below the inguinal ligament describe *Leriche's syndrome*. When aortoiliac disease is associated with femoropopliteal disease, the predominant symptom may be severe calf

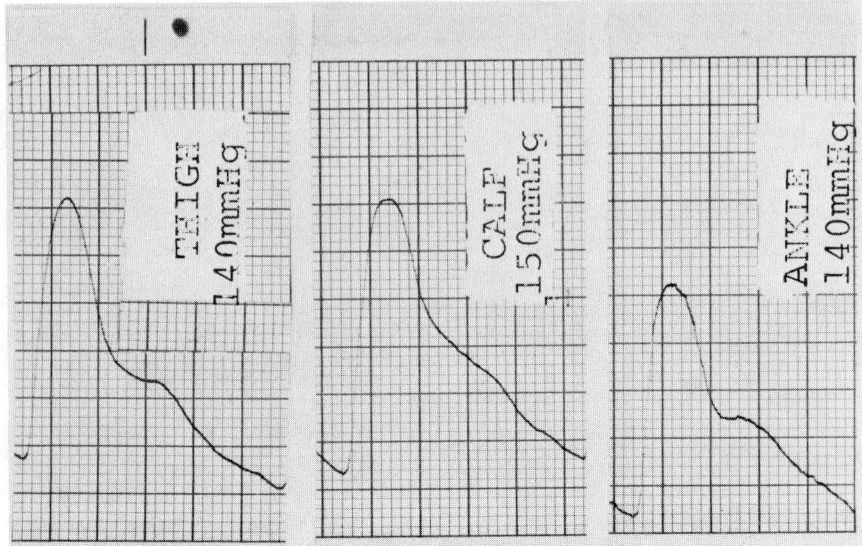

Figure 7-3. Pulse volume recording (PVR)—normal study.

claudication or symptoms due to severe perfusion deficit such as rest pain, ischemic ulcerations, focal gangrene, numbness, and paresthesias of the lower extremities.

Intermittent claudication due to aortoiliac disease may have to be differentiated from pain of neurogenic etiology. In general, a thorough physical examination and noninvasive studies should accurately determine the presence or absence of vascular disease.

The patient's past medical history and other current symptoms should be evaluated, as they may interfere with or alter future diagnostic or therapeutic decisions.

Physical Examination

Complete examination of the vascular system is essential. Specific diagnostic information can be obtained by palpation of the femoral, popliteal, and distal pulses, as well as by auscultation over both groins. The quality of the femoral pulses offers a very good assessment of the circulation through the aortoiliac segment. Absent or diminished pulses indicate the presence of significant proximal stenosis or complete occlusion. A strong femoral pulse usually indicates that the proximal vessels are free of hemodynamically significant disease. A strong but broad pulse should raise the suspicion of a femoral artery aneurysm. Auscultation over both groins and the lower abdomen may reveal bruits, which are strongly suggestive of a significant proximal stenosis.

The physical examination should include cardiorespiratory evaluation because diseases of these systems may modify the approach to treatment of the patient's problem.

Noninvasive Studies

An objective measurement of the blood flow in the lower extremity is now visible with the use of the *Doppler ultrasonic flowmeter* and the *pulse volume recorder.* This mode of evaluation is valuable because it can be reproduced, can be performed at rest or after exercise with the treadmill, and can be recorded on paper for future reference.

Segmental Doppler pressures are measured at three different levels with blood pressure cuffs applied around the thigh, the upper calf, and the ankle. The monitoring Doppler probe detects signals over the popliteal pedis dorsalis or posterior tibial arteries. The segmental pulse volume recordings are also obtained from the thigh, the upper calf, and the ankle (Fig. 7–3). The systemic blood pressure should be also measured simultaneously in the arm; evaluation of ankle/arm pressure index should be done. These two tests, when used in combination, can easily demonstrate an existing flow deficit in the lower extremity; however, they cannot reliably differentiate between aortoiliac and superficial femoral artery disease. This problem exists because all measurements are made below the bifurcation of the common femoral artery. With the recent advances in ultrasonic technology, new instruments have been developed that can reliably describe the flow characteristics of the femoral artery and project this information in a waveform that can be analyzed.

When the results of the noninvasive studies have been considered in conjunction with the findings of the physical examination and the patient's history, the level of an arterial occlusion or stenosis can accurately be determined.

Arteriography

All patients with aortoiliac disease who are considered for surgical intervention should have an arteriogram performed. The femoral route is preferred, but the transaxillary or even the translumbar approach may have to be used when neither femoral pulse is present. The arteriogram should demonstrate the arterial supply to both kidneys, the aortoiliac segment with the existing collateral vessels, the femoral bifurcation with attention to the takeoff of the deep femoral artery, and the distal vessels below the knee. Since the blood may flow to the lower extremities through collateral vessels, delayed films are essential. Occasionally, in patients with occlusion of the distal aorta, the tip of the catheter may have to be positioned higher in the thoracic aorta or even in the aortic arch so that the dye will enter the intercostal or internal mammary collateral vessels and will so enable visualization of the femoral arteries.

It is also essential to measure through the arteriography catheter pressures in the distal aorta and the common femoral artery. This information will be helpful to the surgeon in selecting the appropriate surgical procedure.

TREATMENT

Decision Making

Various surgical procedures have been successfully applied in the treatment of aortoiliac occlusive disease. The surgeon's goal is to revascularize ischemic extremities effectively and, if possible, to reperfuse the pelvic structures with a low operative risk and a low morbidity. This can be accomplished either by an anatomic reconstruction such as (1) endarterectomy, (2) aortoiliac or aortofemoral bypass, or (3) by an extra-anatomic reconstruction such as femorofemoral cross-over or axillofemoral bypass.

The primary indications for surgery are disabling claudication in 65 percent of patients and impeding tissue loss in 35 percent of the patients. The decison to use one procedure over another should be reached with consideration given to sex, age, activity level, and general cardiopulmonary condition of the patient; intra-arterial flow pressure measurements; arteriographic findings; and the surgeon's experience. The patency rate is generally superior with an anatomic reconstruction (Fig. 7–4), but other important factors may favor an extra-anatomic route.

In many patients, aortoiliac disease may be associated with disease of the arteries below the inguinal ligament. In these cases, proximal reconstruction is done first, and, if needed, distal revascularization subsequently follows. Simultaneous performance of both operations has a higher success rate but carries with it increased mortality and morbidity rates. However, simultaneous secondary procedure is indicated in the case of a needed profundoplasty or if the runoff of the distal vascular bed is so poor that there is a strong possibility of early failure of the aortoiliac reconstruction.

The grafts that are used for bypass procedures in large-lumen blood vessels are synthetic, made of Dacron and polytetrafluoroethylene (PTFE), and are used either as bifurcating or as straight grafts. The preferred suture material is monofilament polypropelene, 3–0 for the aortic anastomosis and 5–0 for the anastomosis to the axillary or femoral arteries.

Preoperative Preparation

All patients who undergo aortoiliac reconstruction should be in optimal cardiorespiratory status. Mechanical bowel preparation is preferable when a laparotomy is contemplated. A shower or a bath with betadine soap is recommended the night prior to surgery in order to decrease the number of the skin contaminants. Shaving and prepping are done in the morning of the operation

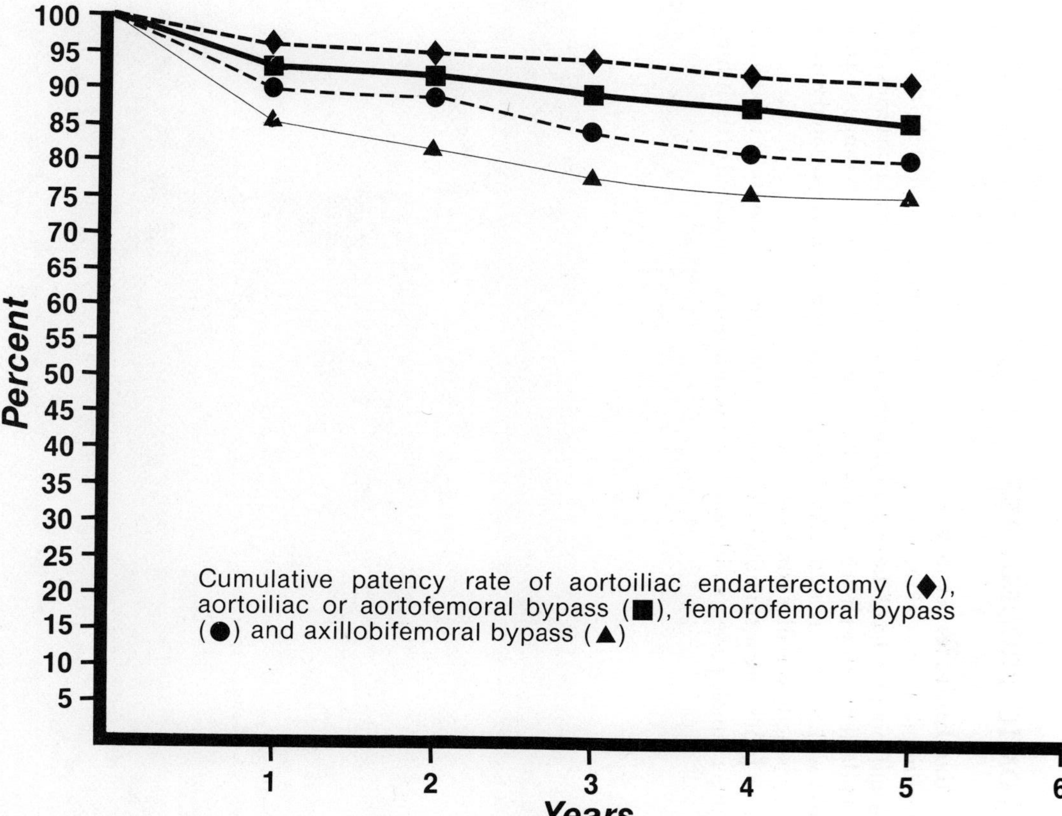

Figure 7-4. Patency of various aortoiliac reconstructions.

day. A broad-spectrum antibiotic effective against staphylococci, usually a first-generation cephalosporin, is started preoperatively and is continued for 48 hours postoperatively.

ANATOMIC PROCEDURES

Aortoiliac Endarterectomy

This technique of arterial reconstruction applies to the removal of the diseased intima and inner media of the distal aorta and/or the common iliac arteries. Aortoiliac endarterectomy has a 5-year patency rate in the 90 percent range and does not carry with it the increased risk of infectious complications associated with the use of prosthetic vascular conduits.

This procedure is suitable in less than 10 percent of patients. It is indicated in younger female patients with short, segmental lesions proximal to the bifurca-

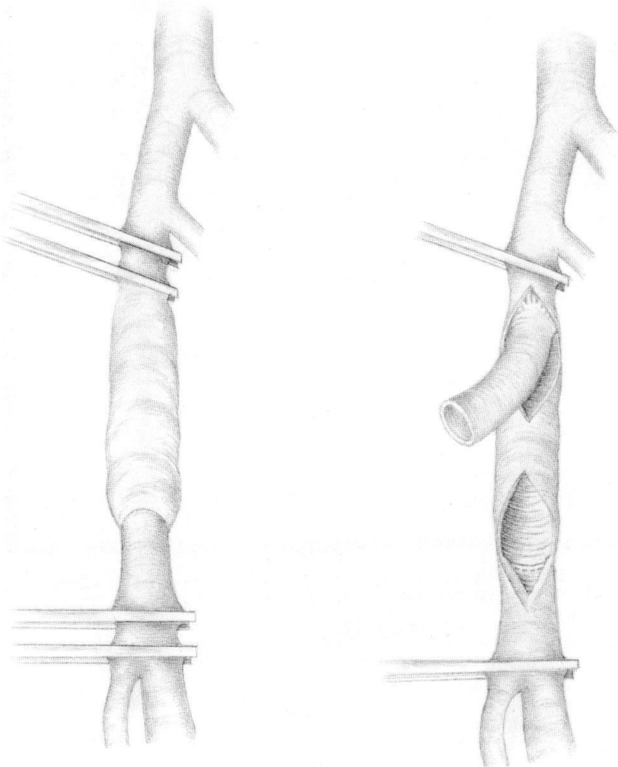

Figure 7–5. Gas endarterectomy.

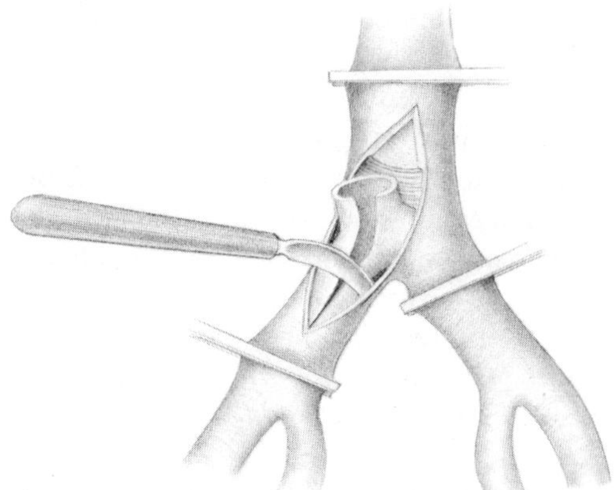

Figure 7-6. Aortoiliac endarterectomy.

tion of the common iliac arteries. When performed in male patients, it may be followed by sexual dysfunction secondary to disruption of sympathetic fibers. More extensive lesions are best treated with bypass procedures because extended endarterectomy requires more operative time and special surgical skills, including the use of various dissecting instruments or gas dissection (Fig. 7-5). Aortoiliac endarterectomy may also be performed for the establishment of vascular continuity in patients who have had an infected aortofemoral graft removed.

Contraindications for the performance of this procedure are (1) aneurysmal degeneration of the aortic wall, (2) complete occlusion of the aorta just below the renal arteries, and (3) extension of the disease in the external iliac artery. For these type of lesions, bypass procedures have lower mortality and failure rates.

Operative Technique. The terminal aorta and common iliac arteries are exposed through a long midline incision. Once the aorta is dissected, the lumbar and inferior mesenteric arteries should be isolated and controlled with small vascular clamps. After systemic heparinization (5000 units) and appropriate proximal and distal control, a longitudinal arteriotomy is performed in the area of the planned endarterectomy. A dissection plane is started on one side, separating the diseased inner layers from the outer media and adventitia (Fig. 7-6). This dissection is advanced circumferentially as well as proximally and distally to normal-appearing vessel walls. The proximal and distal line of separation is accomplished either with gentle traction or with an incision. The endarterectomy should be performed with caution so that it will not result in tears of the aortic wall. Distal intimal flaps should be avoided; if present, they should be tacked down with interrupted sutures. Following completion of the endarterectomy, the arteriotomy is closed, all vascular clamps are removed, and flow is reestablished. Pulsatile flow should be verified in the distal vessels. After reperitonealization, the abdomen is closed in layers.

Aortoiliac and Aortofemoral Bypass

A bypass procedure from the distal aorta to the iliac or femoral arteries is the most frequently performed reconstruction for aortoiliac occlusive disease. The low mortality rate of 2 percent and the excellent 5-year patency of *85 percent* have established this procedure in the treatment of aortoiliac disease. The results are generally better if (1) there is no significant disease below the inguinal ligament, (2) if an occluded superficial femoral artery is compensated by a well-developed deep femoral artery collateral network, and (3) there is no significant trifurcation disease.

The proximal anastomosis between the infrarenal aorta and the graft can be performed either as an end-to-end or as an end-to-side onlay patch. An *end-to-end* anastomosis is associated with a lower incidence of late failure due to recurrent disease in the aorta and allows a more complete tissue interposition between the graft and the duodenum. For these reasons, it is preferable to the end-to-side technique, which offers the theoretical advantage of preserving collateral circulation through the lumbar vessels. The distal anastomosis is usually done in an end-to-side fashion between the graft and the external iliac or common femoral arteries. An *aortoiliac* bypass has advantages because (1) it is faster, as it can be done through a single laparotomy incision, (2) has a lower incidence of graft infection, as the groins are not entered, and (3) the graft does not cross the hip joint. However, an *aortofemoral* graft bypasses all of the disease of the iliac vessels and allows evaluation and possibly correction of problems at the origin of the deep femoral artery, as it is often seen in diabetic patients. Both procedures have an equally good patency rate when applied to the properly selected patients.

Operative Technique. The lower chest, abdomen, and both groins are prepped and appropriately draped. The abdomen is entered through a long midline laparotomy incision. The intestines are eviscerated, and the aorta as well as the iliac arteries are dissected free. Damage of the sympathetic fibers crossing over the aortic bifurcation should be avoided in the male patient. The area of the aorta that seems more suitable for an anastomosis is selected. The iliac arteries are evaluated by direct observation and palpation. A decision is made as to the site of the distal anastomosis, considering the intraoperative findings along with the arteriogram. If an aortofemoral bypass has to be done, the groins are opened at this stage. Tunnels for the limbs of the graft are dissected behind the ureters. A graft of proper size is chosen and preclotted if it is knitted Dacron. The patient is systemically heparinized and diuresis is induced with 40 mg furosemide. For systemic heparinization we use 70 IU of heparin/kgm body weight as initial dose. In prolonged procedures PTT or ACT are checked and supplemented as appropriate. The infrarenal aorta is cross-clamped and divided distally to the level of clamping. The distal stump is oversewn with continuous suture of 3–0 prolene. The proximal, end-to-end anastomosis is constructed between the proximal aorta and the bifurcating prosthetic graft, using a continuous suture of 3–0 prolene. The limbs of the graft are passed through the appropriate tunnels and are anastomosed end to side to the external iliac or common femoral artery. The less diseased side is done first, and flow to this extremity is established through the graft. Sequential clamp release should be done, as will be described in the chapter on aortic aneurysms. If the distal anastomosis is carried down to the common femoral artery and if the superficial femoral artery is occluded, the arteriotomy should be placed in the direction of the takeoff of the deep femoral artery. This allows direct inspection and assessment of the caliber of the femoral artery, with sized arterial dilators up to a

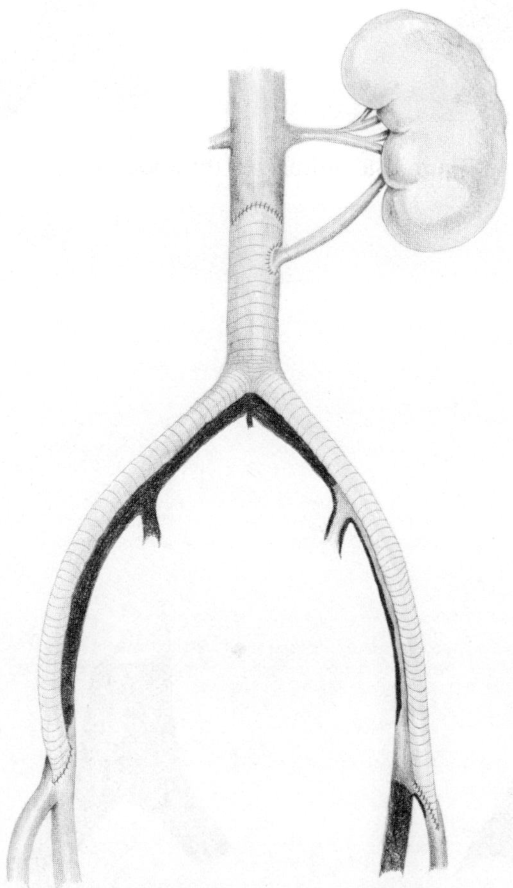

Figure 7–7. Aortobifemoral bypass with profundoplasty.

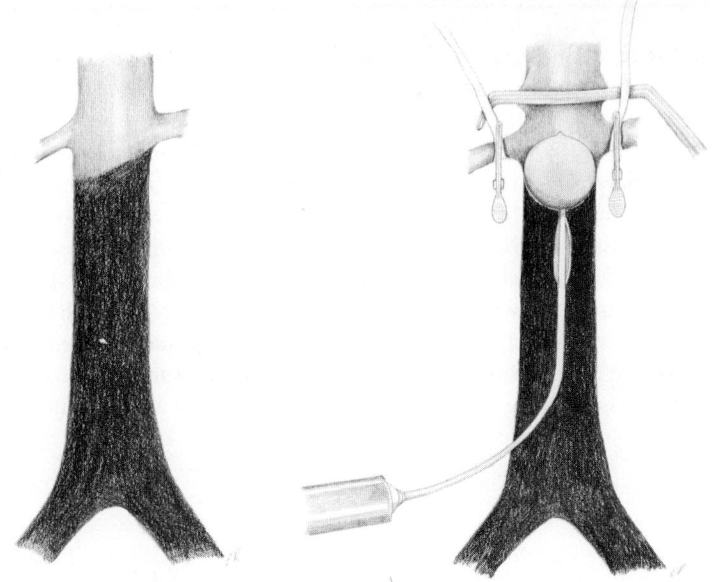

Figure 7-8. Infrarenal thrombectomy.

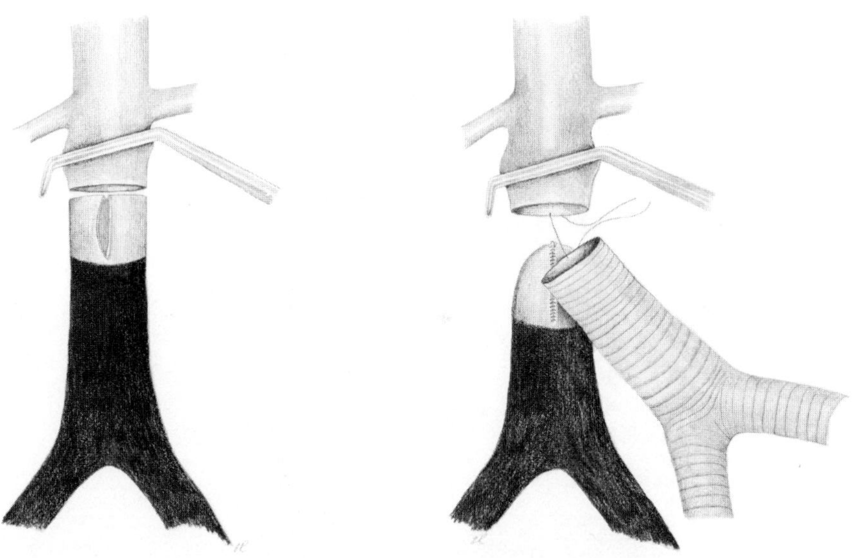

Figure 7-9. Infrarenal thrombectomy.

No. 4F. If stenosis is suspected, the arteriotomy is extended distally, and the tongue of the graft is used for a limited profundoplasty (Fig. 7–7). When indicated and when circumstances allow, an attempt should be made to restore blood flow to at least one internal iliac artery to treat or avoid impotence of vascular etiology.

Accessory renal arteries or a large inferior mesenteric artery should be reimplanted with the aortic cuff technique. Complete occlusion of the infrarenal aorta just below the renal arteries presents a particularly challenging problem. Other procedures have been applied to this situation, such as an axillobifemoral or a thoracic-aortobifemoral bypass. However, a segmental aortic thromboendarterectomy and aortofemoral bypass can be safely accomplished in this patient. The suprarenal aorta is temporarily cross-clamped, and the renal arterial flow is controlled with silastic vessel loops. Through a lower aortic arteriotomy, a proximal segmental thrombectomy is performed with a venous occlusion Fogarty catheter (Fig. 7–8). The infrarenal thrombectomized aorta is cleaned of debris and cross-clamped just below the origin of the renal arteries. The proximal clamp is then removed, and the kidneys are reperfused. The graft is placed as previously described (Fig. 7–9). After proper tissue coverage of the graft and reperitonealization, the abdomen is closed in layers.

EXTRA–ANATOMICAL PROCEDURES

Aortoiliac occlusive disease with ischemia of both lower extremities is best treated by conventional anatomic procedures. However, in the high-risk group of patients with severe pulmonary or cardiac disease, direct aortic reconstruction carries an unacceptably high mortality rate. For these patients, the surgeon's task is to relieve their ischemic symptoms with a reasonable risk. This compromise is accomplished with an extra-anatomical bypass procedure such as an axillofemoral or a femorofemoral bypass.

Axillofemoral Bypass

This procedure is designed to direct blood flow from one axillary artery to one or both lower extremities via a prosthetic graft placed subcutaneously. It can be performed under light general anesthesia and has a mortality rate of 2 to 3 percent. The indications for an axillofemoral bypass are: (1) aortoiliac disease in patients who are *poor risks* for conventional procedures; (2) reconstruction of vascular continuity after removal of an *infected* aortic prosthesis; and (3) as part of the *nonresectional* treatment of large abdominal aortic aneurysms (Fig. 7–10).

The reported patency rates have been as low as 50 percent for a 2-year or as high as 89 percent for a 5-year follow-up period. It seems that axillo*bifemoral*

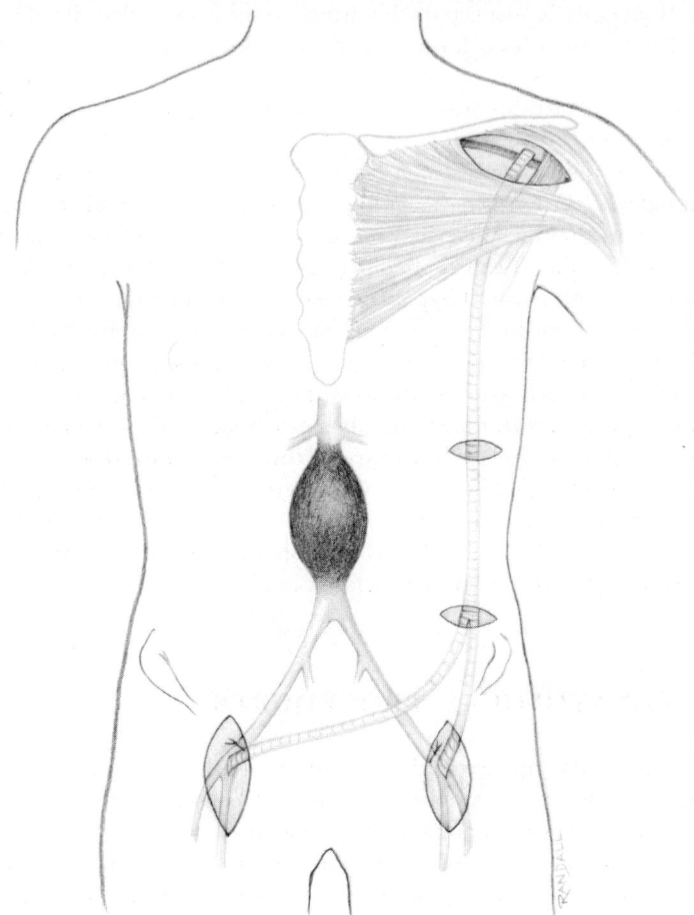

Figure 7-10. Axillobifemoral bypass in the treatment of an abdominal aortic aneurysm.

grafts generally have a better patency rate than unilateral grafts and that the surgeon should promptly attempt a thrombectomy or revision of a recently occluded graft. The cumulative patency rates so achieved are remarkable. In order to assure good flow through the graft and prevent possible steal symptoms, the donor axillary artery should be clinically evaluated preoperatively. It is essential to assure a strong axillary pulse, a good systolic arm pressure, and the lack of bruits in the subclavian region.

Operative Technique.   The neck, chest, abdomen, and both groins are prepped and draped. Each groin is entered through a longitudinal incision. The common, superficial, and deep femoral arteries are dissected and encircled with vessel loops.

The selected axillary artery is approached through a 3-inch-long infraclavicular skin incision. The incision is deepened down, through the subcutaneous tissue, to the fascia of the pectoralis major muscle. Once the fascia is incised, the muscle fibers are separated in their direction, exposing the clavicopectoral fascia. A self-returning retractor with deep blades helps to keep the wound open. The clavicopectoral fascia is incised, and the axillary artery is then localized with gentle exploration. Injury to the adjacent axillary vein and brachial plexus should be avoided. Two or three venous branches that cross over the artery should be ligated and divided (Fig. 7–11). The artery is now exposed, and occasionally division of pectoralis minor is necessary to gain more length for adequate control. Further mobilization can be accomplished if two or three arterial branches are ligated and divided. At this point, a tunnel is created under the pectoralis major muscle and is continued subcutaneously along the anterior axillary line to the ipsilateral groin. A small accessory incision on the chest wall facilitates the creation of the tunnel (Fig. 7–12). The patient is then systemically heparinized. The axillary artery is clamped, and an anterior arteriotomy is performed. The synthetic graft is cut with a short bevel and anastomosed with the artery with a continuous suture of 5–0 prolene. When the end-to-side

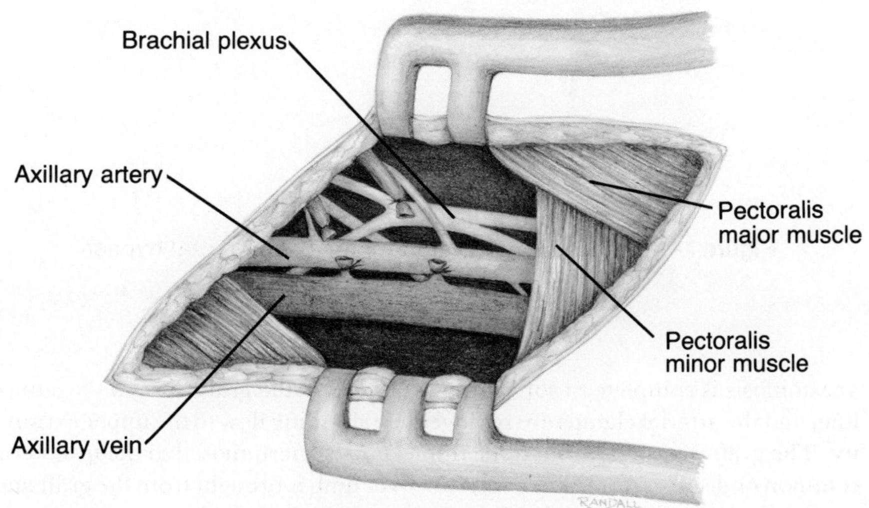

Figure 7–11. Exposure of the axillary artery.

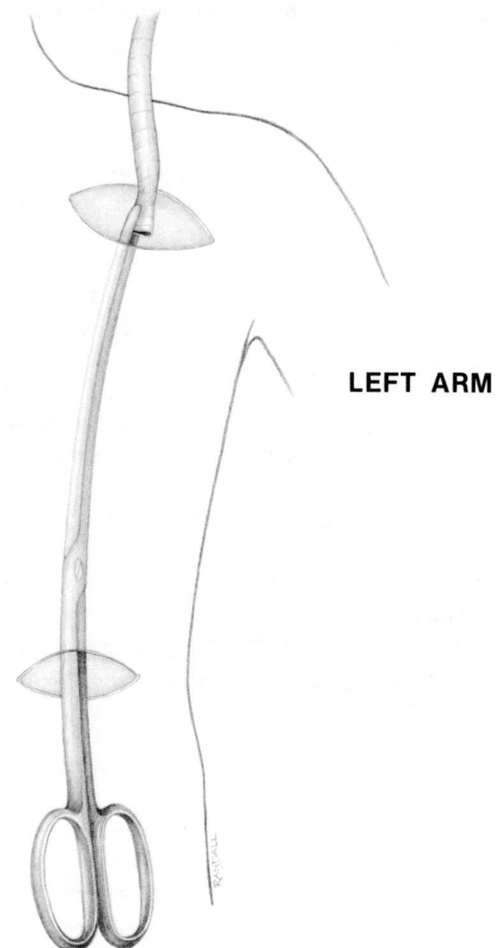

Figure 7-12. Accessory incision for an axillofemoral bypass.

anastomosis is complete, a soft clamp is applied to the graft close to the suture line, and the arterial clamps are removed, establishing flow to the upper extremity. The graft is passed through the tunnel and is anastomosed to the ipsilateral common or deep femoral artery. A cross-over limb is brought from the graft and is anastomosed to the contralateral common or deep femoral artery. The clamp is removed from the graft, and flow is established to both lower extremities. All incisions are closed in layers.

Femorofemoral Cross-Over Graft

Femorofemoral bypass is an extra-anatomical bypass procedure that diverts blood flow from one femoral artery (donor) to the other (recipient) (Fig. 7–13). The donor femoral artery should be free of significant disease, as demonstrated by arteriography, and should have an intraluminal systolic pressure close to the systolic arm pressure. The mean pressure in the recipient femoral artery should also be at least 40 to 50 mm Hg lower than the donor site, so that a pressure gradient will exist, assuring flow through the graft.

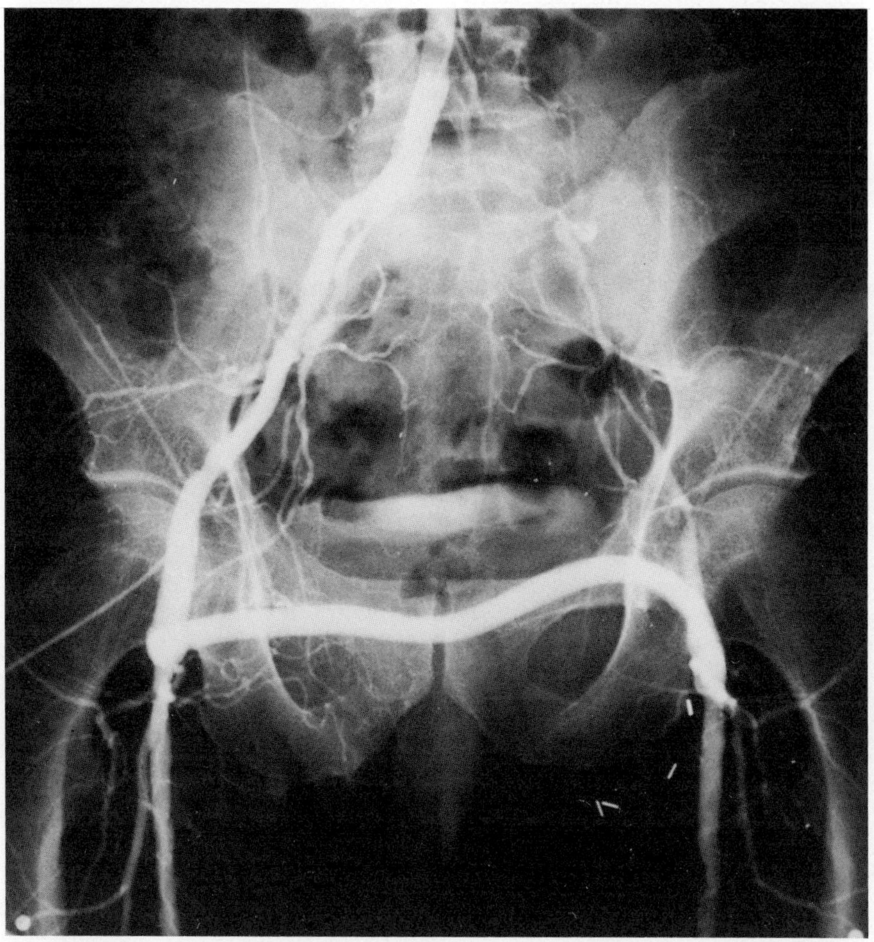

Figure 7–13. Femorofemoral bypass.

The indications for this procedure are (1) unilateral stenosis or occlusion of the common or external iliac artery or (2) unilateral occlusion of one limb of an aortofemoral bypass. Although this procedure was initially designed as a compromise for the poor-risk patient, it is now considered to be the procedure of choice over a unilateral aortofemoral bypass. It is proven to be a durable procedure with a cumulative 5-year patency rate of 80 percent. It offers the advantage of not requiring a laparotomy, and it can be performed under regional or even local anesthesia. It also seems to *protect the donor artery* from further disease, probably by increasing the total flow through this vessel. Steal, as manifested with appearance of ischemic symptoms in the extremity of the donor side, is rare and has been seen during exercise in patients with stenosis of the donor femoral artery.

Variants of this procedure are the extraperitoneal placement of an external iliac-femoral cross-over bypass and external iliac cross-over bypass (Fig. 7–14). The latter procedure has the disadvantage of not allowing evaluation and possibly correction of problems at the takeoff of the deep and superficial femoral arteries.

Operative Technique. Excellent anesthesia is accomplished with epidural or spinal regional anesthesia. In the poor-risk patient, the procedure may even be done under local anesthesia. Both groins are prepped, draped, and entered

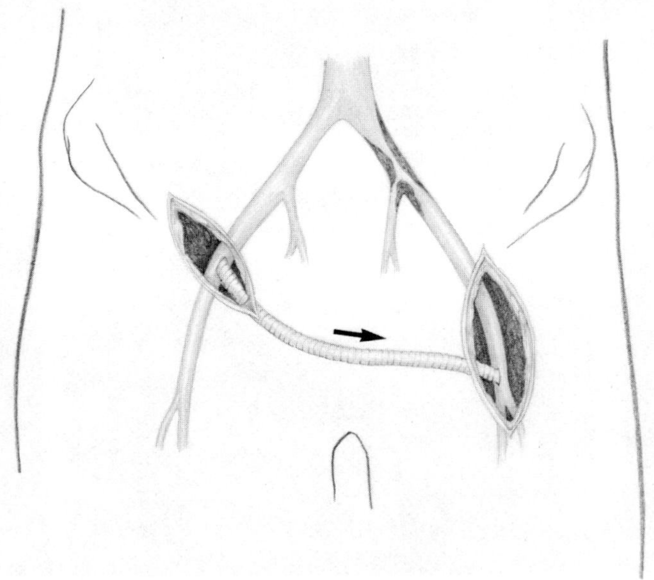

Figure 7–14. External iliac-femoral bypass.

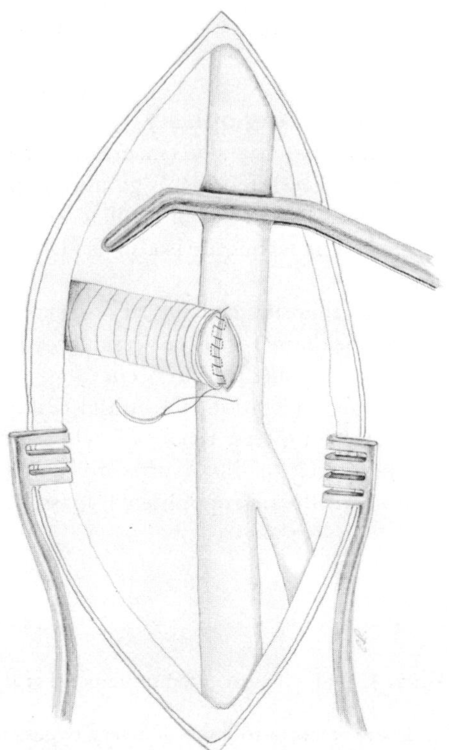

Figure 7-15. Transverse mattress suture.

through two separate longitudinal incisions. The common superficial and deep femoral arteries are dissected and isolated. Intra-arterial pressure is measured in both common femoral arteries. After the vascular clamps are applied, an arteriotomy is made on the donor common femoral artery and the selected graft is sutured in place with continuous suture of 5–0 prolene. If the donor site is the patent limb of an aortofemoral bypass, an oval window should be made on the wall of the donor graft. A soft Fogarty clamp is applied on the graft, next to the anastomosis, and the circulation is reestablished in the extremity of the inflow side. The graft is then passed through a subcutaneous suprapubic tunnel. On the recipient side, the graft is anastomosed with the common femoral artery unless there is stenosis of the origin of the superficial or deep femoral artery. In this case, the longitudinal arteriotomy is extended through the stenotic segment, and the graft is tailored so that a patch angioplasty will result. The posterior row of the outflow anastomosis is easily done from the inside of the vessel, and a transverse matress continuous suture will assure complete eversion of the graft and the vessel wall (Fig. 7–15). Once the anastomosis is complete, all clamps are removed, and flow is established through the cross-over graft. The wounds are then irrigated and closed in layers.

Percutaneous Transluminal Angioplasty

This technique, which includes percutaneous insertion if special balloon-tipped catheters to dilate areas of localized stenosis, is gaining popularity. It could be used in this situation to dilate narrowing of an iliac artery to increase blood flows to the lower extremity. The technique is also used for localized superficial artery stenosis.

It is presumed that the atheroma causing stenosis is compressed and flattened, therefore increasing the diameter of the vessel. However, it has also been reported that actual break in the calcification occurs.

When used in the proper indication, the initial results of this technique seem promising; however, the long-term results remain to be seen. Another use of this technique is intraoperatively to dilate a proximal iliac artery stenosis to increase inflow in association with temero-popliteal bypass.

BIBLIOGRAPHY

Brief DK, Brener BJ, Alpert J, et al: Crossover femorofemoral grafts followed up to five years or more. *Arch Surg* 110:1294, 1975.

Cevese PG, Gallucci V: Thoracic aorta-to-femoral artery bypass (for the treatment of complete obstruction of the abdominal aorta at the level of the renal arteries). *J Cardiovasc Surg* 16:432, 1975.

Dardik H, Ibrahim IM, et al: Synchronous aortofemoral or iliofemoral bypass with revascularization of the lower extremity. *Surg Gynecol Obstet* 149:676, 1979.

Darling RC, Brewster DC, Hallett JW, et al: Aortoiliac reconstruction. *Surg Clin North Am* 59:565, 1979.

DePalma RG, Levine SB, Feldman S: Preservation of erectile function after aortoiliac reconstruction. *Arch Surg* 113:958, 1978.

Eugene J, Goldstone J, Moore WS: Fifteen year experience with subcutaneous bypass grafts for lower extremity ischemia. *Ann Surg* 177, 1977.

Foster JH: Arteriography. Cornerstone of vascular surgery. *Arch Surg* 109:605, 1974.

Gaspar, MR, Morris JH: Aortoiliac thromboendarterectomy, technique and results. *Am J Surg* 111:457, 1966.

Leriche R, Morel A: The syndrome of thrombotic obliteration of the aortic bifurcation. *Ann Surg* 127:193, 1948.

LoGerfo FW, Johnson WC, Corson JD, et al: A comparison of the late patency rates of axillobilateral femoral and axillounilateral femoral grafts. *Surgery* 81:33, 1977.

Malone JM, Moore WS, Goldstone J: The natural history of bilateral aorto-femoral bypass grafts for ischemia of the lower extremities. *Arch Surg* 110:1300, 1975.

May AG, DeWeese JA, Rob CG: Changes in sexual function following operation on the abdominal aorta. *Surgery* 65:41, 1969.

Perdue GD, Smith RB, Veazey CR, et al: Revascularization for severe limb ischemia. *Arch Surg* 115:168, 1980.

Plecha FR, Pories WJ: Extraanatomic bypasses for aortoiliac disease in high-risk patients. *Surgery* 80:480, 1976.

Raines JK, Darling RC, et al: Vascular laboratory criteria for the management of peripheral vascular disease of the lower extremities. *Surgery* 71:21, 1976.

Sumner DS, Strandness DE, Jr: The hemodynamics of the femoro-femoral shunt. *Surg Gynec Obstet* 134:629, 1972.

CHAPTER EIGHT

Abdominal Aortic Aneurysms

INTRODUCTION

Aneurysms of the abdominal aorta are predominantly a disease of the elderly male and presents with an incidence of 2 percent in the general population aged 50 years or older. Seventy percent of the patients have associated heart, cerebrovascular, renal, or pulmonary disease. Of the true abdominal aortic aneurysms, 96 percent are of arteriosclerotic origin, and their vast majority are fusiform aneurysms below the renal arteries. Four percent are mycotic, traumatic, or congenital. Two percent of the aneurysms are suprarenal, most as part of a thoracoabdominal aneurysm.

The natural history of abdominal aortic aneurysm was first reported in 1950. It was discovered that the 5-year survival rate was 19.8 percent and that *63.8 percent* of the patients with known cause of death died of ruptured aneurysms. The surgical management of this problem made great strides over the next few years. In 1951, DuBost reported the successful replacement of an abdominal aortic aneurysm with a homograft. Studies soon followed, reporting early surgical intervention as a feasible means of correcting abdominal aortic aneurysms and preventing the potentially fatal complication of rupture. The initially utilized homografts were later replaced by synthetic grafts as the ideal conduit for replacement of the aorta.

Various studies have reported the incidence of rupture to be in the 4 to 6 percent range. However, in a recent study from South Africa, the incidence of rupture was reported to be 47.5 percent. It was thought that this was related to the lack of early diagnosis of abdominal aortic aneurysms, the misdiagnosis of impending rupture of an abdominal aortic aneurysm, and late referral of patients.

The mortality rate of elective aneurysmectomy has decreased over the years, but the mortality rate of aneurysmectomy for rupture is still high, from 50–60 percent. It appears reasonable that prevention of rupture by selection of patients for *elective aneurysmectomy* would decrease the total number of patients who die because of rupture.

Atherosclerotic aneurysms demonstrate loss of the normal architecture with replacement of the intima with atheromatous debris and clot. The media loses its orderly arrangement of elastic fibers, collagen, and smooth muscle. The collagen strength of the aneurysm is mainly found in the adventitia. Rupture occurs when (1) the intraluminal pressure exceeds the strength of this layer, which occurs as the radius of the aneurysm increases according to LaPlace's law or (2) the aneurysmal wall weakens. The mural thrombus may fragment with resulting distal embolization.

DIAGNOSIS

More than half of all patients with abdominal aortic aneurysms are asymptomatic, and these lesions are discovered either on physical examination or with varous studies done for other reasons.

When symptoms are present, they vary from vague abdominal discomfort and mild back pain for stationary aneurysms to acute severe and often excruciating back, flank, or abdominal pain associated with acutely expanding, leaking, or ruptured aneurysms. The pain often radiates to one or both groins.

The physical examination should reveal a pulsatile epigastric or midabdominal mass that *expands* with each heart beat. A bruit may also be heard. Complete vascular evaluation may reveal aneurysms elsewhere in the body or evidence of coexisting occlusive disease.

A plain film of the abdomen may demonstrate the presence of an unsuspected aneurysm (Fig. 8–1). Oblique and cross-table lateral views are helpful in the evaluation of the size of an aneurysm. Bony erosion is characteristic of a mycotic aneurysm. However, the diagnostic modalities that will accurately delineate the size, lumen, and proximal extension of an abdominal aortic aneurysm are: (1) ultrasonography (Fig. 8–2), (2) computerized tomography (Fig. 8–3), and (3) arteriography. We believe that it is essential for the complete preoperative evaluation of the vascular architecture. It will demonstrate the presence of accessory renal arteries, patency or occlusion of the inferior

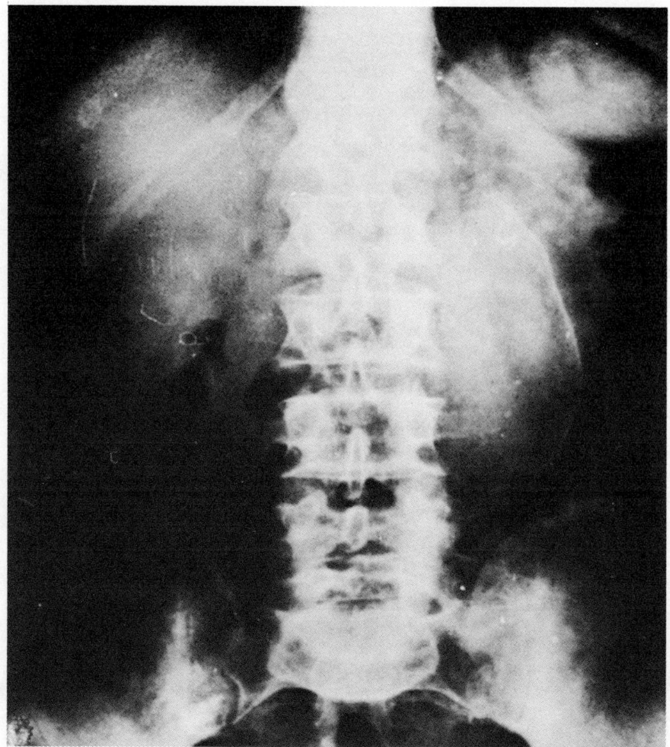

Figure 8-1. Abdominal aortic aneurysms: Mural calcifications.

mesenteric artery, ulcerated lesions of the iliac arteries, as well as disease of the distal vessels.

TREATMENT

Decision Making

Although every patient should be individualized, it seems that surgery is indicated if the maximum diameter of the aneurysm is 6 cm. Smaller aneurysms may be resected if patient is in good condition.

However, the only accepted treatment for abdominal aortic aneurysms at this time is resection and placement with a Dacron prosthesis. If the aneurysm is small and the patient is a poor risk, continuing observation may be indicated. Survival of patients with untreated abdominal aortic aneurysms is decreased.

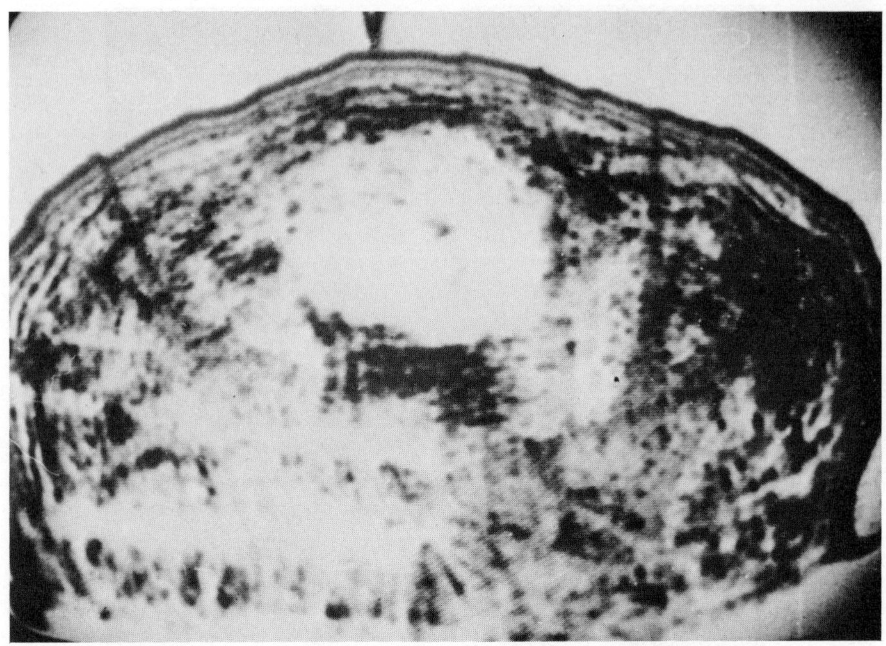

Figure 8–2. Abdominal aortic aneurysms: ultrasonography.

Surgery should be performed in all patients when the operative risk is well below the disease-associated mortality.

The available information from several studies indicates that the size of the aneurysm and the presence or absence of cardiopulmonary disease should determine the therapeutic decisions. In patients without significant associated disease, the operative risk is less than 5 percent, and all aneurysms should be surgically treated. When coronary artery, renal, or pulmonary disease complicates the presence of an abdominal aortic aneurysm, it is the severity of the disease and the size of the aneurysm, as estimated by sonography, that should determine the advisability of an operation.

All patients in whom the diagnosis of a ruptured aneurysm is strongly suspected should be operated on immediately.

Preoperative Care

All associated medical problems should be under optimal control. Prior to the arteriogram, the patient should be well hydrated in order to prevent impairment of the renal function induced by the dye. A mechanical bowel preparation is necessary. It has been demonstrated that the large intestines tolerate ischemia better if they are mechanically prepared. Antibiotics are administered just

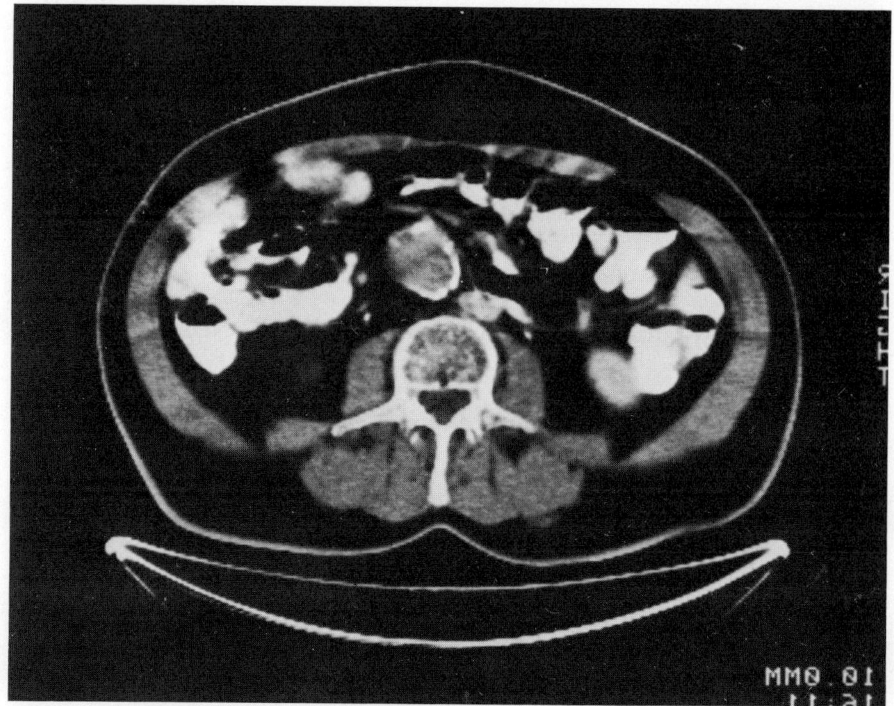

Figure 8-3. Abdominal aortic aneurysm—CAT scan.

preoperatively during surgery and for 24 hours postoperatively. In the patients with compromised cardiopulmonary function, a Swan-Ganz catheter is inserted preoperatively. This will allow precise intraoperative and postoperative monitoring of the function of the diseased heart.

Aneurysmectomy—Operative Technique

For an adequate exposure of an abdominal aortic aneurysm, a long xyphoid-to-pubis middle line incision is necessary. Both groins should also be prepped and draped. Once the abdomen is entered, an exploration should be performed because the presence of other intra-abdominal pathology may alter the operative plan. The aneurysm should not be roughly manipulated until the external iliac arteries are clamped at their origin, after systemic heparinization. Gentle manipulation and minimal dissection are essential. This will effectively protect from distal embolization. The small bowel mesentery, the cecum, and the distal duodenum are mobilized, after incising the peritoneum, medially to the inferior mesenteric vein. The entire small bowel may now be placed in a plastic bag with the help of the surgeon's hand, inserted through an opening at the top corner.

Once the aneurysm is exposed, the neck is identified and dissected from the surrounding structures with sharp and blunt dissection in a plane developed right on the aortic wall. The dissection is usually started on the caval side and advanced posteriorly, with care, so as not to injure any of the lumbar vessels. On the left side of the neck, the dissection ought to be more meticulous, as small retroperitoneal veins may be injured with resultant bothersome bleeding. Digital manipulation of the neck should be avoided during this dissection. The aortic bifurcation is not routinely dissected or incised when the aneurysmal sac is entered. *This is done in an attempt to preserve the sympathetic innervation of the pelvic structures.*

An assessment of the bifurcation and the iliac vessels is then performed. If the distal aorta at the bifurcation is not involved in the aneurysm and the iliac vessels have not significant disease, a tube graft should be considered (Fig. 8–4). In most cases, however, a bifurcation graft has to be utilized, with an end-to-end anastomosis to the common iliac arteries or an end-to-end anastomosis to the external iliac or femoral arteries. When dissecting the common iliac arteries, it should be remembered that they are closely adherent to the iliac veins and that

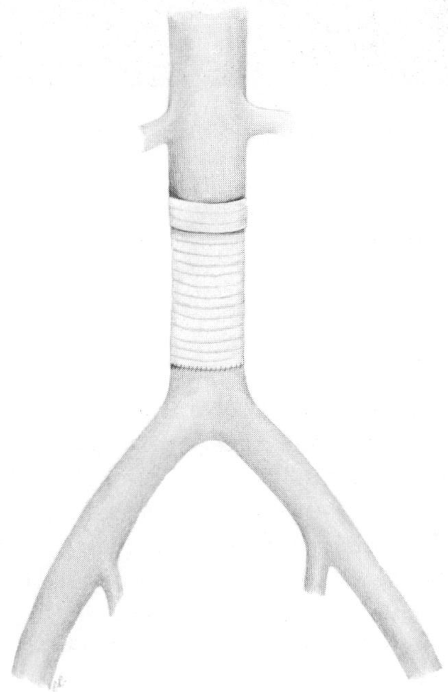

Figure 8–4. Resection of abdominal aortic aneurysm with tube graft.

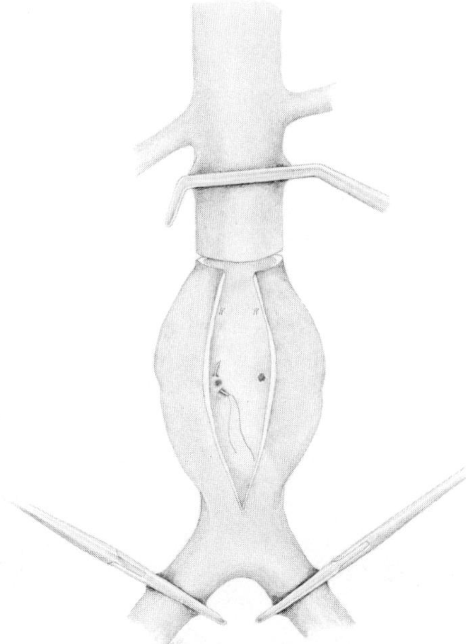

Figure 8–5. Oversewing of lumbar artery.

the bifurcation may be rotated with one iliac artery overlying the other. When the femoral arteries are considered for the distal anastomosis, they should be exposed at this stage. The inferior mesenteric artery and any possible accessory renal arteries are also dissected free, close to their takeoff from the aneurysmal wall. In order to avoid a renal infarct, reimplanation of all accessory renal arteries is advisable.

The use of a *knitted double velour Dacron graft* is preferred except in the case of a disorder of hemostasis or significant blood loss, as with ruptured aneurysms when woven Dacron graft is used instead. When knitted Dacron is used, pre-clotting of the graft with blood aspirated from the aneurysm cavity, before systemic heparinization, is done. Consideration should be given to a PTFE straight or bifurcation graft. The patient is then heparinized systemically. At this point, diuresis is induced with 12.5 gm of mannitol and 40 mg. of furosemide. The infrarenal aorta and the iliac arteries are now clamped at the previously selected places, the aneurysm is opened longitudinally, and the mural thrombus is evacuated. The openings of the lumbar arteries are oversewn with figure-eight sutures of 0–0 silk (Fig. 8–5). The opening of the inferior mesenteric artery (IMA) is inspected for backbleeding after the occluding clamp is released. If the artery was not visualized in the angiogram, the vessel is ligated. If it is patent and

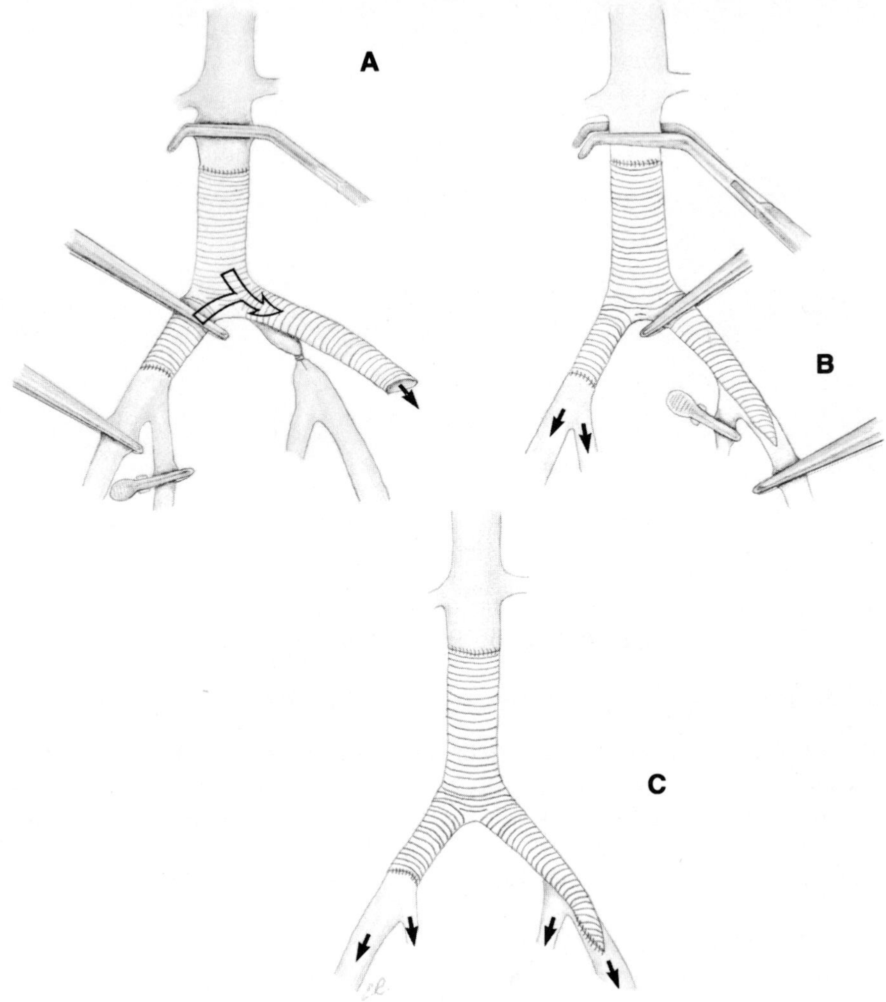

Figure 8-6. Sequential clamp release.

there is brisk backbleeding, ligation can be done with impunity. However, if the IMA is visualized and the backbleeding is poor, consideration is given to reimplantation.

The proximal aortic cuff is then trimmed to the start of the aneurysmal sac and tailored for an end-to-end anastomosis with the graft using continuous suture of 3–0 prolene. When the posterior wall of the aorta is completely divided, a cuff of the graft can be used to later cover the anastomotic line. When a tube graft is used the aortic bifurcation is appropriately tailored to accommodate the distal end of the graft. For an aorto-common iliac graft, the common iliac artery is transected, and an end-to-end anastomosis is performed with 4–0 prolene continuous suture. Otherwise, the common iliac arteries are ligated, and a more distal, end-to-side anastomosis is performed so that perfusion of the lower extremity as well as the pelvic structures are maintained. Before completion of the distal anastomosis, the arteries are let to backbleed, and the graft is flashed in order, as illustrated, to prevent debris from embolizing in the leg (Fig. 8–6). Once hemostasis is confirmed, the incised aneurysmal wall that was left in place is now sutured over the graft in an attempt to separate completely the graft and the proximal anastomosis from the duodenum. If further tissue interposition is required, a piece of omentum may be passed through a tunnel penetrating the gastrocolic ligament and the root of the transverse mesocolon (Fig. 8–7). Following adequate reperitonealization, the abdomen is closed in layers. No drains are used.

Special Problems

Inflammatory Aneurysms.   They are rather rare and are characterized by dense desmoplastic reaction enveloping the arteriosclerotic aortic wall and surround-

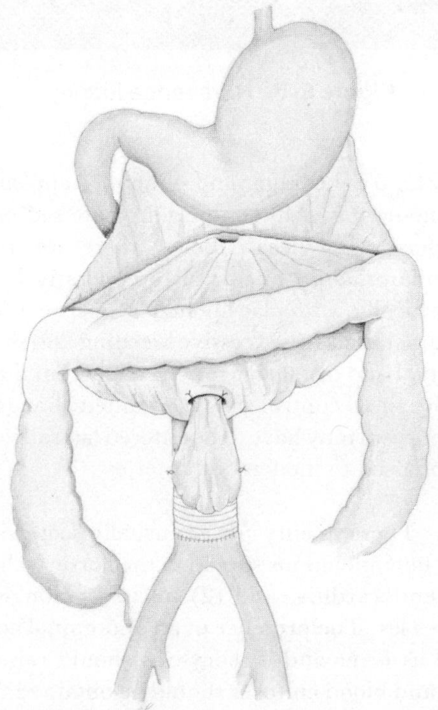

Figure 8–7. Interposition of the omentum.

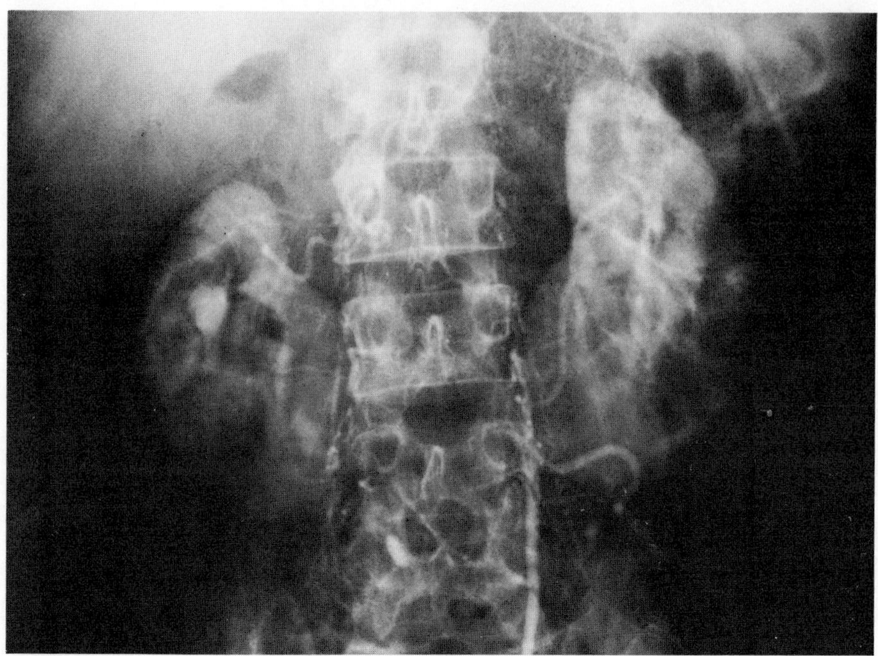

Figure 8-8. Horseshoe kidney.

ing structures. They tend to be larger and symptoms appear more often than in noninflammatory aneurysms. Although erythrocyte sedimentation rates may be elevated in 50 percent of these patients, there are no reliable means of distinguishing an inflammatory aneurysm preoperatively. These aneurysms should be treated surgically, with placement of a Dacron graft. The retroperitoneal dissection is characterized by excessive bleeding and should be limited only to the areas of proximal and distal control. The adherent duodenum should not be mobilized, and proximal control can be obtained above the third part of the duodenum. The aneurysm may have to be entered laterally, and the limbs of the graft are best anastomosed to the femoral arteries.

Mycotic Aneurysms. These aneurysms are usually seen with (1) a preexisting source of sepsis and hematogenous spread to the aortic wall, as may occur with subacute bacterial endocarditis, and (2) in association with mediastinal or retroperitoneal abscesses. The presence of an abdominal aortic aneurysm with signs of sepsis such as fever and leukocytosis should raise the suspicion of a mycotic aneurysm, and blood cultures should be obtained. The organisms that are usually isolated are *Staphylococcus, Salmonella,* and *Streptococcus.*

Once the diagnosis is established, proper antibiotics should be started. The aneurysm should be completely excised, including the *posterior wall*. Both proximal and distal ends should be oversewn, and the vascular continuity should be reestablished via an extra-anatomic route such as an axillobifemoral bypass graft.

Horseshoe Kidney. In a patient with a horseshoe or ectopic kidney, the problem is the preservation of the blood supply to the kidney. Whenever the diagnosis is entertained preoperatively, angiography is indicated in order to delineate accurately the usually multiple vessels that supply this kidney (Fig. 8–8). If this is discovered intraoperatively, both lateral walls of the aneurysm should be carefully dissected and all renal arteries identified. If the corresponding segment of the kidney becomes ischemic when an accessory renal artery is clamped, it has to be reimplanted in a buttonhole of the prosthetic graft. Ectopic veins may also be present and, if possible, should be preserved. In most instances, the graft has to be brought over the fused lower poles of the horseshoe kidney.

Left Renal Vein. Although the left renal vein can usually be retracted for exposure of the infrarenal aorta, it should be emphasized that if it is necessary, this vessel can be divided with impunity close to the inferior vena cava. The adrenal and gonadal veins provide collateral pathways for drainage of the left kidney (Fig. 8–9). Some temporary elevation of the serum creatinine may occur

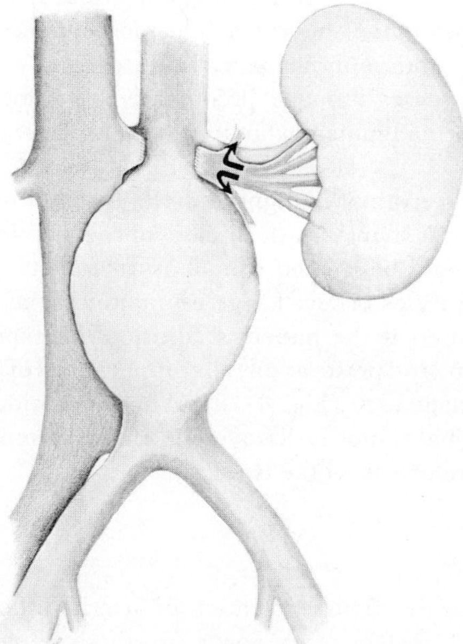

Figure 8–9. The left renal vein.

postoperatively; in general, however, it returns to normal in a few days. As with all major veins, a transfixion suture should be placed on each end. Division of the renal vein creates a regional venous hypertension, and some retroperitoneal bleeding may be seen. It is imperative that complete hemostasis is secured before this vessel is divided.

Aortocaval Fistula. This develops in 1 percent of abdominal aortic aneurysms by gradual erosion and eventual rupture of the aneurysm into the inferior vena cava, creating a high-flow arteriovenous fistula. The usual presentation is that of a patient with an abdominal aortic aneurysm and *high-output cardiac failure.* A machinerylike bruit is audible over the epigastrium. The veins of the lower extremity are engorged secondary to the venous hypertension, and the liver may be enlarged. When the size of the fistula is larger than 1.5 cm, cardiac decompensation follows.

Surgical correction is accomplished through an approach similar to that for an uncomplicated aneurysm. Dissection in the area of the fistula should not be done. When the aneurysmal sac is incised, backbleeding from the inferior vena cava is controlled with manual compression from the outside or with the surgeon's finger from the inside. The defect of the caval wall is sutured from the *inside of the sac* with interrupted sutures.

Coexisting Malignancy. It is estimated that 4 percent of patients with abdominal aortic aneurysms harbor a malignant tumor before, simultaneously with, or after diagnosis of the aneurysm. The most common malignant tumors are colorectal, lung, and genitourinary. In 35 percent of these patients, the diagnosis of both diseases is made preoperatively. Another 40 percent are patients with known malignancy who are found to have an abdominal aortic aneurysm.

No patient with terminal malignant disease should have resection of an aneurysm. In patients with metastatic disease, only expanding, leaking, or ruptured aneurysms should be treated. Small asymptomatic aneurysms are left alone unless complications occur. Large asymptomatic aneurysms should be considered for resection if the patient's adjusted life expectancy justifies it. Bleeding, obstruction, and perforation, all complications of a malignant tumor, have priority in management (Fig. 8–10). When operating for an aneurysm, and an intra-abdominal tumor is discovered, consideration should be given in dealing with the more urgent of the two first.

Complications

Declamping Hypotension. The restoration of arterial inflow in the lower extremities after the placement of an aortic prosthesis is often associated with

Aneurysms → Cancer ↓	small: <6 cm	large: >6 cm	symptomatic or ruptured
Curable Disease	treat only the cancer	treat both	treat aneurysm first then cancer
Metastatic Disease	do not treat aneurysm	do not treat aneurysm	treat aneurysm
Complications	treat complication	treat complication first	treat both
Terminal Disease	do not treat aneurysm	do not treat aneurysm	do not treat aneurysm

Figure 8–10. Abdominal aortic aneurysm and malignancy.

significant temporary hypotension, which, in turn, may result in a period of dangerous myocardial and cerebral ischemia.

Various mechanisms have been suggested in the etiology of declamping hypotension. These are (1) increased capacity of the vascular bed below the occlusion, secondary to ischemia induced *vasodilatation*. As the volume remains the same, the vascular capacity increases due to decreased resistance, and the pressure drops. (2) Liberation of *vasoactive substances* and bradykinin from the ischemic tissues. Once the flow is reestablished, these substances circulate and cause generalized vasodilatation. (3) Acute *blood loss* either at the site of the vascular anastomosis or through a poorly preclotted graft. If this occurs, the aorta is temporarily reclamped so that leaking points can be sutured and additional fibrin can be deposited in the prosthetic graft.

The measures to prevent this from happening are: (1) sequential restoration of flow to one and later to the other extremity; (2) repletion of blood volume just prior to declamping; (3) placing the OR table in a Trendelenburg position; (4) if concominant sympathectomy is considered, it should not be done prior to the placement of the graft.

Ileus. Retroperitoneal dissection, prolonged evisceration, and anesthesia contribute to the development of postoperative ileus. A nasogastric tube has to stay in place for 2 to 4 days. If ileus develops, it responds well to prolonged nasogastric suction and N. P. O.

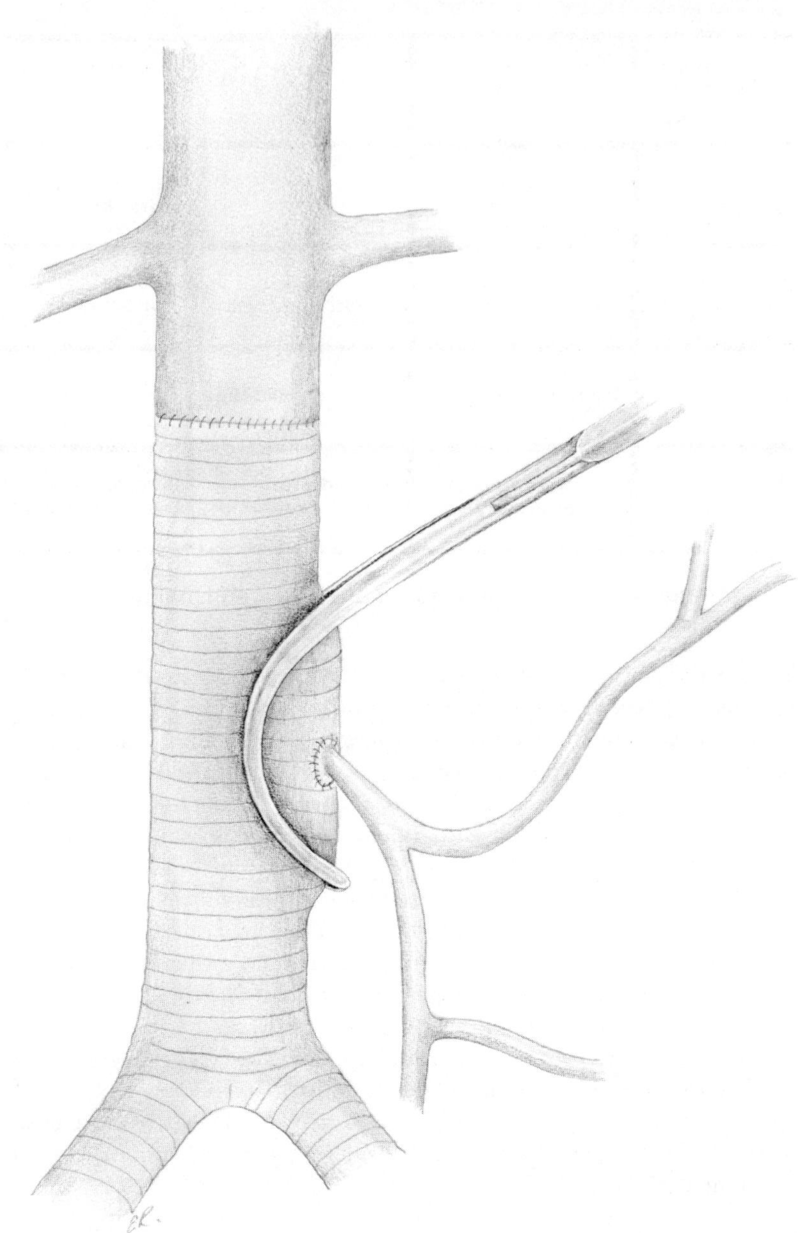

Figure 8–11. Reimplantation of the inferior mesenteric artery.

Ischemic Gut Syndrome. Ischemic gut syndrome develops secondary to ligation of the inferior mesenteric artery and/or exclusion of blood flow into the pelvic vasculature. It may present as bloody diarrhea or even colonic gangrene. It is mandatory to prep the large bowel preoperatively, as clean colon tolerates ischemia better.

Simple diarrhea is controlled with medications. Some bleeding may occur as ischemic mucosa slough off, which may lead to future stricture formation. Acute abdomen, with localization in the left lower quadrant, indicates perforation, and emergency surgery is necessary for resection of the ischemic colon and colostomy. Extraperitoneal perforation usually makes the graft removal mandatory.

This complication is preventable. With a good pulse in the superior mesenteric and direct revascularization of the pelvis, the inferior mesenteric artery can be ligated. Whenever the hypogastric arteries are significantly diseased or the distal anastomosis is done at the femoral level, the inferior mesenteric artery should be considered for reimplantation in a buttonhole of the graft. A 2-to 3-mm rim of the aortic wall should be preserved (Fig. 8–11).

Trash Foot Syndrome. This syndrome is caused by distal embolization during aortic surgery. It usually involves the smaller distal vessels, and once it occurs, embolectomy is extremely difficult. Every attempt should be made to limit perianeurysmal dissection and avoid digital manipulation of the aneurysm or its neck. If the dissection of the neck is difficult, the *external iliac arteries* must be *cross-clamped* first. This will divert any debris and thrombi in the hypogastric arteries. This maneuver is generally safe, except in the case of a thin-wall aneurysm.

Paraplegia. A rare but distressing problem, paraplegia is the result of interruption of flow in the *arteria radicularis magna,* also known as the artery of Adamkiewicz. This vessel originates somewhere in the upper lumbar or lower thoracic portion of the aorta between T8–L4.

Sexual Disturbances. Postoperative impotence may be the result either of interruption of the preaortic sympathetic plexus or exclusion of the hypogastric vessels from the reconstruction. Such a complication should be avoided by all means in male patients, which implies that the bifurcation will not be dissected or incised and that adequate flow will be reestablished into the pelvic vascular bed. However, all patients should be told that impotence may still occur.

Sepsis. Graft sepsis is an infrequent, delayed complication with high mortality. In most instances, it is associated with an aortoenteric fistula and manifests itself with fever, leukocytosis, and intermittent gastrointestinal bleeding. Computerized tomography and ultrasonography are very helpful in the diagnosis of retroperitoneal sepsis by demonstrating a collection of fluid around the graft. Angiograms may delineate the fistula.

Once the diagnosis is strongly suspected, urgent surgery should be performed. The graft is removed, the aorta is oversewn, the iliac arteries are ligated, and an extra-anatomic axillobifemoral bypass is performed. If an aortoduodenal fistula exists, the duodenum should be débrided, closed, and patched with a loop of jejunum.

Ruptured Abdominal Aortic Aneurysms

Preparation. Once the diagnosis of a ruptured aortic aneurysm is made, immediate preparations are made to take the patient to the operating suite. Many aneurysms are easily palpable, but it may be necessary to perform cross-table lateral abdominal X-ray to confirm the presence of an abdominal aortic aneurysm. Arteriograms, ultrasound, and CAT scans are rarely required in the work-up of a ruptured abdominal aortic aneurysm. The time between diagnosis and surgery should be minimal. Blood is drawn for type and cross match and routine studies. Large-bore venous access is obtained, and a central venous pressure or a Swan-Ganz catheter is inserted. Antibiotics and fluids are administered, and an indwelling Foley catheter is inserted. Obviously, if the patient presents with hypotension and the diagnosis is evident, the patient should immediately be taken to the operating suite, with work-up and preparation completed as the operation proceeds.

It should be mentioned that the use of the *blood retransfusion apparatus,* which can be prepared preoperatively, could reduce the amount of bank blood transfused and provide a quick supply of blood for autotransfusion without the hazards of transfused, banked blood. It does require additional personnel to centrifuge the blood, but this can be easily handled by the anesthesia personnel or a trained circulating nurse.

In addition, the use of the new ring retractors can provide excellent exposure with involvement of fewer assistants. This would be most helpful in settings and times when assistants are not available.

Operative Management. The patient is prepped and draped prior to the induction of anesthesia, and the surgeon and his assistants are ready to make the incision. A xyphoid-to-pubis midline incision is made, and control of the aorta is obtained. It may be necessary to obtain this control temporarily at the level of the diaphragm until infrarenal aortic control can be achieved. Other writers have advocated a left thoracotomy to gain initial control of the aorta. This practice is based on the observation that opening the abdomen may relieve the tamponading effect of the intra-abdominal pressure and result in exsanquination. This is best applied to obese patients and those patients in profound shock and cardiac arrest because transthoracic aortic control can be obtained in minutes. After temporary control, the aorta below the renal arteries is isolated and clamped. Frequently, the hematoma will facilitate the dissection in this area for the placement of an infrarenal aortic clamp. Once this control is obtained, the previously placed clamp is removed in an effort to reduce the time that the kidneys and bowel are not perfused. Many vascular surgeons do not use systemic heparin in this situation. However, once control of bleeding is obtained, regional heparin flush of the distal circulation by direct injection into iliac arteries is recommended. Additional heparin is instilled locally into the iliac arteries, which are also dissected and clamped next in order to eliminate back-bleeding.

When free rupture into the peritoneal cavity occurs, a 30-cc balloon Foley catheter may be inserted into the proximal aorta to obtain control of blood loss until the aorta can be clamped. Fogarty venous-occlusion catheters can be inserted distally to obtain similar control, if necessary. One can also use an aortic compression clamp to maintain control by compressing the aorta against the vertebral column until the infrarenal aorta can be clamped.

Once aortic and iliac artery control is obtained, the approach essentially reverts to an elective aneurysmectomy. The aneurysm is opened, and lumbar arteries that bleed are suture ligated with figure-eight stitches. Laminated clot is removed from within the aneurysm. The aorta may or may not be divided below the renal arteries, and an approximately sized and shaped *woven Dacron* graft is anastomosed to the proximal aorta. If the iliac arteries are not involved with atherosclerotic changes, then a tube graft is inserted. If it is not feasible to insert a tube graft, then a bifurcation graft is selected. The graft is completed to the iliac or femoral level, depending on associated atherosclerotic disease at respective levels. When the anastomoses are completed and flow is reestablished, the graft is covered by the aneurysmal wall. Special attention is made to be certain that the graft is separated from any contact with the duodenum. If the aneurysmal wall or retroperitoneal tissue is insufficient to cover the graft, then the tongue of omentum is tailored to cover the graft. The peritoneum is then closed, if possible.

It should be emphasized that patients with aneurysms may have other intra-abdominal problems that may be mistaken as a symptomatic aneurysm. Exploration of the abdomen should be performed if a leak or rupture is not obvious, for disastrous complications can occur if a graft is inserted in the presence of a contaminated intra-abdominal process such as diverticulitis or appendicitis.

Postoperatively, the patient should be transferred to an intensive care unit and monitored closely for changes in vital signs, urinary output, and cardiac function. Fluid and drug administration are determined by the various modes of monitoring, as mentioned previously.

Mortality and Morbidity. The mortality rate for ruptured abdominal aortic aneurysms varies but the average is 50–60 percent and sometimes higher. This is considerably higher than that of elective aneurysmectomy. It has been shown that the mortality rate is related to the age of the patient and the volume of blood lost and replaced. The amount of blood loss indirectly reflects the number of patients who present in shock. It is strongly suggested to consider all patients as operative candidates on an elective basis in spite of age and other factors. As technical advances have been made, fewer contraindications to elective aneurysmectomy should exist. With the knowledge of the increased mortality rate with ruptured aneurysms, the number of elective aneurysmectomies performed should aid in decreasing the number of human lives that are lost because of this disease.

The morbidity rate associated with emergency repair involve cardiac, respiratory, renal, and cerebrovascular complications; emboli, hemorrhage, paraplegia, and wound problems have also been encountered. Late complications include false aneurysm and aortoenteric fistulas.

The major cause of death determined by the long-term follow-up of patients who have undergone abdominal aortic aneurysmectomy is myocardial infarction. It seems reasonable to consider these patients candidates for coronary arteriography either pre- or postoperatively to determine which patients would benefit from coronary artery bypass in an attempt to decrease the late mortality. Currently, studies are being performed to attempt to make clear the topic of improved life expectancy of patients who have undergone aneurysmectomy and coronary artery bypass.

BIBLIOGRAPHY

Baker AF, Sharzer LA, Ehrenhaft JL: Aortocaval fistula as a complication of abdominal aortic aneurysms. *Surgery* 72:933, 1972.

Brener BJ, Darling RC, et al: Major venous anomalies complicating abdominal aortic surgery. *Arch Surg* 108:159–165, 1974.

Chang FC, Smith JL, Rahbar A, et al: Abdominal aortic aneurysms: a comparative analysis of surgical treatment of symptomatic and asymptomatic patients. *Am J Surg* 136:705, 1978.

DuBost D, Allary M, Oeconomos NA: A propos du traitement des aneurysmes de l'aorte. *Mem Acad Chis* 77:381, 1951.

Estes JE Jr: Abdominal aortic aneurysm: a study of one hundred two cases. *Circulation* 2:258, 1950.

Ezzet F, Dorazio R, Herzberg R: Horseshoe and pelvic kidneys associated with abdominal aortic aneurysms. *Am J Surg* 134:196, 1977.

Gaylis H, Kesshe E: Ruptured aortic aneurysm. *Surgery* 87:300, 1980.

Golden GT, Sears HF, Wellons HA Jr, et al: Paraplegia complicating resection of aneurysms of the infrarenal aorta. *Surgery* 73:91, 1973.

Goldstone J, Malone JM, Moore WS: Inflammatory aneurysms of the abdominal aorta. *Surgery* 83:425, 1978.

Hardy JD, Timmis HH: Abdominal aortic aneurysms: special problems. *Am Surg* 173:945, 1971.

Imparato AM, Berman IR, et al: Avoidance of shock and peripheral embolism during surgery of the abdominal aorta. *Surgery* 73:68, 1973.

Lawrie GM, Morris GG Jr, Crawford ES, et al: Improved results of operations for ruptured abdominal aortic aneurysms. *Surgery* 85:483, 1979.

Leopold GR, Goldberger LE, Bernstein EF: Ultrasonic detection and evaluation of abdominal aortic aneurysms. *Surgery* 72:939, 1972.

Mittal VK, Bodzin JH: Ruptured abdominal aortic aneurysms. *Int Surg* 85:483, 1979.

Stokes J, Butcher HR Jr: Abdominal aortic aneurysms. Factors influencing operative mortality and criteria of operability. *Arch Surg* 107:279, 1973.

Szilagyi DE, Rodriguez FJ, Smith RF, et al: Late fate of arterial allografts: observations 6 to 15 years after implantation. *Arch Surg* 101:721, 1970.

Thompson JE, Hollier LH, et al: Surgical management of abdominal aortic aneurysms: factors influencing mortality and morbidity—a 20 year experience. *Am Surg* 181:654, 1975.

CHAPTER NINE

Diseases of the Femoropopliteal Segment

Femoropopliteal occlusive disease

INTRODUCTION

The last three decades have seen many advances in the surgical treatment of femoropopliteal occlusive disease. Various operations have been designed in an attempt to revascularize a critically ischemic lower extremity. Most of these are now bypass procedures that extend to the distal popliteal or tibial arteries. The graft material of choice is autogenous saphenous vein. However, as a saphenous vein of good size is not always available, other vascular conduits have to be utilized. Umbilical vein homografts and polytetrafluoroethylene and Dacron synthetic grafts have been used with varying degrees of success. Profundoplasty and lumbar sympathectomy have proven to be beneficial in a selected group of patients.

The pattern of the disease varies from segmental stenosis of the distal superficial femoral artery to complete occlusion of the superficial femoral, popliteal, and tibial arteries (Fig. 9-1). Compensation is achieved through collateral pathways via the deep femoral artery and the descending branch of the circumflex iliac artery to the genicular network and recurrent tibial tributaries.

The clinical presentation will depend on the distribution of the disease and the efficiency of the collateral circulation. In patients with intermittent claudica-

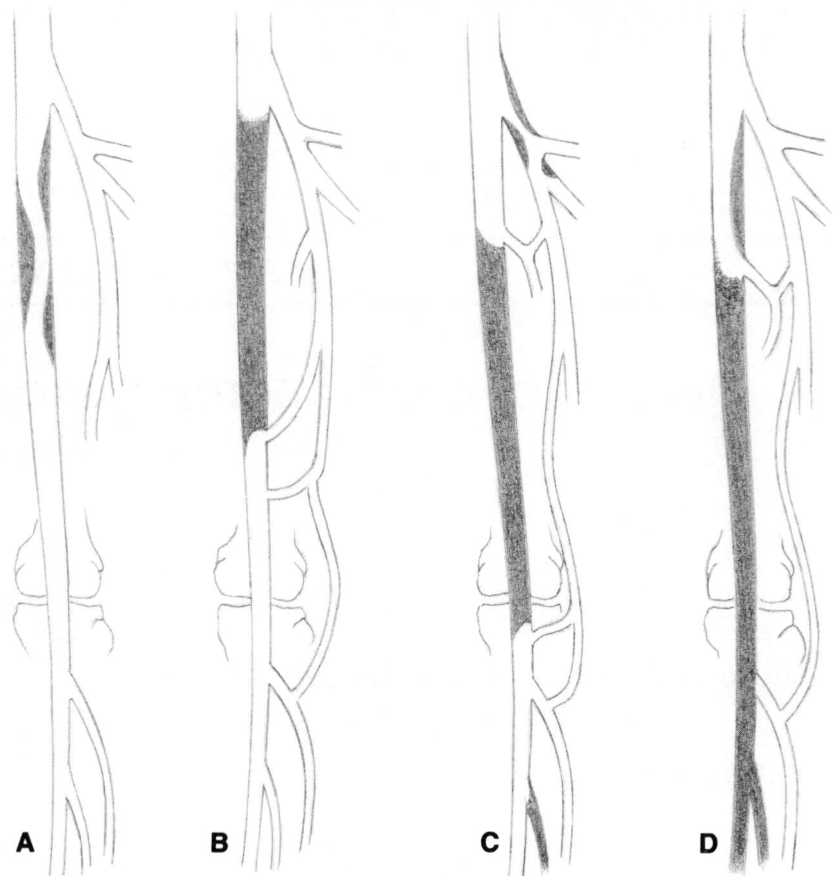

Figure 9-1. Patterns of femoropopliteal disease.

tion, adequate compensation has occurred. In the majority of these patients (90 percent), the disease remains stable or even improves. The patients who present with ischemic symptoms at rest should be treated aggressively because their disease is unstable and will invariably result in significant tissue loss if left untreated.

Many limbs are now salvaged, and the quality of life of these patients is much improved. The toll paid for reconstructive procedures is in the range of 2 to 5 percent, substantially lower than the 10 percent mortality of a primary amputation. However, not all ischemic extremities can be salvaged, and 5 percent of them will have to be amputated either because of advanced frank gangrene or uncontrolled sepsis. In this selected group of patients, an amputation should be considered as a procedure aiming toward converting a diseased extremity to a functional unit.

DIAGNOSIS

History

Most patients with femoropopliteal occlusive disease will present initially with intermittent claudication of the calf, relieved with rest. The severity of the claudication is classically described by the number of blocks, or yards, that the patient can walk before symptoms appear. More advanced stages of the disease present with rest pain or ischemic lesions. Rest pain is constant, involves the toes and forefoot, and improves on dependency. Ischemic lesions may be areas of focal gangrene or nonhealing ulcerations. Unless successful arterial reconstruction is performed, these limbs will eventually be lost.

Medical and social histories are of great importance. Coexisting physical or mental disorders as well as the ambulatory status of the patient are important considerations in the patient's management.

Physical Examination

Inspection alone can give a reasonably accurate impression of the degree of the existing ischemia. Trophic changes of the skin, pallor on elevation, rubor on dependency, ulcerations, and areas of gangrene should be detected. The lack or presence of distal pulses should be recorded. The popliteal fossae should always be palpated so that popliteal aneurysms will not be missed. Assessment of the venous refill and capillary filling will yield reliable information. The range of motion of the different joints should be examined, and any existing muscular contractions should be detected.

The physical examination should include complete cardiac, respiratory, and cerebrovascular evaluation.

Noninvasive Studies

The vascular laboratory is able to supply objective and accurate information with regard to the degree of an existent hemodynamic deficit. The use of the Doppler ultrasonic flowmeter allows (1) measurement of the segmental systolic arterial pressure at the levels of the thigh, upper calf, and ankle and (2) detection of arterial flow in the posterior tibial and dorsalis pedis arteries, indicative of patency of these vessels. The pulse volume recorder detects segmental total flow at different levels. A strong femoral pulse in combination with decreased Doppler pressures and abnormal plethysmographic recordings indicate the presence of superficial femoral artery disease. Significant differences between the recordings and the pressures from the thigh, the upper calf, or the ankle strongly suggests significant disease of trifurcation and all tibial vessels (Fig. 9–2).

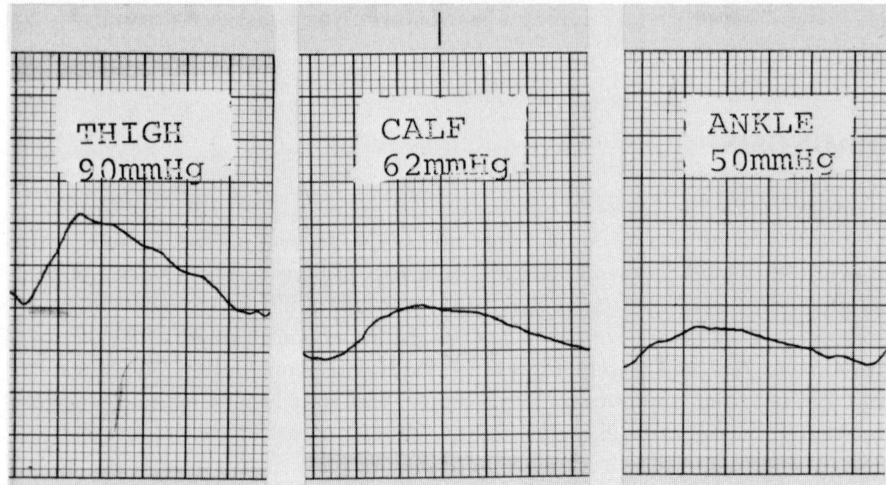

Figure 9-2. Pulse volume recording (PVR)—abnormal study.

In the evaluation of claudication, the above studies are performed at rest and after exercise on the treadmill. Exercise testing will disclose the hemodynamic significance of an existent flow deficit. It also provides reliable baseline information in the follow-up of the patient with intermittent claudication. However, this should not be done with patients with history of myocardial infarction or angina because the exercise may induce significant symptomatic myocardial ischemia. Pulse volume recorder information and measurement of segmental arterial pressures are also valuable in the postoperative follow-up of patients who undergo an arterial reconstruction in the lower extremities.

Arteriography

If the disease seems to be unilateral, a needle puncture arteriogram may be adequate. Otherwise, the retrograde catheter technique is used, which has the advantage of evaluating the aortoiliac segment as well as both extremities. Oblique views of the groin, as well as iliac vessels, are essential for the evaluation of the inflow and takeoff of the deep femoral artery (Fig. 9-3). The trifurcation and the distal tibial vessels, as well as the arterial pedal and plantar arch, should also be visualized. A successful operation can be designed only on the basis of a good-quality arteriogram. Occasionally, the preoperative arteriogram is unsatisfactory. In this case, the vessel in question can be selectively explored during surgery and an intraoperative arteriogram can be obtained with a small catheter inserted through an arteriotomy.

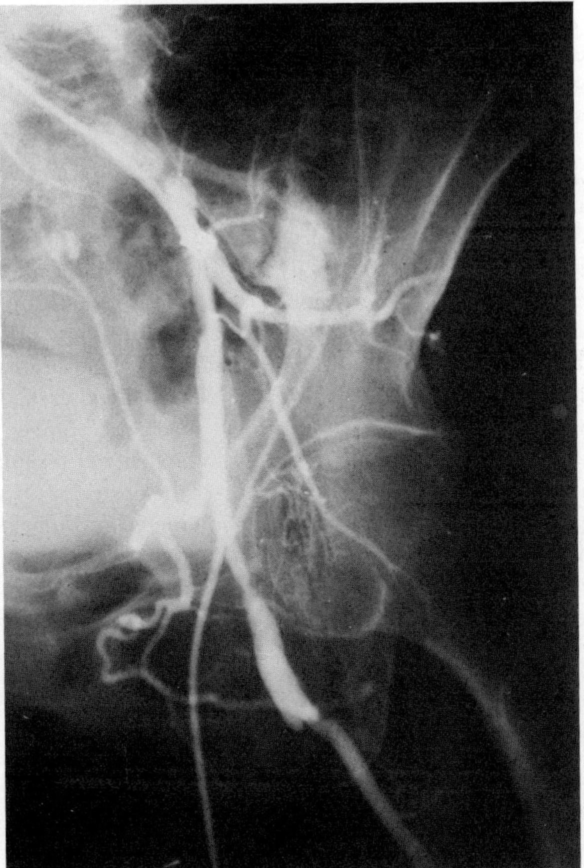

Figure 9-3. Deep femoral artery.

TREATMENT

Decision Making

Most patients with intermittent claudication will respond to conservative measures such as exercise to tolerance, diet, cessation of smoking, and control of hypertension and diabetes. These patients learn to modify their activity and live with their disease. Only 10 to 15 percent of the patients with claudication will come to surgery either because it is of a disabling nature or because of progression to the ischemic stage. Patients with ischemic symptoms such as rest pain, focal gangrene, or nonhealing ulcerations are all considered for revascularization. The decision to operate should be made between the involved physicians, the patient, and his family. Once this decision is reached, further invasive investigation is warranted. Arteriograms should not serve as a ''baseline study'' but as a ''roadmap'' for the operating surgeon so that the proper procedure will be performed.

Preoperative Care

Patients who are scheduled for femoropopliteal reconstruction should have all associated diseases under control. If any ulcerations are present, they should be cleaned preoperatively with daily local care. Appropriate antibiotics given preoperatively are essential in order to sterilize the lymphatics that drain areas with potentially infected ulcerations. The choice of an antibiotic is based on results of culture and sensitivity testing from the involved area.

The day before surgery, all patients have a bath or a shower with betadine soap. After this, the patient should stand up. The ipsilateral saphenous vein is marked with permanent marker. The position of the posterior tibial and dorsalis pedis arteries is detected with the Doppler flowmeter and marked in order to serve for an intraoperative reference. Prophylactic antibiotics are given 1 hour preoperatively to assure high circulating levels during the surgical procedure. The lower abdomen, the pubis, and the entire lower extremity are shaved and prepped the morning of surgery.

Vascular Grafts

Autogenous Vein Graft. The superiority of the autogenous vein as an arterial substitute is well established. A good vein should have a luminal size of 4 mm or more and no evidence of ectasia or phlebitic changes.

When periadventitial constrictions are present, they should be carefully resected with fine vascular instruments. Twisting of the vein inside the tunnel may occur, and it is usually recognized intraoperatively because of marked decrease or absence of pulsatile flow through the graft. If this occurs, the proximal anastomosis should be done over again after untwisting of the vein. In doubtful cases, arteriography is very helpful. Late complications of a vein graft are myointimal hyperplasia and arteriosclerosis of the graft. Though infections may occur, they are usually well tolerated in the presence of autogenous saphenous vein. The only disadvantage of this graft is that the time required to harvest the vein prolongs the operative procedure.

If the saphenous vein is unavailable or unsatisfactory or if the surgeon desires to shorten the operative time because of a high-risk patient, one of the following grafts may be used. It should also be mentioned that a short segment of vein may be combined with other grafts as a composite or a sequential graft, especially across the knee joint (Fig. 9–4).

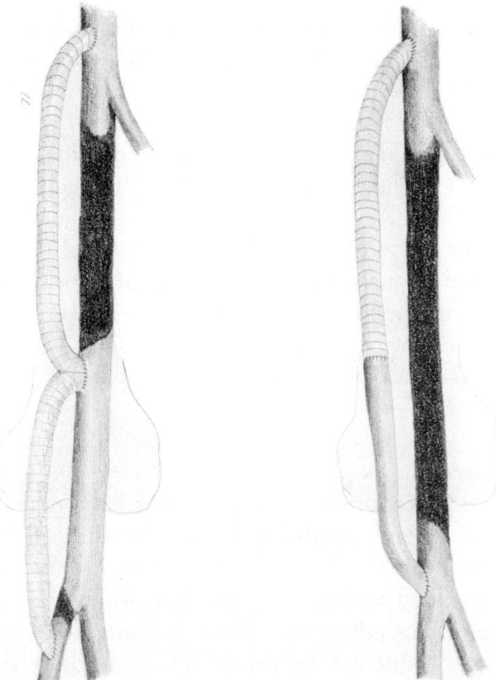

Figure 9-4. Composite and sequential grafts.

Polytetrafluoroethylene (PTFE) Graft. The PTFE graft has been successfully used in both above- and below- knee femoropopliteal reconstructions. It has the advantage of instant availability and needs no preparation before its use. Its behavior across the knee joint is satisfactory, and it may be used when a good vein graft is not available. When placed subcutaneously, it can be easily thrombectomized under local anesthesia. A certain degree of experience is required in handling, tailoring, aligning, and suturing this graft.

The porosity of this graft allows controlled tissue ingrowth with thin neointima formation. The development of intramural neocapillaries increases its resistance to infection. The increased fibrinolytic activator activity prevents neointimal proliferation and reduces the thrombogenicity of the graft. The reinforced PTFE has an outer layer that reinforces the inner tube. This increases the tensile strength and reduces the incidence of aneurysmal dilation.

PTFE grafts have hydrophobic properties, and irrigations of this conduit with saline solution should be avoided. If this is done, an area of tissue induration resembling cellulitis may be noted over the graft. This complication is due to plasma exudation through the graft wall. It is self-limiting and subsides in 7 to 10 days without sequelae.

Dacron Graft. Dacron graft is falling out of favor for reconstructions below the inguinal ligament. It is available in woven and knitted forms; the latter have to be preclotted. It resists infection poorly, and once thrombosed, it cannot be salvaged as easily as the PTFE graft.

A Dacron graft with a coil, a design for use across the knee joint, has been recently introduced. Clinical experience with it is limited.

Umbilical Vein Graft. The glutaraldehyde-tanned umbilical vein homograft has also been successfully used for femoropopliteal reconstructions. It is reinforced with a fine Dacron mesh that prevents aneurysmal dilation. It maintains a good patency rate for infrapopliteal reconstructions and in general is an easy graft to work with. Its disadvantages are its high cost and the need for copious irrigation before it is used.

Surgical Procedures

Most reconstructive procedures for femoropopliteal disease are based on the bypass principle. It is well established that the best graft material is an autogenous saphenous vein that has a diameter of 4 mm or more. The vein has to be harvested and reversed so that the blood flow will not be obstructed by the venous valves. The vein can then be used for a bypass either in its entirety or as part of a composite or sequential bypass. If a vein is not available, a synthetic graft (PTFE, Dacron) or an umbilical vein homograft can be used.

Saphenectomy. Once the femoral artery is exposed, the saphenous vein can be found medially and superficially to the fascia that covers the femoral triangle. All its branches in the groin are doubly ligated and divided. The dissection is advanced distally either with one continuous incision or through multiple segmental skin incisions (Fig. 9–5). This should be done with caution in order to avoid injury to the vein. All distal tributaries are doubly ligated and divided. The ligatures should not be placed too closely to the main vessel, as this may result in segmental construction. The vein is dissected as far distally as the size remains satisfactory and the length is adequate for the planned procedure. Occasionally, the vein may become extremely small in the area around the knee. This finding should terminate further dissection.

If there is difficulty in identifying the vein in its groin position, a long Fogarty catheter may be passed cephalad through a small saphenous venotomy just anteriorly to the medial malleolus (Fig. 9–6). Once the vein is harvested, it is kept in heparinized saline solution with its orientation marked. The graft is irrigated under moderate pressure, and any leaking point is controlled with fine sutures.

Femoropopliteal Bypass. Femoropopliteal bypass is designed to reestablish adequate flow in the leg and foot through the popliteal artery and its branches.

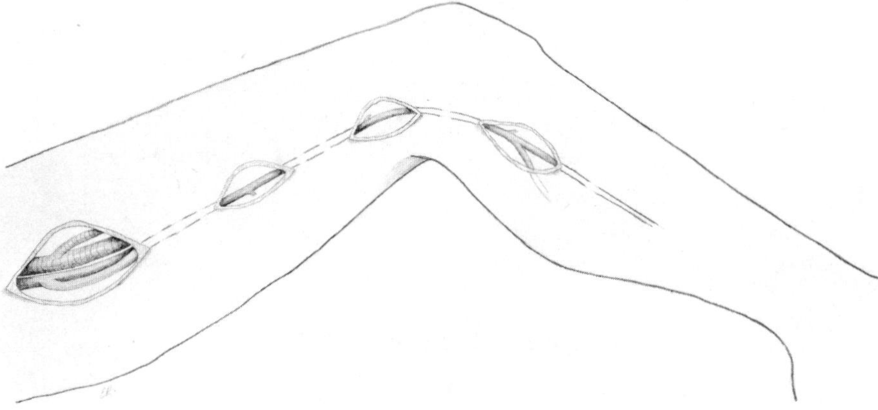

Figure 9–5. Saphenectomy.

Depending on the anatomic distribution of the occlusive disease, the proximal or the distal, the below-the-knee portion of the popliteal artery may be used. Placement of the distal anastomosis above the knee joint seems to prolong the life of the graft. When this procedure is used for limb salvage, the early results show a success rate of over 90 percent. The 5-year patency rate is over 70 percent for reconstructions performed with autogenous vein. When a synthetic graft is used, this patency rate falls significantly.

The reasons for the early failure of a femoropopliteal bypass are: (1) technical errors (twisting of the graft, intimal flaps), (2) unrecognized poor inflow, and (3) poor runoff. Reasons for late failure are: (1) progression of the disease in

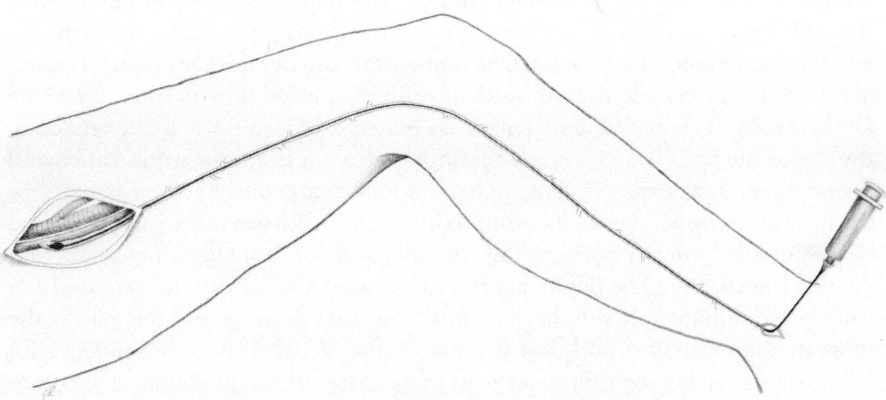

Figure 9–6. Saphenectomy with Fogarty catheter.

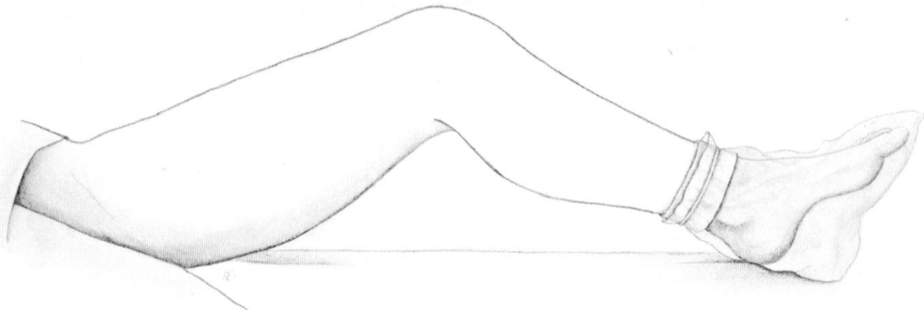

Figure 9–7. Draping of the foot.

the inflow or runoff vessels, (2) intimal hyperplasia, and (3) arteriosclerosis of the vein graft.

Operative Technique.　　The lower abdomen, the pubis, and the entire lower extremity are prepped and exposed in a wide sterile field. Although the foot itself is not prepped, it is covered with a transparent intestinal bag that allows monitoring of skin color changes (Fig. 9–7). The groin incision is made first and is deepened down to the femoral triangle. Lymph nodes that are transected are best removed, and their vascular pedicle is ligated. Similarly, all lymphatics that are injured should be ligated. These two steps are essential in the prevention of the annoying and occasionally disastrous complication of a lymphocele. The common, superficial, and deep femoral arteries are dissected and controlled with vessel loops. The point of the femoral bifurcation is usually recognized by the change of vessel size as the common femoral runs into the superficial femoral artery. The deep femoral artery has a posterolateral orientation, and as the vessel's wall is rather thin, it should be handled with care. With the knee semiflexed and the hip externally rotated, the popliteal artery is approached through a medial vertical incision placed in the groove created by the sartorius and the vastus medialis muscles. The saphenous vein lies farther posteriorly, but occasionally it may get injured by an improperly placed skin incision. Once the fascia is seen, it is incised, and a plane is created just posteriorly to the tendon of the vastus medialis muscle. A self-retaining retractor keeps the wound open and the popliteal fossa exposed. The saphenous nerve can now be seen crossing sub-fascially in the upper part of the wound (Fig. 9–8). Injury to this structure should be avoided in order to prevent the complications of saphenous neuralgia and patellar anesthesia. The popliteal artery is located medially to the vein and can usually be palpated. It should be pointed out that occasionally the vein is the most medial structure and that it may consist of two venae comitantes with tributaries crossing over the artery. In these cases, dissection ought to be more precise, and absolute hemostasis is imperative. The popliteal artery is dissected for a distance of 4 to 5 cm, provided that this portion of the artery is rather soft

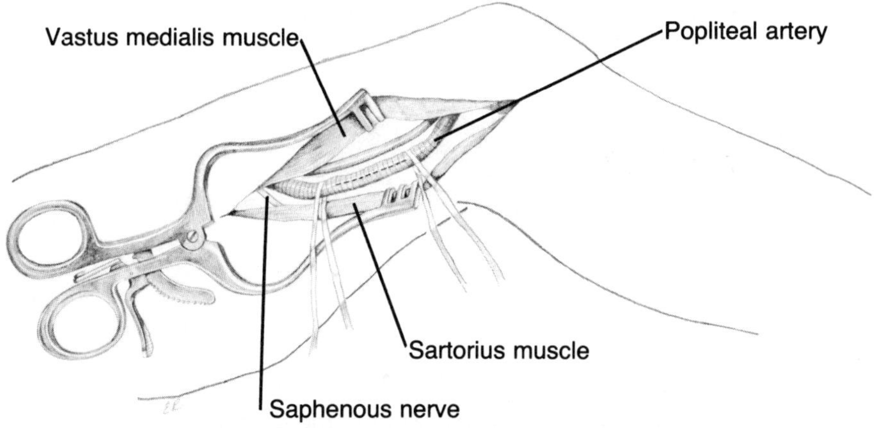

Figure 9–8. Exposure of the popliteal artery.

and suitable for an anastomosis. The genicular branches of the artery should be preserved. If the proximal popliteal artery is unsatisfactory, the medial head of the gastrocnemius muscle may be transected, exposing the more distal portion of the vessel at the level of the knee joint.

The saphenous vein is now harvested and prepared. A subsartorial tunnel is created, and its continuity is secured with a sterile nasogastric tube that is passed through it. The patient is systemically heparinized with 5000 units of heparin. The area of the proposed arteriotomy in the popliteal artery is selected, and proximal and distal control is accomplished with soft vascular clamps. The arteriotomy is made long enough to accommodate the beveled proximal end of the saphenous vein. Backbleeding is verified, and the distal clamp is reapplied. An anastomosis is then performed using a continuous suture of 6–0 prolene. Once the distal anastomosis is completed, the vein graft is passed through the tunnel. The risks of this passage are twisting of the graft and friction injury inside a poorly developed tunnel. These are best avoided by checking the orientation of the graft in its distended condition and by passing the graft through a tunnel sheath, as a bronchoscope or a chest tube container (Fig. 9–9). The proximal anastomosis is performed between the common femoral artery and the vein graft with use of continuous suture of 5–0 prolene. It is important that the takeoff of the deep femoral artery is visualized and calibrated through the femoral arteriotomy (Fig. 9–10). All clamps and loops are removed, and flow is established through the graft. It is essential to verify pulsations in the distal popliteal artery as well as the graft and to observe skin-color changes in the foot.

If the below-knee portion of the popliteal artery is to be exposed, a medial incision is made just posteriorly to the tibia. The fascia of the gastrocnemius muscle is divided close to the bone, and a plane is created between the soleus and gastrocnemius muscles. If necessary, the medial head of the gastrocnemius may

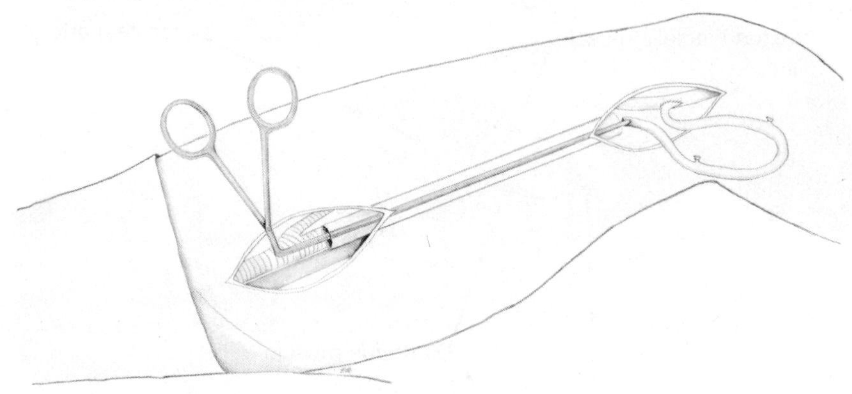

Figure 9-9. The vein graft in the tunnel.

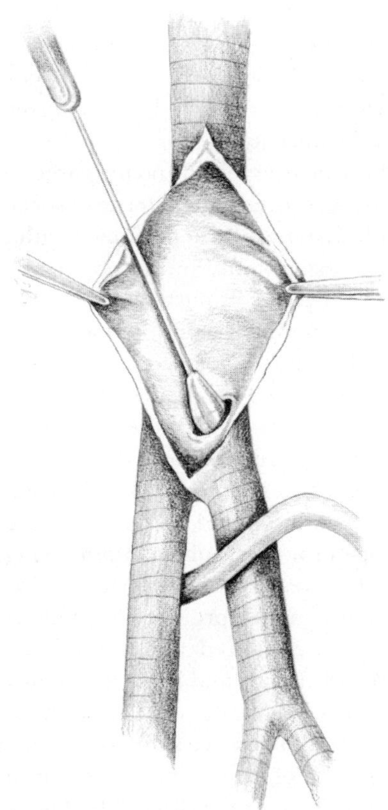

Figure 9-10. Calibration of the takeoff of the deep femoral artery.

be divided to improve the exposure. For a below-knee femoropopliteal bypass, another smaller incision is necessary above the knee in order to facilitate the creation of a tunnel under the sartorius and between the two heads of the gastrocnemius muscles. The proper tailoring of the graft is done with temporary straightening of the knee joint. The anastomoses are performed as previously described. All wounds are irrigated and closed in layers.

Femorotibial Bypass. A femoropopliteal bypass is the ideal procedure provided that the distal popliteal and proximal tibial arteries are open. Whenever this prerequisite is not present, bypasses to the more distal tibial arteries are necessary for revascularization of a critically ischemic extremity. This can be accomplished either with a long femorotibial bypass or a sequential femoropopliteal-tibial bypass. Autogenous vein, PTFE, or umbilical vein grafts can be used. The distal anastomosis may be done anywhere from the trifurcation down to the foot. It is essential that the recipient tibial vessel communicate directly to the pedal or plantar arch.

The durability of a femorotibial bypass, as estimated by the patency and limb salvage rate, is inferior to that of a femoropopliteal bypass but clearly superior to a femoroperoneal reconstruction. The mortality rate of these procedures is in the range of 3 to 5 percent. Operative techniques for an anterior tibial and a posterior tibial reconstruction will be discussed separately.

Femoroanterior Tibial Bypass. The anterior tibial artery is best exposed through a lateral approach. With the hip internally rotated and the knee flexed 30 degrees, a longitudinal incision is made, or an imaginary line bisecting the thumb, when it is pressed against the arch by the tibia and fibula, is created. The fascia is incised at the same line, and the muscles of the anterior compartment are visualized. The curving plane between the tibialis anterior and the extensor longus muscles is then entered, and with digital dissection the muscles are separated, exposing the neurovascular bundle that rests on the interosseous membrane. The anterior tibial artery is dissected for a distance of 3 cm (Fig. 9–11). Caution is necessary to avoid injury to the deep peroneal nerve (anterior tibial nerve) and to the veins that invest the artery. When the femoral vessels are exposed, two medial incisions are made, one above and one below the knee, to facilitate the creation of the tunnel. This is started subsartoriously, advances between the two heads of the gastrocnemius muscle in the popliteal fossa, and then pierces through the interosseous membrane. Division of an adequate strip of the interosseous membrane at the level of the proposed distal anastomosis is essential for an unconstricting tunnel. When a subcutaneous tunnel is preferred, the lateral route is appropriate. Small atraumatic vascular clips (Edward clips) or looped silastic tapes are used for vascular control of the tibial vessels. The distal and then the proximal anastomosis are performed in that order, establishing flow through the graft. In the lateral incision, only the subcutaneous tissue and the skin are closed. All other wounds are closed in layers.

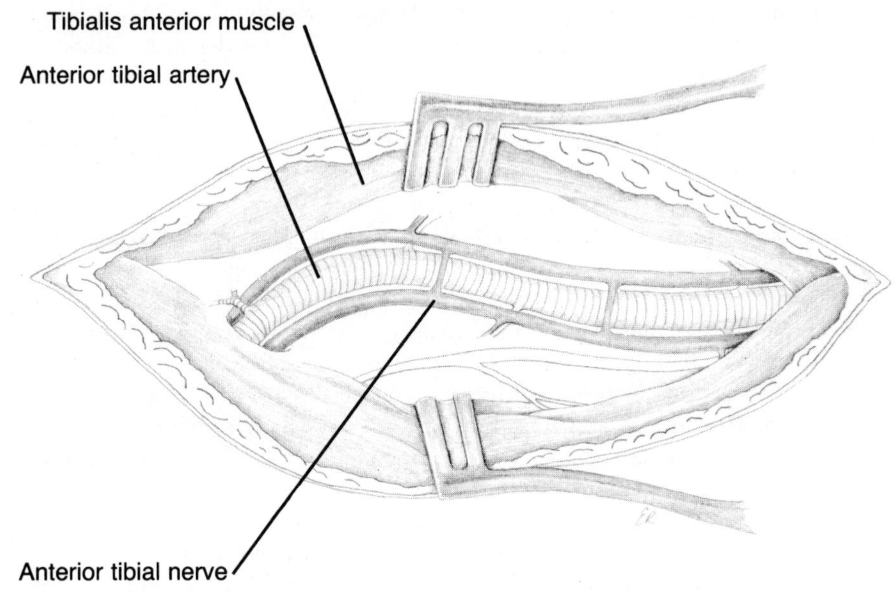

Figure 9–11. Exposure of the anterior tibial artery.

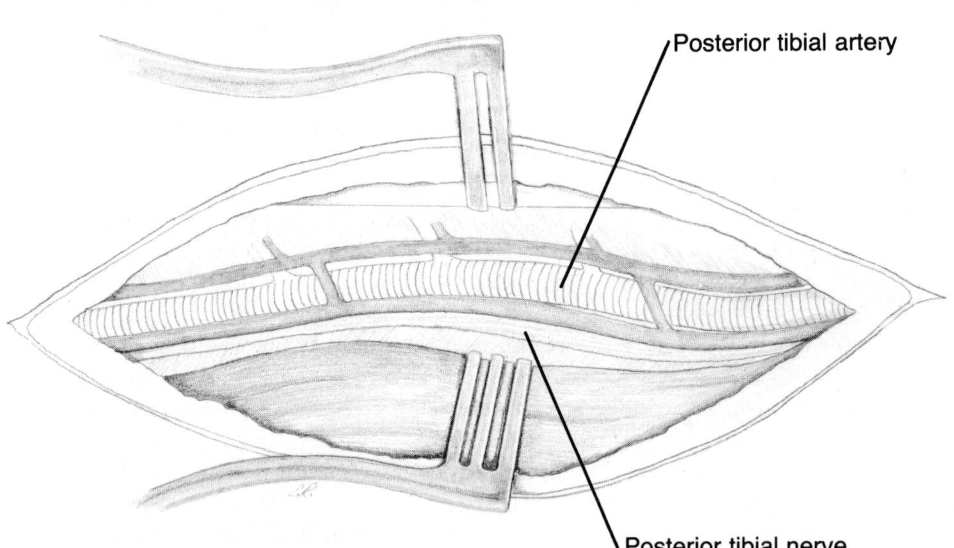

Figure 9–12. Posterior tibial artery—medical exposure.

The distal anterior tibial artery can be approached through a skin incision placed 1 cm lateral to the tibia. A plane is created between the tendon of the tibialis anterior and the extensor muscles. For a femoropedis dorsalis bypass, the distal artery is exposed at the dorsum of the foot, and a lateral subcutaneous tunnel is used.

Femoroposterior Tibial Bypass. The posterior tibial artery is exposed through the medial approach. The skin incision is placed close to the posterior edge of the tibia. The fascia is incised, and the gastrocnemius muscle is reflected posteriorly. The tibial attachments of the soleus muscle are then severed, and the muscle is turned back, exposing the posterior tibial neurovascular bundle that lies on the tibialis posterior muscle (Fig. 9–12). If the very proximal portion of the artery is to be exposed, the medial attachment of the soleus arch is divided and reflected posteriorly. The artery is invested between the veins, and the dissection should be done with caution, ligating all venous tributaries. The tunnel is formed under the sartorius muscle, through the popliteal fossa, and inside the soleus arch. The medial subcutaneous route may also be used. The latter is especially preferred when the distal posterior tibial artery is exposed behind the medial maleolus. After heparinization and proximal and distal control, the distal anastomosis is performed. The heel and the toe of the graft are best secured with interrupted sutures of 6–0 prolene (Fig. 9–13). The anastomosis is then completed with a continuous suture of 6–0 prolene. As with all infrapopliteal reconstructions, magnifying loops are helpful. Once the femoral anastomosis is completed, all clamps are removed, and flow is established through the graft.

Femoroperoneal Bypass. Peroneal arterial reconstruction is indicated only as a limb salvage procedure in patients with rest pain or ischemic lesions in lieu of primary amputation. The peroneal artery should be the only patent or the dominant vessel in a distal arteriogram, and the presence of reconstructible disease of the deep femoral artery should be excluded. Essentials for the success of this operation are: (1) the presence of a pedal or plantar arch communicating with the peroneal artery, (2) a good luminal diameter of the artery, and (3) the

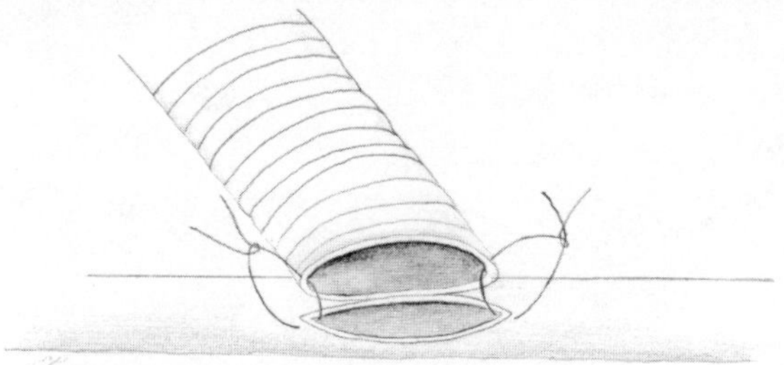

Figure 9–13. The toe and heel sutures.

absence of mural calcifications. It seems that early postoperative occlusion of the graft predisposes to failure, and further attempts to reestablish flow should be abandoned. The 2-year patency rate is in the range of 40 percent, and the incidence of limb salvage is somewhat increased. This is due to the fact that grafts that eventually fail stay open for a long enough time to permit healing of ischemic lesions. In general, the results of peroneal artery reconstructions are inferior to those of other infrapopliteal bypasses.

Operative Technique. The peroneal artery is exposed through a lateral approach with segmental fibulectomy. The medial approach has also been used successfully. After the femoral vessels are exposed and dissected, the hip is internally rotated, and the knee is flexed. A skin incision is made over the middle third of the fibula and is carried down until the bone is encountered. The peroneal muscles are retracted anteriorly and the soleus muscles posteriorly. With the help of a periosteum elevator, all muscular attachments to the fibula are severed, and an 8 to 10-cm segment of the bone is removed. If the upper portion of the peroneal artery is exposed, caution is essential to avoid injury of the peroneal nerve as it crosses over the fibular. The peroneal vessels overlying the flexor hallucis longus muscle are now visualized (Fig. 9–14). The artery is carefully dissected from the accompanying veins for a distance of 3 to 4 cm. A tunnel is created subsartoriously, then through the heads of the gastrocnemius, and finally it crosses over medially to laterally, under the soleus muscle. An alternative lateral subcutaneous route may be used. Once the tunnel is complete, the graft is

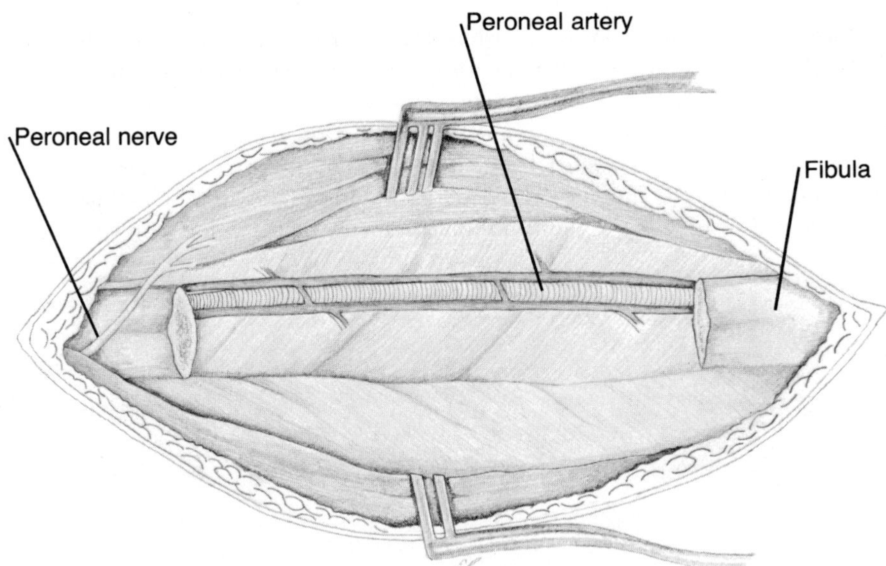

Figure 9–14. Exposure of the peroneal artery.

passed through, and the distal anastomosis is done first. Control of the peroneal artery is best accomplished with small atraumatic vascular clips (Edward clips), and the anastomosis is performed with 6–0 continuous prolene suture. The proximal anastomosis is done next, and flow through the graft is established. Meticulous, atraumatic technique is necessary for the success of distal anastomosis. The use of a closed suction catheter for 24 hours should be considered.

Profundoplasty. The deep femoral artery provides the main collateral pathway of blood flow in limbs with femoropopliteal occlusive disease. This route of compensation is successful in eliminating rest symptoms in a great number of patients. However, when the disease progresses distally or involves the deep femoral artery, the compensation is inadequate and distal ischemia is apparent. Restoration of flow and pressure in the diseased deep femoral artery by means of a profundoplasty will improve distal perfusion and salvage many limbs. This is accomplished by the development of more efficient collateral routes. For this reason, the maximum effect of this procedure is realized a few weeks postoperatively.

Oblique arteriographic views are essential for the demonstration of the takeoff of the profunda femoris artery. Significant stenosis is often seen in diabetic patients with femoropopliteal occlusion. An extended arteriotomy with endarterectomy and possibly angioplasty will effectively increase the flow pressure in the descending branch of the deep femoral artery and subsequently to the lower leg and foot. A profundoplasty may be performed either as a primary procedure for limb salvage or in combination with proximal reconstruction, as discussed in the chapter of aortoiliac disease. When done for limb salvage, the early success rate is over 80 percent, and it represents a reasonable alternative to long bypass procedures.

Operative Technique. A long, longitudinal skin incision is made over the femoral triangle. The common, superficial, and deep femoral arteries are dissected and controlled with silastic vessel loops. The dissection is then advanced alongside the profunda femoris artery until the second or third branch of this vessel is encountered. Two or three veins cross over the artery at a 1- to 6-cm distance from the takeoff of the artery. These veins should be securely ligated and divided so that the entire deep femoral artery will be well exposed. The saphenous nerve is also seen lateral to the artery, and caution is necessary to avoid injuring it during dissection and placement of a self-retaining retractor. All arterial branches should be controlled with vessel loops. If the size of the artery is rather small, a patch angioplasty will be necessary. A piece of saphenous vein is harvested at this stage. If a vein is unavailable, the proximal superficial femoral artery may be removed, thromboendarterectomized, and used as autogenous tissue patch. After the patient is systemically heparinized and the vessels are controlled, a long arteriotomy is performed. An open endarterec-

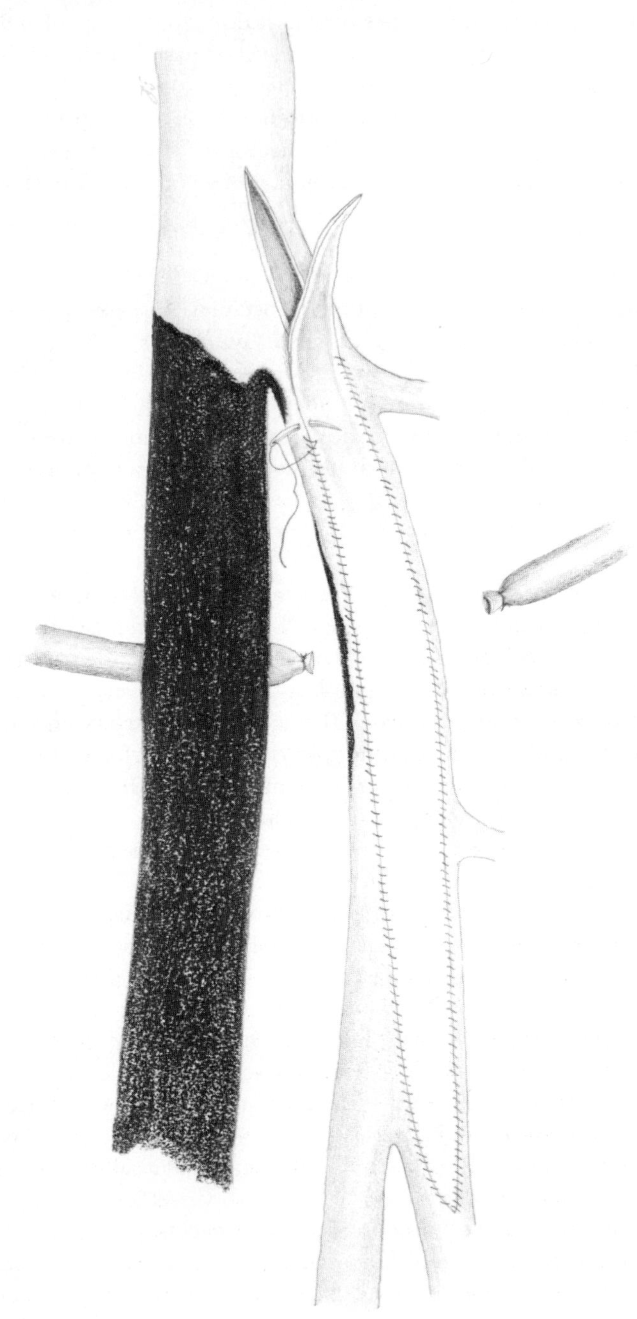

Figure 9-15. Extended profundoplasty.

tomy of the profunda femoris artery is then done. The previously prepared patch is sutured in place with continuous 6–0 prolene sutures (Fig. 9–15). The wound is irrigated and closed in layers.

Endarterectomy. Although not as frequently used nowadays as in the past in favor of bypass procedures, endarterectomy of limited areas of narrowing of common, superficial of deep femeral artery may still be of value in such situations.

In Situ Saphenous Vein Graft. The use of in situ saphenous vein for bypass procedures have been recently reported. The technique involves rendering the venous valves incompetent by a special scissors. The early results of this technique have been comparable to the use of reversed venous grafts. It offers the advantage of maintaining the vein in its bed, minimizing trauma to the vein and using the appropriate sized end for its corresponding arterial size. The long-term results of this method remain to be seen.

In revasculization techniques of the lower extremity, we recommend routine on-table arteriogram at the termination of the procedure. Although it is estimated that only about 5 percent of the cases will visualize technical problems, it is certainly advantageous that this can be corrected immediately.

Transluminal Arterial Dilatation. Segmental stenosis of the superficial femoral artery may be corrected with the use of a transluminal dilatation. This is done either percutaneously or through a small incision. This procedure was initially performed with stiff catheters. The recent introduction of the balloon angioplasty (Gruntzig) catheters has generated new interest in the procedure. Extreme care and experience are necessary for the safe application of this mode of treatment. Dislodgement of an arteriosclerotic plaque, creation of false lumen, and injury to the arterial wall are some of the complications associated with the procedure of transluminal arterial dilatation.

Lesions of the Popliteal Artery

POPLITEAL ANEURYSMS

Introduction

Aneurysms of the popliteal artery are the most common peripheral arterial aneurysms. They are usually bilateral and are often associated with aneurysms elsewhere in the body. Their peak incidence is in the fifth to sixth decade, and they are predominantly seen in males. They are associated with significant morbidity that may lead to limb loss. Prompt diagnosis and treatment are essential.

Diagnosis

Arteriosclerotic popliteal aneurysms are usually asymptomatic and are mostly detected because of a secondary complication. Unlike abdominal aortic aneurysms, they rarely rupture but often thrombose and embolize. Aneurysmal debris causes distal *embolization* that presents either as petechiae of the leg or as areas of focal gangrene in the toes. Acute *thrombosis* of a popliteal aneurysm is an emergency. Acute occlusion results in severe peripheral ischemia, as the collateral vessels are not well developed yet. Rarely symptoms may arise because of pressure on the popliteal vein or tibial nerve.

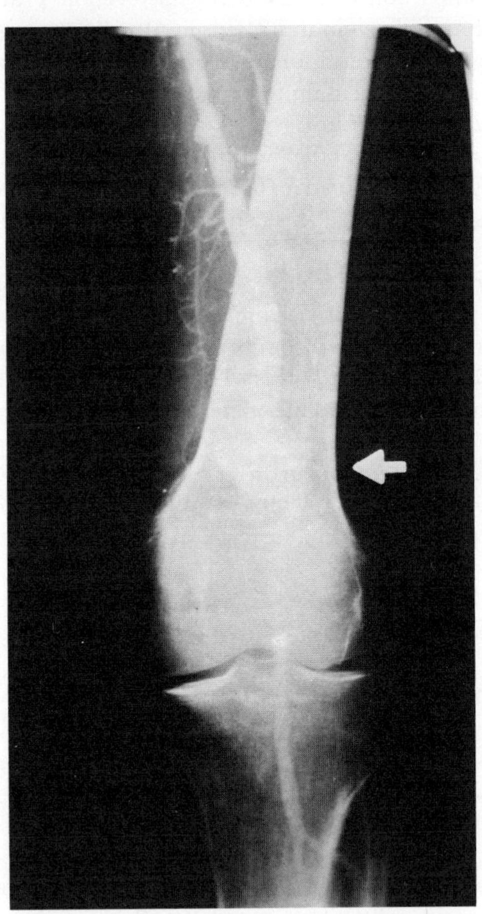

Figure 9–16. Popliteal artery aneurysm.

On physical examination, a pulsatile mass is found in the popliteal fossa unless thrombosis has occurred. In the latter situation, palpation of the controlateral side may reveal an aneurysm, a finding highly suggestive of a thrombosed aneurysm in the acutely symptomatic limb. Complete vascular examination should be performed.

Angiography will delineate a nonthrombosed aneurysm (Fig 9–16), it will reveal other coexisting lesions, and it will visualize the distal vessels. This information is necessary for successful reconstruction if surgery is considered. *Ultrasonography* has also been used recently for the evaluation of peripheral aneurysms. It will easily differentiate prominent pulsations from aneurysms and will detect associated abdominal aortic aneurysms.

Treatment

All complicated aneurysms should be treated. Asymptomatic lesions should also be treated unless the life expectancy is short or severe cardiopulmonary disease coexists. Resection need not be done to cure this lesion. The procedure of choice is *exclusion* of the aneurysm with proximal and distal ligation and *bypass graft* using autogenous saphenous vein. This can be accomplished through a medial approach with two short separate incisions (Fig. 9–17). When suspected thrombosis of a popliteal aneurysm is confirmed by arteriography, full heparinization should be initiated, and the patient should be operated on promptly. A thrombectomy of the distal popliteal may have to be performed, and intraoperative angiography with delayed views is occasionally necessary for the evaluation of the distal circulation. The distal end of the bypass graft may have to be connected to one of the tibial vessels. Due to prolonged ischemia of the leg muscles, a compartment syndrome may develop. For this reason, routine *fasciotomy* is recommended in those patients who suffered acute thrombosis of a popliteal aneurysm. In delayed cases, irreversible tissue necrosis should be managed with an amputation.

CYSTIC ADVENTITIAL DISEASE

Cystic adventitial disease of the popliteal artery is a rare lesion that occurs usually in young males and presents with intermittent claudication. It is due to the development of *subadventitial cysts* that compress the intima and cause stenosis or even complete occlusion of the lumen. These cysts are filled with clear viscous fluid. The etiology is unknown.

Angiography will demonstrate tapering stenosis or complete occlusion of the popliteal artery. These lesions can be treated either with operative cyst evacuation or with a saphenous vein graft bypassing the involved segment of the artery.

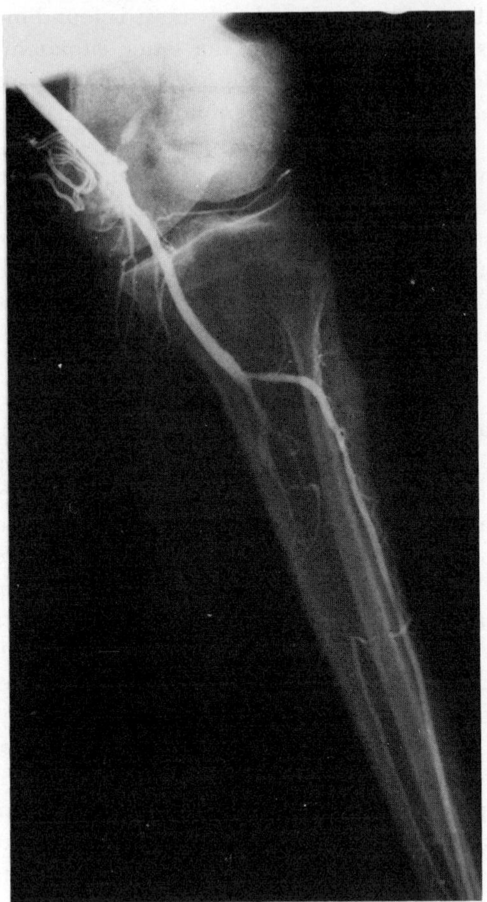

Figure 9-17. Popliteal artery aneurysm.

POPLITEAL ENTRAPMENT SYNDROME

This is a rare syndrome that is seen in young athletic males and is due to displacement of the popliteal artery around the medial head of the *gastrocnemius* muscle (Fig. 9-18). It causes stenosis and eventual occlusion of the popliteal artery. The presenting symptom is claudication. The characteristic sign is that on dorsiflexion of the foot the distal pulses diminish or disappear.

The treatment of this condition involves division of the muscle fibers so that the popliteal artery can return in the popliteal fossa. If the vessel is occluded, a bypass is necessary.

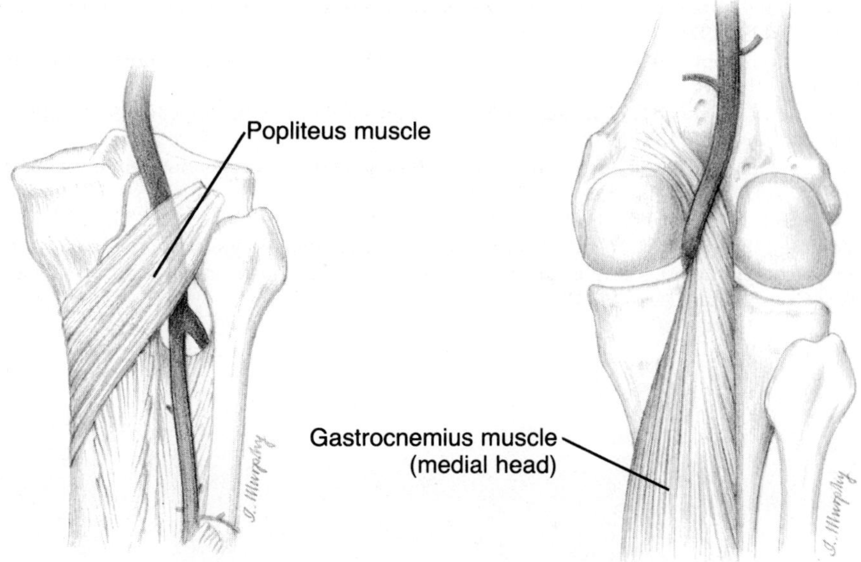

Figure 9–18. Popliteal entrapment syndrome.

BIBLIOGRAPHY

Bernhard VM, Militello JM, Geringer AM: Repair of the profunda femoris artery. *Am J Surg* 127:676, 1974.

Buda JA, et al: The results of treatment of popliteal artery aneurysms: a follow-up study of 86 aneurysms. *J Cardiovasc Surg* 15:615, 1974.

Dale WA, DeWeese JA: Autogenous venous graft for arterial repair. *Surgery* 55:870, 1964.

Dardik H, Ibrahim IM, et al: Routine intraoperative angiography: an essential adjunct in vascular surgery. *Arch Surg* 110:184, 1975.

Dardik H, Ibrahim IM, et al: Glutaraldehyde-stabilized umbilical vein prosthesis for revascularization of the legs. Three year's results by life table analysis. *Am J Surg* 138:234, 1979.

DeWeese JA, Rob CG: Autogenous venous grafts ten years later. *Surgery* 82:755, 1977.

Dotter CT, Rosch J, Judkins MP: Transluminal dilatation of atherosclerotic stenosis, *Surg Gynecol Obstet* 127:794, 1968.

Friedmann P, DeLaurentis DA, Rhee SW: The sequential femoropopliteal bypass graft. *Am J Surg* 131:452, 1976.

Hildreth DH: Cystic adventitial disease of the common femoral artery. *Am J Surg* 130:92, 1975.

Kempczinski RF: Physical characteristics of implanted polytetrafluoroethylene grafts: a preliminary report. *Arch Surg* 114:917, 1979.

Linton RR, Wirthlin LS: Femoropopliteal composite Dacron and autogenous vein bypass grafts. *Arch Surg* 107:184, 1975.

Reichle FA, Tyson RR: Comparison of long-term results of 364 femoropopliteal and femorotibial bypasses for revascularization of severely ischemic lower extremities. *Ann Surg* 182:449, 1975.

Rich NM: Popliteal vascular entrapment (PVE): its increasing interest. *Arch Surg* 114:1377, 1979.

Robert PL, Powers SR, Karmody AM: A reappraisal of in situ saphenous vein arterial bypass. *Surgery* 86:453, 1979.

Szilagyi DE, Elliot JP, Hageman JH, et al: Biologic fate of autogenous vein implants as arterial substitutes. *Ann Surg* 178:232, 1973.

Tyson RR, Reichle FA: Technique for femorotibial bypass. *Surgery* 68:730, 1970.

Veith FJ, Moss CM, et al: Comparison of expanded polytetrafluoroethylene and autologous saphenous vein grafts in high risks arterial reconstructions for limb salvage. *Surg Gynecol Obstet* 147:749, 1978.

CHAPTER TEN

Sympathectomy

Lumbar sympathectomy was first employed in the treatment of muscular rigidity associated with certain neurologic disorders. The observation that the skin of the extremities was rendered warm and hyperemic introduced this procedure in the treatment of vascular diseases. Until the development of modern techniques of direct vascular reconstruction, sympathectomy had been the only procedure in the treatment of *occlusive and vasospastic disorders*. Its value has been strongly challenged for some time by many authors. However, when certain strict indications exist, sympathectomy has proved to be a useful therapeutic alternative in lieu of amputation. Although the role of sympathectomy in the treatment of arterial occlusive disease is rather limited, it seems to be the value in the surgical treatment of certain vasospastic disorders of the upper and lower extremities.

Certain anatomic considerations are essential in the understanding of the effect of a sympathectomy. The efferent sympathetic fibers originate from cells of the *C-8 to L-2 or L-3* segments of the anteromediolateral columns of the spinal cord. They are preganglionic myelinated neural axons that exit via the anterior nerve roots and synapse with cells of the sympathetic ganglia. This innervation is derived from C-8 to T-3 for the upper extremity, and from T-10 to L-2 or L-3 for the lower extremity. The *paravertebral ganglia* supplies postganglionic non-myelinated fibers that reenter the anterior nerve roots and supply the skin with (1) vasomotor, (2) sudomotor, and (3) pilomotor fibers (Fig. 10–1). The prevertebral ganglia give directly postganglionic fibers to the smooth muscle and

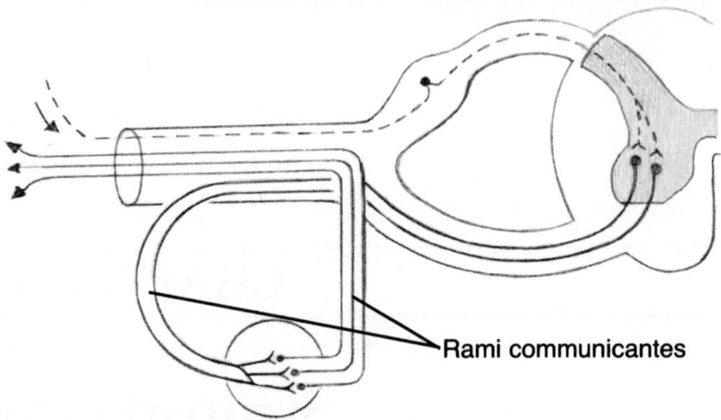

Figure 10-1. Paravertebral sympathetic ganglion.

blood vessels of various viscera. All ganglia are connected to each other by nerve trunks and to the anterior spinal roots with the *rami communicantes*.

Sympathectomy results in (1) denervation of the small vessels of the skin and increased cutaneous blood flow through arteriovenous fistulas, (2) cessation of sweating, and (3) lack of piloerection. These changes, except the last, are manifested by increased warmth and dryness with improved pink color of the skin. It appears to have no significant direct effect on the blood vessels of the muscles. The increased cutaneous blood flow does not necessarily reflect increased total flow but rather a diversion of blood from the muscles to the skin through open arteriovenous fistulas. With these physiologic data, there is little justification in performing a sympathectomy for the treatment of intermittent claudication without skin changes.

The effect of sympathectomy is manifested immediately. Within the following 10 postoperative days, there may be a temporary return of the vascular tone due to adrenergic sensitization of the sympathetic fibers.

Lumbar Sympathectomy

INTRODUCTION

Lumbar sympathectomy has a definite place in the armamentarium of the vascular surgeon. All patients with advanced stages of ischemia, as manifested by impending or frank *gangrene,* skin *ulcerations,* and *rest pain,* should be properly investigated with noninvasive testing and angiography. If no direct surgical revascularization seems visible, these patients should be considered for sympathectomy. Diabetic patients with unreconstructible disease, with or without peripheral neuropathy, should also be considered as surgical candidates. Approximately 50 to 60 percent of patients with rest pain or superficial ischemic ulcerations of the foot respond favorably to this procedure. Gangrenous lesion of the toes may heal or mumify and slough off in approximately 30 percent of patients. However, ischemic ulcerations of the leg and heel, as well as gangrenous lesions of the proximal foot, do not ultimately show a significant benefit derived from lumbar sympathectomy. It is generally agreed that there is no place for performance of sympathectomy for the relief of claudication.

Healing of ischemic lesions and relief of rest pain result in salvage of limbs that would otherwise be amputated. This is accomplished with a low mortality rate in the range of *3 to 6 percent*. But if sympathectomy fails, there is no evidence that this procedure may alter the ultimate level of an amputation, above or below the knee.

Occasionally, a lumbar sympathectomy is performed in conjunction with an arterial reconstruction. This practice is based on the assumption that a vascular bed with decreased resistance will maintain a higher flow through a graft and possibly prolong the life of the graft. Although it is demonstrated that concomitant sympathectomy effectively decreases the vasomotor tone of the foot, there is still no conclusive evidence of improved graft survival.

The current results of lumbar sympathectomy are satisfactory. However, proper selection of the patients that are likely to benefit from this operation is essential. In this selection process, certain tests may help the clinician improve his overall success rate.

PREDICTIVE TESTS

(1) The *vasomotor tone*, (2) the *degree of ischemia*, and (3) the adequacy of *compensation* through the collateral circulation have all been investigated in an attempt to foresee the result of lumbar sympathectomy.

Elimination of the vasomotor activity can be achieved with spinal anesthesia, lumbar paravertebral, epidural, or posterior tibial nerve blocks. The response to these tests is evaluated immediately with skin temperature changes, alteration of the appearance of the skin, and segmental volume plethysmography. Positive vasomotor tests are associated with a 70 percent response to lumbar sympathectomy.

The degree of existing ischemia and the adequacy of the collateral circulation seem to have a significant predictive value. The presence of gangrenous lesions proximal to the forefoot may be a contraindication to sympathectomy. The measurement of the ankle systolic pressure by the Doppler ultrasonic technique has been shown to be a valuable test. With the blood pressure cuff around the ankle, flow is detected at the posterior tibial or dorsalis pedis arteries. The systolic pressure is then compared to the systolic brachial pressure. If the ratio is above *0.35,* these limbs will generally show a good response to sympathectomy. If the index is *0.20* or less, it is very unlikely that an amputation will be avoided. In these hopeless patients, the performance of a sympathectomy must be critically evaluated.

The above tests are not absolute and should be considered in association with the clinical picture, the ambulatory status of the patient, and the personal experience of the surgeon.

OPERATIVE TECHNIQUE

Sympathetic innervation of the entire lower extremity is derived from the first, second, and third lumbar ganglia (Fig. 10–2). Exposure of the paravertebral sympathetic chain allows visualization of L-2, L-3, and L-4 between the diaphragmatic crus and the ipsilateral iliac vessels. Removal of the *L-2 and L-3* ganglia assures complete sympathetic ablation of the lower leg and foot.

The patient is positioned supine on the operating table with the ipsilateral lower chest and flank elevated. An incision is made on a line from the umbilicus to the tip of the eleventh rib. It starts from the *lateral edge of the rectus muscle* and extends laterally for a length of 10 to 12 cm. A muscle-splitting incision is then performed with all muscular layers well undermined. Once the transversalis

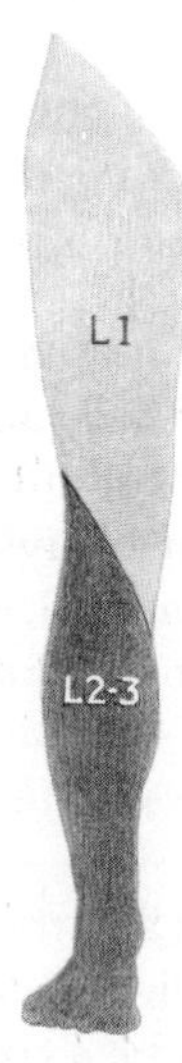

Figure 10–2. Sympathetic innervation to the skin of the lower extremity.

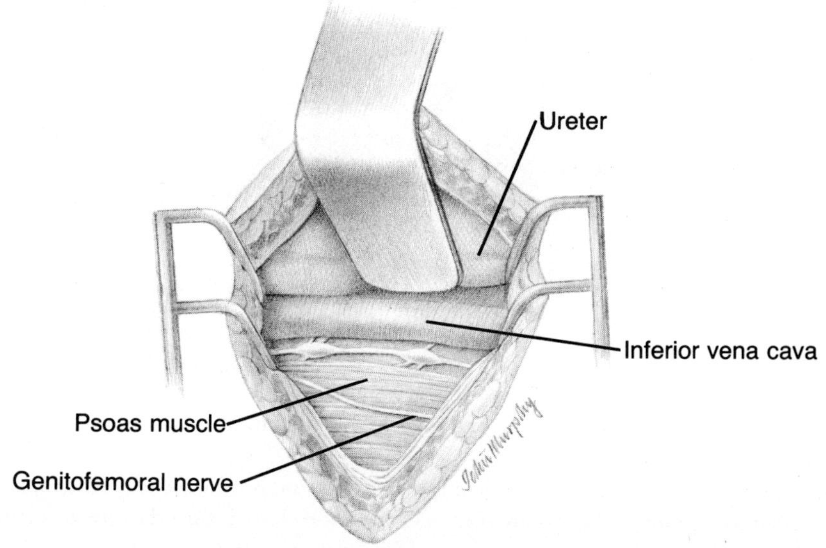

Figure 10–3. Lumbar sympathectomy.

fascia is incised, the peritoneum and its contents are mobilized medially with blunt subfascial dissection. If the peritoneum is injured, it should be repaired before any further dissection. When the retroperitoneal fatty tissue is encountered, the dissection should advance in a plane, between the fat and the peritoneum, that will guide the surgeon's fingers *on the anterior surface of the psoas muscle.* If the wrong plane is followed between the fatty tissue and the lumbar fascia, annoying bleeding will occur, and the surgeon will find himself behind the psoas muscle. The ureter is well visualized and kept behind the retractor. The sympathetic chain is identified by palpation of firm ganglia at their paravertebral location, medial to the psoas muscle and the genitofemoral nerve (Fig. 10–3). It is usually the L-3 ganglion that is palpated first and guides to the full exposure of the sympathetic chain from the crus of the diaphragm to the iliac vessels. On the right side, the inferior vena cava may be medially retracted with the retractor placed firmly against the vertebra and stabilized. This should be done with caution to avoid disturbing bleeding from the lumbar veins.

With the L-2, L-3, and L-4 ganglia exposed, the chain is severed distally (Fig. 10–4). It is then reflected cephalad, and all communicating rami are hemoclipped and divided. Once the mobilization has reached proximal to the L-2 ganglion, the preganglionic fibers are hemoclipped and severed. If the surgeon has any doubt about the tissue obtained, the specimen then must be submitted to pathology for frozen section. *The ganglionic tissue is whitish and rubbery*

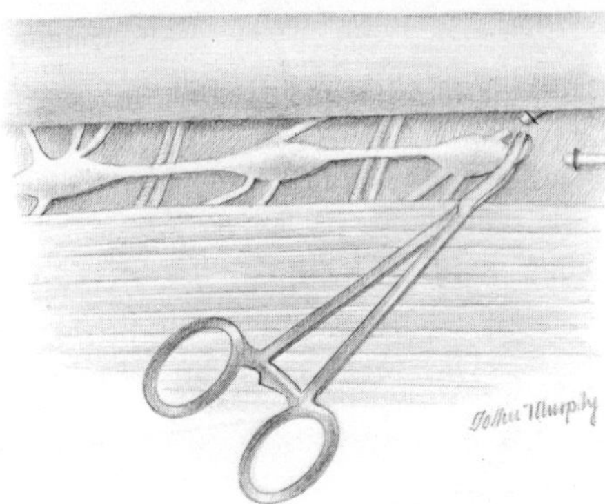

Figure 10–4. Lumbar sympathetic chain.

hard in consistency, and an experienced surgeon should not confuse it with adjacent lymph nodes or any other tissue. On occasion, the chain is found more anteriorly to the psoas muscle and very rarely inside the muscle fibers. Systematic and anatomic visual search in the paravertebral area will invariably demonstrate the sympathetic chain. Hemostasis is confirmed in the retroperitoneal space, and the wound is closed in layers. There is no need for drainage.

COMPLICATIONS

Various complications may be associated with the performance of a lumbar sympathectomy. The overall morbidity rate is in the range of 5 to 10 percent, and the mortality is usually associated with cardiac or respiratory complications.

Venous Injuries

The inferior vena cava, the common iliac vein, and various lumbar branches may be injured during dissection and retraction. All major venous injuries should be repaired with fine vascular sutures after good exposure of the area. This can be accomplished with compression of the vessel above and below the injury. This maneuver makes the field bloodless and allows precise repair.

Peripheral Emboli

This may occur on a left lumbar sympathectomy, and it is caused by undue manipulation of the aorta or iliac arteries that may have ulcerated atheromatous lesions.

Paradoxical Gangrene

This term applies to the development of gangrene following a lumbar sympathectomy. It may be the result of disease progression, blood flow redistribution, peripheral emboli, or interruption of collateral pathways of the abdominal wall with the sympathectomy incision. Whatever the etiology, this complication is seen infrequently and the exact cause is not known.

Retroperitoneal Hematoma

A retroperitoneal hematoma may be quite extensive and is manifested with a drop of the hemoglobin value, tachycardia, hypotension, and discoloration of the flank and the incisional wound. It is easily preventable if complete hemostasis is secured before closure and with preoperative exclusion of patients with coagulopathy.

Neuralgia

Postsympathectomy neuralgia is often nocturnal and mainly involves the thigh. It may appear 1 to 2 weeks postoperatively and usually subsides within 2 to 3 months. *Diphenylhydantion (Dilantin)* or narcotic analgesics are usually effective in the management of this neuralgia.

Ureteral Injuries

Once they occur, they should be immediately repaired with or without a stent. The area should be properly drained.

Sexual Complications

Bilateral removal of L-1 ganglia is associated with *retrograde ejaculation*. Although erection is not a function of the sympathetic systems, impotence could occur in certain patients.

Paralytic Ileus

This is occasionally seen after lumbar sympathectomy. All patients should be kept NPO (given nothing by mouth) until intestinal peristalsis resumes. If ileus occurs, it responds well to nasogastric suction.

Cervical Sympathectomy

INTRODUCTION

Ischemia of the hands and digits may be due to either organic obstruction or functional vasomotor disturbances. Patients with symptomatic acute or chronic proximal arterial occlusion are best treated with thromboembolectomy or bypass surgery.

If the disease is localized distally in the hands and fingers, arteriography is essential in the differential diagnosis of the various *ischemic hand-digit syndromes.* Demonstration of recent small emboli in the distal vessels is treated with anticoagulation. Chronic distal arterial occlusive lesions have been shown to respond well to thoracocervical sympathectomy. Vasospastic disorders without an organic component are treated conservatively with avoidance of exposure to cold, restoration of emotional stability, cessation of smoking, and discontinuation of any offending medications. If the above measures do not have a favorable result, pharmacologic therapy should be attempted. This includes intra-arterial injections of *reserpine* and oral administration of *guanethidine* alone or in combination with phenoxybenzamine. In the few cases of *Raynaud's disease* in which patients either fail to respond to this therapy or develop significant hypotension while on the above agents, a cervical sympathectomy is in order.

Other indications for thoracocervical sympathectomy include posttraumatic causalgia, hyperhidrosis, and frostbite in the early stage. A reliable predictive test performed in an attempt to foresee the postoperative result of a sympathectomy is a block of the stellate ganglion. It is emphasized that failure to respond to a stellate ganglion block does not exclude a cervical sympathectomy. However, a good response is an indication that the surgical result will be favorable.

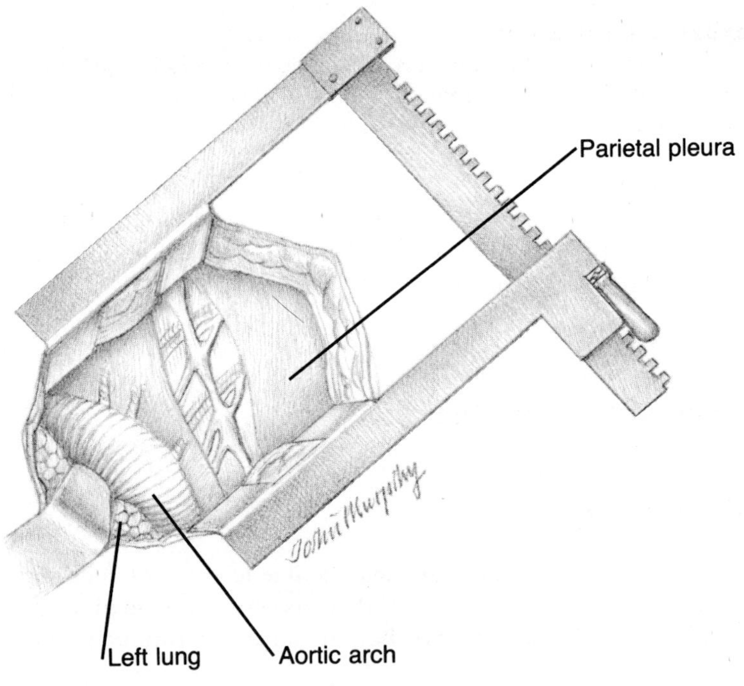

Figure 10–5. Thoracic sympathectomy.

OPERATIVE TECHNIQUE: AXILLARY APPROACH

An effective thoracocervical sympathectomy should include the T-1 to T-3 sympathetic ganglia. The upper half of the stellate ganglion should be preserved in an attempt to prevent the development of a permanent *Horner's* syndrome.

General anesthesia is necessary. The patient is placed on the operating table in the lateral position with the arm hyperabducted, resting on an overhead arm rest. A 3- to 4-inch transverse incision is made in the normal skin lines below the inferior border of the axillary hair stubble and extending from the border of the latissimus dorsi muscle to the edge of the pectoralis major muscle, anteriorly. The incision is deepened down through the subcutaneous tissue to the serattus anterior muscle. Care must be taken to avoid injury to the nerve of the latissimus dorsi, which lies in the posterior limit of the wound. The fibers of the serratus anterior muscle are separated, and the *second intercostal space* is exposed. The intercostal muscle and pleura are incised, and the pleural cavity is entered. A rib-spreading retractor is applied, and the space is gradually enlarged (Fig. 10–5). With optimal light, the apex of the lung is retracted inferiorly, and the sympathetic chain is visualized distinctly in its posteromedial location. The *stellate ganglion* is identified by its dumbbell shape, overlying the lower edge of the first rib (Fig. 10–6). The T-3 ganglion is also identified, and the overlying pleura is incised, exposing the sympathetic chain. The fibers past the T-3 ganglion are severed between hemoclips. The dissection is then advanced cephalad, raising the gânglionic chain from the thoracic wall. All rami are hemoclipped and di-

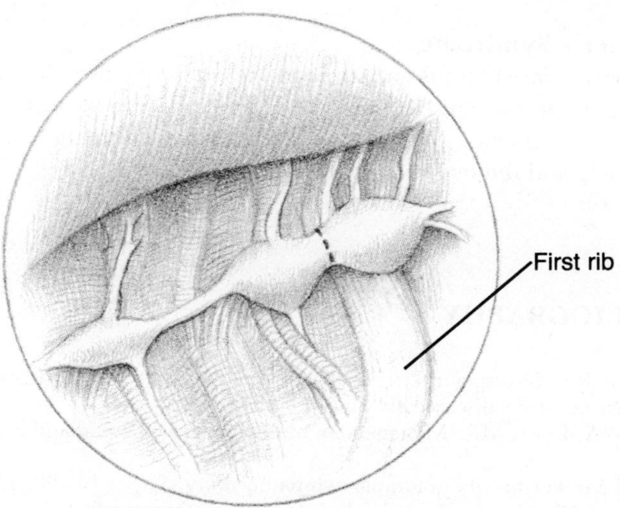

Figure 10–6. Stellate ganglion.

vided. The stellate ganglion is transected so that only the lower half is removed. Hemostasis is secured. The pleura need not be closed. A chest tube is left in the chest cavity for 24 hours. The lung is reexpanded, and the chest is closed in layers.

Transaxillary sympathectomy offers a good cosmetic result with good exposure. Its hazards are possible injury to the thoracodorsal, the long thoracic and the *intercostobrachial* cutaneous nerves. The latter can be injured as it pierces through the second intercostal space, supplying *sensory* fibers to the axilla and the inner portion of the upper arm. The above hazards can be eliminated with a standard *anterolateral thoracotomy* approach.

COMPLICATIONS

Respiratory Problems

Pulmonary problems occur in 5 to 10 percent of patients undergoing trans-axillary or transthoracic sympathectomy. These are mainly due to incomplete expansion of the ipsilateral upper lobe or hemothorax. The latter is due to inadequate hemostasis and usually responds to drainage and transfusions.

Nerve Injuries

Injuries to the thoracodorsal and intercostobrachial nerves are not associated with significant morbidity; however, *injury* of the *long thoracic* nerve is associated with winging of the scapula. Precise knowledge of the anatomy of the area is essential.

Horner's Syndrome

The occurrence of transient *Horner's syndrome* is not infrequent; however, the incidence of permanent Horner's syndrome is low, in the range of 3 to 5 percent. This low incidence is due to insistence on identifying the stellate ganglion routinely and remove only the lower half of it.

BIBLIOGRAPHY

Berardi RS, Siroospour D: Lumbar sympathectomy in the treatment of peripheral vascular occlusive disease. *Am J Surg* 130:309, 1975.
Dale WA, Lewis MR: Management of ischemia of the hand and fingers. *Surgery* 67:62, 1970.
Ewing M: The history of lumbar sympathectomy. *Surgery* 70:790, 1971.
Golding MR, Matinez A, et al: The role of sympathectomy in frostbite with a review of 68 cases. *Surgery* 57:774, 1965.

Jochimsen PR, Hartfall WG: Per axillary upper extremity sympathectomy: technique reviewed and clinical experience. *Surgery* 71:686, 1972.

Kim GE, Ibrahim IM, Imparato AM: Lumbar sympathectomy in the end stage arterial occlusive disease. *Ann Surg* 183:157, 1976.

Moore WS, Hall AD: Effects of lumbar sympathectomy on skin capillary blood flow in arterial occlusive disease. *J Surg Res* 14:151, 1973.

Patman RD, Thompson JE, Persson AV: Management of posttraumatic pain syndromes: report of 113 cases. *Ann Surg* 177:780, 1973.

Sanik GD, Ford J, Hayes AC, et al: Pedal vasomotor tone following aortofemoral reconstructions: a randomized study of concomitant lumbar sympathectomy. *Ann Surg* 183:136, 1976.

Szilagyi ED, Smith RF, Scerpilla JR, et al: Lumbar sympathectomy: current role in the treatment of arteriosclerotic occlusive disease. *Arch Surg* 95:753, 1967.

Yao JST, Bergan JJ: Predictability of vascular reactivity relative to sympathetic ablation. *Arch Surg* 107:676, 1973.

CHAPTER ELEVEN

Amputations

INTRODUCTION

When ischemic lesions fail to heal or the extremity remains in a stage of rest pain in spite of attempted reconstructive arterial surgery and/or sympathectomy, the only existing therapeutic solution is an amputation. This seems to delineate the current role of a major amputation in the treatment of arterial occlusive disease. However, the indications were much broader some decades ago. As many suffering limbs are now salvaged, the need for a primary amputation has markedly decreased, but there are definite situations in which the presence of extensive, frank gangrene with advancing sepsis precludes any revascularization procedures and requires a major primary amputation.

Another interesting change in the last two decades is the trend to *lower* the level of amputation, preferably below the knee, and in so doing, to facilitate the rehabilitation of many amputees. The great majority of unilateral below-knee amputees are walking with a leg prosthesis; even some bilateral amputees have been successfully rehabilitated. However, the knee joint cannot always be preserved. An above-knee amputation has an inferior rehabilitation potential but assures primary healing. Recent modifications in the surgical technique and improved preoperative and postoperative care have significantly decreased both the morbidity and the mortality of a below-knee amputation. This means that more amputees survive and have a well-healed below-the-knee stump on which they can walk.

Primary toe, ray, or transmetatarsal amputations may be indicated in patients, often diabetic, with focal distal gangrene or infection. Restorative vascular procedures, when properly applied, may also improve the healing of distal amputations performed for the removal of demarcated necrotic tissue.

The goals of an amputation should be (1) preservation of the patient's life and (2) restoration of *function* of the extremity with minimal anatomic loss. Amputation should be viewed as a reconstructive procedure, with rehabilitation and ultimate restoration of function in mind.

DISTAL AMPUTATIONS

Distal amputations for the removal of gangrenous or infected tissue of the toes or the forefoot are usually performed on diabetic patients with small vessel disease who frequently have *palpable pulses* in the foot. If infection is present, it should be treated with antibiotics according to the results of culture and sensitivity testing. *Osteomyelitis* should be detected clinically by insertion of a metal probe to the depth of the sinus or the ulcer. Radiographic demonstration of osteomyelitis is confirmatory, but a negative radiograph does not rule out bone involvement. Joint infections may also be recognized when clear synovial fluid drains from the ulcer or the sinus. Bone or joint infection requires amputation of at least the involved digit.

Elective distal amputations have an excellent healing rate of over 90 percent. When a digital amputation fails to heal, a transmetatarsal or a below-knee amputation should follow promptly, before a spreading space infection occurs.

Toe Amputation

Toe amputation can be performed either by direct surgical intervention or by allowance of a dry gangrenous segment of a toe to autoamputate. *Autoamputation* requires a long period of epithelization and meticulous care of the ischemic foot by the patient. The presence of infection makes surgical removal of the toe mandatory. Before attempting a digital amputation, one should be reasonably certain that there is good circulation of the skin proximal to the demarcation line. A toe amputation is contraindicated when the gangrene extends toward the metatarsal crease and when there is dependent rubor and/or rest pain of the foot.

The procedure is done under light general anesthesia. A circular skin incision is made proximal to the necrotic tissue and is carried down to the bone (Fig. 11–1). The bone is divided and rongeured proximally to the skin incision but distal to the joint space. This will allow transverse closure of the wound without tension. Simple sutures of monofilament material are used for the skin closure. Primary healing usually occurs within 2 weeks. When the *big toe* is amputated, it

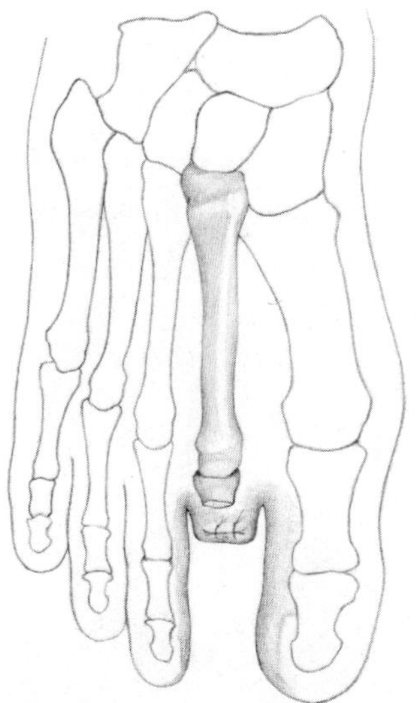

Figure 11-1. Toe amputation.

is extemely important to perform the amputation transdigitally, preserving the head of the first metatarsal bone and, in so doing, maintaining the balance of the foot. The functional disability of a digital amputation is minimal.

Occasionally, a toe amputation has to be done as an emergency procedure in an attempt to control sepsis. In such a case, the wound is left open for drainage. A definite procedure is usually needed in the future.

Ray Amputation

A transmetatarsal digital amputation is indicated when the gangrenous process extends to the base of a minor toe or when infection extends into the proximal forefoot. This amputation requires good blood supply and is especially useful in diabetic patients with *digital osteomyelitis* and intact distal pulses. It may also be performed in association with a successful proximal reconstruction.

The technique combines a circular incision at the base of the involved toe with a dorsal linear extension down to the level of the metatarsal bone (Fig. 11-2). The bone is divided and rongeured. The wound is left open for secondary healing. The functional results from a ray amputation of a minor toe are excellent.

Transmetatarsal Amputation

Transmetatarsal amputation is indicated if three or more toes are gangrenous or if the entire big toe is involved in the gangrenous process. Adequate skin blood flow and good plantar skin are essential for successful healing. The presence of

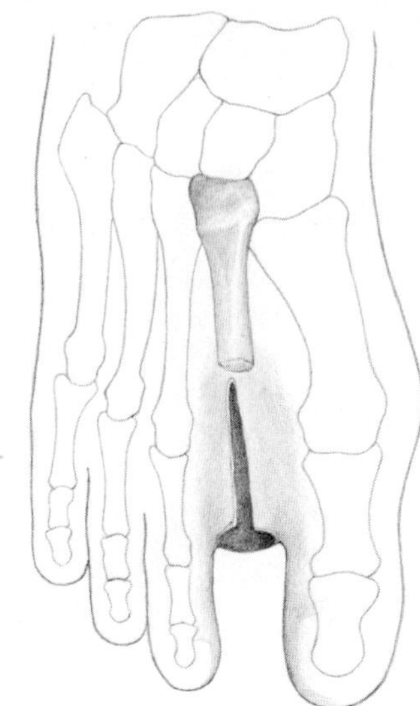

Figure 11–2. Ray amputation.

(1) infection extending into the metatarsal spaces, (2) rest pain, (3) skin rubor, and (4) plantar skin neuropathy are definite contraindications for a transmetatarsal amputation. Ideal candidates are diabetic patients with intact pedal pulses.

The procedure is performed through a skin incision that creates a plantar skin flap and no dorsal flap (Fig. 11–3). The incision is carried down to the metatarsal bones that are severed, somewhat cephalad to the dorsal part of the skin incision. All tendons, excess fat, and necrotic tissue are removed from the plantar flap. This flap is then brought up over the amputated stump and is sutured to the dorsal skin. A well-padded dressing and a posterior splint are used to protect the amputated foot, which stays immobilized for 2 weeks.

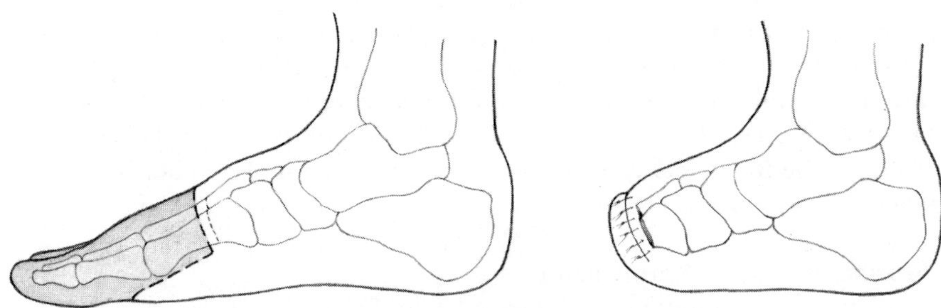

Figure 11–3. Transmetatarsal amputation.

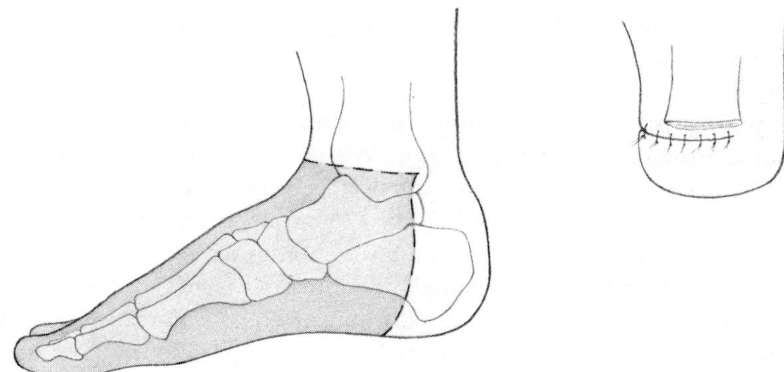

Figure 11–4. Syme's amputation.

No special prosthesis is needed. However, a stainless steel *plantar shank* may be inserted into the sole of the shoe to restore spring to the gait. Also, a styrofoam or balsa wood block inserted into the toe of the shoe prevents collapse of the leather against the amputation stump. The functional result is excellent, and only minimal gait training is required.

Syme's Amputation

Syme's amputation is of limited value to the patient with peripheral vascular disease. Failed transmetatarsal amputations are best handled with a below-knee amputation. A Syme's amputation involves disarticulation of the tibial-talar joint, removal of the calcaneous, flattening of the tibial articular surface by removal of both maleoli, and coverage of the stump with a heel flap (Fig. 11–4). The contraindications to this procedure are (1) heel-skin neuropathy, (2) lesions of the heel, and (3) rest pain with rubor. Stump problems are frequent. Unlike a below-knee amputation, a Syme's amputation creates an *end-weight* bearing stump.

PROXIMAL AMPUTATIONS

Below-Knee Amputation

Indications. A below-knee amputation is the most frequently performed amputation for ischemic disease of the lower extremity. It is indicated for gangrene and infection of the foot as well as for rest pain in patients who either are not candidates for vascular surgery or have had failed arterial reconstruction. It should *not* be performed in the case of a *knee contracture* of 20 degrees or more and in the case of a *hemiparetic* limb because a below-knee amputation is usually followed by spastic flexion contracture. The presence of ulceration or infection at the level of the proposed skin incision is certainly a contraindication for a below-knee amputation.

A prerequisite for successful healing of a below-knee amputation is adequate flow through the *deep femoral artery*. With arteriographic evidence of good flow in the deep femoral artery, one can perform a below-knee amputation and anticipate an excellent result. When an angiogram is not available, it is the noninvasive studies that may aid in the selection of the ideal candidates for a below-knee amputation. Systolic thigh pressure of *50 mm Hg* or less and absent Doppler flow signals in the posterior tibial or pedis dorsalis arteries are associated with a high failure rate for below-knee amputations.

Operative Technique. In an elective situation, a below-knee amputation should be performed with the technique of a *long posterior flap*. When this technique is compared to the old circular fish-mouth incision, it seems to have a higher primary healing rate. Anterior placement of the scar reduces the incidence of chronically painful scars and facilitates the application of a prosthesis.

The optimal length of the stump is 10 to 15 cm so that the tendons of the extensors and the flexors muscles of the knee joint are left intact. The anterior skin incision is begun 10 cm distal to the tibial tuberosity and is advanced both laterally and medially to the mid-posterior-anterior line. The incision is then curved inferiorly and posteriorly to create a curved posterior flap (Fig. 11–5). The calf muscles are divided at the level of the anterior skin incision (Fig. 11–6). All neurovascular bundles are isolated, and their structures are individually ligated and divided. The tibia is divided at a level just proximal to the anterior skin incision. The anterior portion of the severed bone is tapered to avoid pressure necrosis of the overlying skin. The fibula is divided 1 cm higher than the tibia. The posterior flap, which includes fascia, subcutaneous tissue, and skin, is brought over and sutured anteriorly in two layers. The ischemic skin should not be handled with forceps during the closure, and the skin sutures should only approximate the edges without further compromising the already marginal blood flow. If no immediate prosthesis is applied, the wound is dressed with bulky dressings and wrapped with an Ace bandage. A light posterior splint may be used in elderly patients in order to prevent knee contraction.

Rehabilitation. Advances in prosthetic technology have made possible the ambulation of below-knee amputees. The artificial leg is a *patellar tendon weight-bearing* prosthesis. This is lightweight and easily managed by the elderly patient.

In performing a below-knee amputation, the surgeon has the option of immediate or delayed postoperative prosthesis. For an *immediate prosthesis,* a plaster of Paris cast is applied to the stump in the operating room. If a suction drain is used, it may be brought out through a window in the cast. A pylon device and the

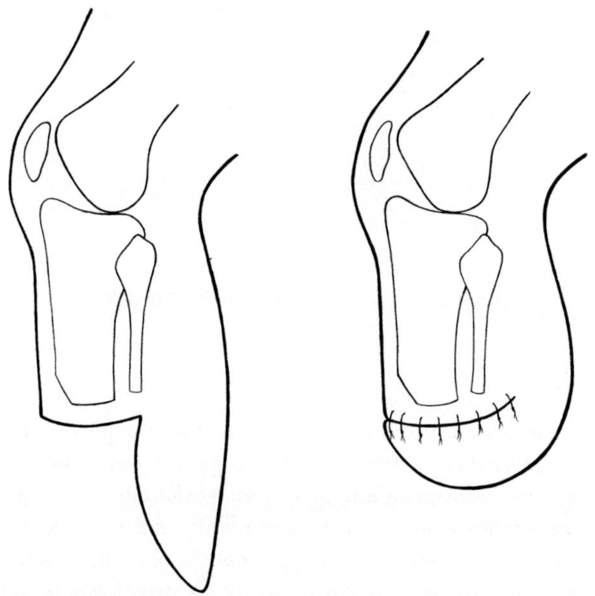

Figure 11-5. Below-the-knee amputation.

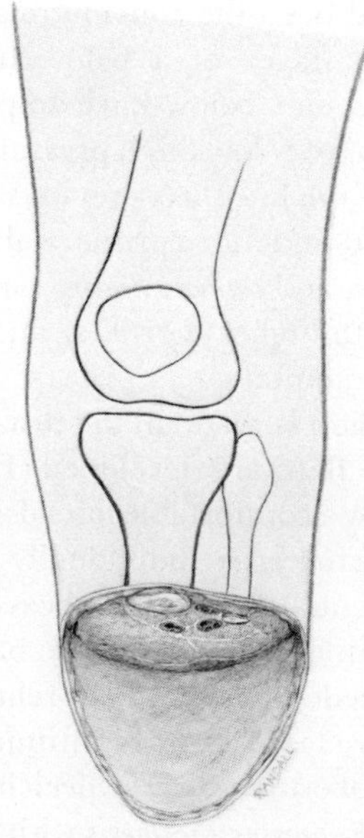

Figure 11-6. Below-the-knee amputation.

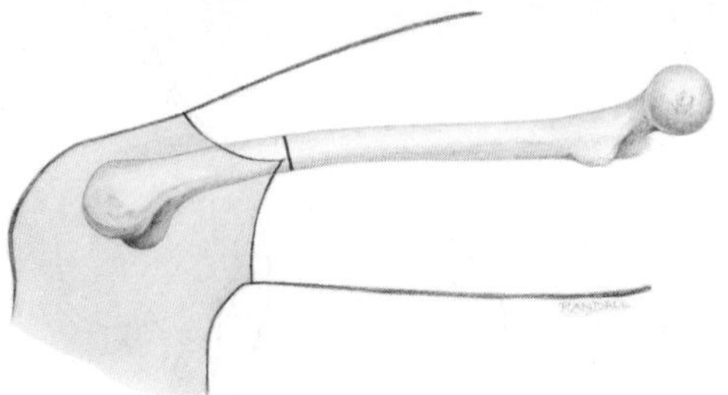

Figure 11–7. Above-the-knee amputation.

prosthetic foot are incorporated into the cast so that the patient can walk in the first few postoperative days. This offers a strong *psychological advantage* for the patient and allows *early ambulation* and *accelerated rehabilitation*. It is postulated that the rigid cast diminishes wound edema and results in improved wound healing. However, many surgeons distrust the application of a rigid cast and favor the conventional amputation with a soft dressing. A prosthesis is then fitted on a well-healed stump.

Above-Knee Amputation

Above-knee amputation had been the conventional lower-extremity amputation before the many advantages of a below-knee amputation were well recognized. It is indicated when a below-knee amputation has failed or is predicted to fail either because of very low thigh pressure of 50 mm Hg or less or extensive tissue damage below the knee. As previously indicated, hemiparetic or contracted extremities should undergo a primary above-knee amputation. This procedure is easy technically, and *primary healing is usual.* However, above-knee amputation is associated with higher mortality and morbidity rates and has a much lower rehabilitation potential.

A fish-mouth skin incision is made in the distal thigh. Short anterior and posterior musculocutaneous flaps are developed (Fig. 11–7). The femur is divided at a higher level to allow a comfortable fascial and skin closure without tension. All neurovascular structures are individually ligated and divided. Gentle handling of the tissues is essential to avoid unnecessary trauma. A well-padded dressing is applied and is reinforced with an Ace bandage.

Extended training is needed for successful rehabilitation of an above-knee amputee. Elderly patients are less eager to continue a prolonged rehabilitation program and prefer the use of crutches or a wheelchair. The artificial extremity that is used is an *ischial weight-bearing prosthesis* with a mechanical knee joint.

BIBLIOGRAPHY

Burgess EM, Romano RL, Zettl JH, et al: Amputation of the leg for peripheral vascular insufficiency. *J Bone Joint Surg (Am)* 53:874, 1971.

Dean RH, Yao JST, Thompson RG, et al: Predictive value of ultrasonically derived arterial pressure in determination of amputation level. *Am Surg* 41:731, 1975.

Eidemiller LR, Awe WC, Peterson CG: Amputation of the ischemic extremity. *Am Surg* 34:491, 1968.

Hunter G, Holliday B: Major amputation following vascular reconstructive procedures (including sympathectomy). *Can J Surg* 21:456, 1978.

Jamienson CW, Hill D: Amputation for vascular disease. *Br J Surg* 63:683, 1976.

Kihn RB, Warren R, Beebe GW: The "geriatric" amputee, *Ann Surg* 176:305, 1972.

Lawson RS: Amputations through the ages. *Aust NZJ. Surg* 42:221, 1973.

Lipp MR, Malone SJ: Group rehabilitation of vascular surgery patients. *Arch Phys Med Rehabil* 57:180, 1976.

Robinson K: Long-posterior-flap myoplastic below-knee amputation in ischemic disease, review of experience in 1967–71, *Lancet* (1) 193, 1972.

Roon AJ, Moore WS, Goldstone J: Below-knee amputation: a modern approach, *Am J Surg* 134:153, 1977.

Sizer, JS, Wheelock FC Jr: Digital amputations in diabetic patients. *Surgery* 72:980, 1972.

Warren R, Kihn RB: A survey of lower extremity amputations for ischemia, *Surgery* 63:107, 1968.

Young AE: Transmetatarsal amputation in the management of peripheral ischemia, *Am J Surg* 133:331, 1977.

CHAPTER TWELVE

Cerebrovascular Disease

Carotid and Vertebro-Basilar Insufficiency

INTRODUCTION

It is now well appreciated that stroke may be caused by both intracranial and extracranial vascular disease. The feasibility of surgical correction of atheromatous lesions of the extracranial vessels has created a new interest in this field. Amaurosis fugax, transient ischemic attack, and symptoms of basilar insufficiency serve as warning signals before the catastrophic event of a completed stroke. The presence of the above symptoms dictates the need for further investigation. Heart disease with possible distal embolization or temporary cerebral perfusion deficits should be ruled out. If there is no cardiac disease that can explain the patient's symptomatology, the possibility of a surgically correctable lesion of the extracranial vessels must be considered.

DIAGNOSIS

Symptoms

Symptoms of cerebrovascular insufficiency of extracranial origin can be attributed either to (1) lesions of the anterior circulation, the common and internal carotid arteries, or to (2) lesions of the posterior circulation, the subclavian, vertebral, and basilar arteries.

Amaurosis fugax is a temporary unilateral loss of vision that occurs rather abruptly, as if a curtain is drawn in front of the visual field of one eye. This event usually clears up within minutes, and it is thought to represent an embolic phenomenon of the ophthalmic artery.

Transient ischemic attack (TIA) represents an event of temporary ischemia of a cerebral hemisphere and may present as a focal motor or sensory deficit. *Aphasia* may be part of the clinical presentation. It is generally accepted that TIA should be followed by complete recovery within 24 hours from its onset. If the recovery is incomplete, the term transient ischemic attack-incomplete recovery (TIA-IR) is used. This should not be mistaken for a completed stroke. The latter will demonstrate the presence of an ischemic infarct on computerized tomography of the brain. The mechanism of a TIA has been attributed to: (1) distal embolization from an ulcerated plaque and (2) critical reduction of cerebral blood flow due to a stenotic lesion of the common or internal carotid artery.

Dizziness, vertigo, *dysphagia,* incoordination, headache, and bilateral visual blurring may represent symptoms of vertebrobasilar insufficiency. The clinical picture of a posterior circulation deficit is somewhat less specific. For this reason, the patient should be questioned about the duration, severity, and possible association of these symptoms with other activities. Even minor exercise of the upper extremity may precipitate these symptoms as they occur in subclavian or innominate steal syndromes.

The medical history of the patient is also very important. *Atrial fibrillation, aortic valvular disease,* and *previous myocardial infarction* may cause the same symptoms in the absence of extracranial vascular disease. Previous injury to the neck and fibromuscular dysplasia may cause a nonatheromatous problem.

Physical Examination

Cardiac evaluation is of importance. Atrial fibrillation and murmurs indicating valvular disease should be excluded. The pulses of the subclavian, carotid, superficial temporal, and facial arteries should be felt bilaterally. Any detected deficit should be recorded. Auscultation of both carotid and subclavian arteries may elicit bruits, indicating the presence of a stenotic lesion. The blood pressure should be taken on both arms and recorded individually. Pressure differences may suggest the presence of occlusive disease in the innominate or subclavian arteries.

Complete vascular examination of the abdomen and lower extremities is important. Existing neurological deficits should also be detected.

Noninvasive Studies

An electrocardiogram may show undetected arrhythmias. Twenty-four-hour cardiac monitoring is occasionally indicated. It is imperative to exclude the heart as the source of emboli or temporary deficits of cerebral perfusion.

Investigation of extracranial carotid disease cannot be complete without the use of the vascular laboratory. Carotid phonangiography (CPA), Doppler ultra-

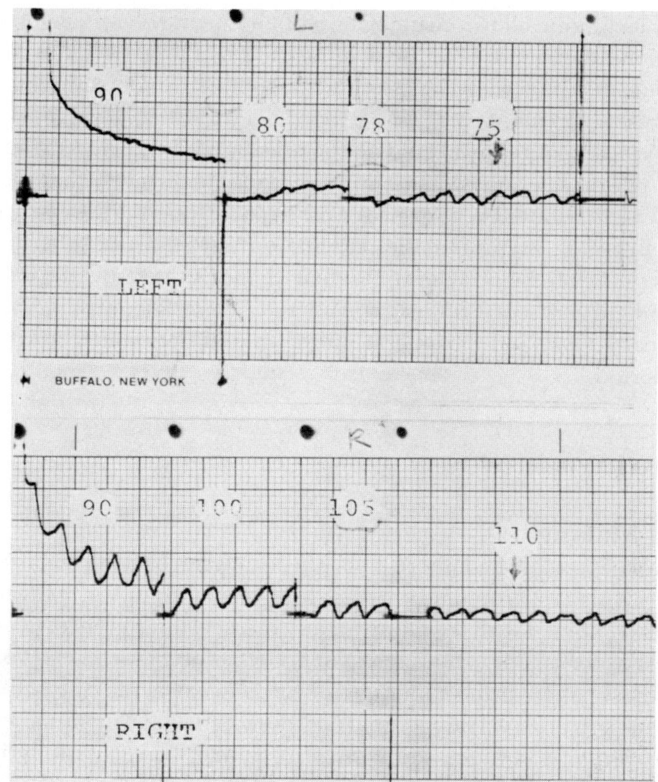

Figure 12-1. Oculoplethysmography (OPG).

sonography, and ocular plethysmography (OPG; Fig. 12-1), when all combined, yield valuable data and, in most instances, accurately demonstrate the presence of occlusive disease in the anterior circulation as well as the degree of the existing compensation. However, a negative study should not be considered as exclusive of disease, and if the clinical picture warrants, further invasive investigation may be needed. It is well appreciated that small, hemodynamically insignificant but ulcerated plaques may cause symptoms of distal embolization. Contrast angiography would detect such lesions.

Computerized tomography of the brain is advised prior to a cerebral angiogram. This may demonstrate (1) space-occupying lesions and (2) an ischemic infarct.

Angiography

Carotid angiography may be done either by "direct stick" or the common carotid artery or by the retrograde, transfemoral, or transaxillary approach.

The latter technique allows visualization of all four extracranial vessels. Selective injections offer a more precise demonstration of stenotic lesions. Visualization of the intracranial vessels is essential for complete understanding of the pattern of cerebral circulation.

Cerebral angiography should not be used as a routine investigative tool. It should be performed only when there is reasonable certainty that the patient's symptoms are attributed to a surgically correctable lesion of the extracranial circulation. Bruits in asymptomatic patients do not justify angiography unless there is significant hemodynamic deficit demonstrated by the noninvasive studies and surgical correction is considered. Postangiography, the patient's neurological status, and peripheral pulses should be monitored closely for a 24-hour period.

TREATMENT

Decision Making

Once a stroke is established, there is very little that can be done medically to alter the course of this catastrophic event. The high mortality and disabling morbidity of a stroke, combined with the failure of any medical interference, have diverted the interest in treatment to an interest in *prevention* of this disease. It is well realized that most patients who suffer a stroke due to extracranial vascular disease have had enough prior warning signals. If these signals alarm the patient and the primary care physician, preventive measures may be successfully instituted. The majority of strokes that occur in a symptomatic patient seem to follow the appearance of symptoms by *only a few months*. Therefore, it is recommended that prophylaxis be properly timed.

Surgical consideration should be given to the following groups of patients:

1. *Symptomatic* patients with recent onset of TIAs and/or amaurosis fugax should be promptly evaluated. Any surgically correctable lesion should be treated without unnecessary delay. In this group of patients, the risk of the disease is clearly higher that the risk of treatment, which involves a 1 percent mortality rate and a 2 to 5 percent incidence of postoperative neurologic deficits.

2. Patients with *asymptomatic* bruits or *asymptomatic* ulcerating carotid lesions present a unique challenge to the treating physicians. Various reports have been published, but the controversy still exists. It seems that the safest and most justifiable approach to this problem is the one that takes into account the hemodynamic significance of the lesion, the general status of the patient, and the life expectancy of the patient. *Compensated lesions* that do not elicit a hemodynamic deficit and should not be treated unless they become symptomatic. If the lesion is hemodynami-

cally significant, surgical correction may be advised after individual consideration.

3. For patients who have suffered a recent *completed stroke* or stroke in progress, it is wise not to surgically interfere. Such an attempt may change an ischemic infarct to a hemorrhagic infarct that is associated with a higher mortality rate. But once a stroke is stable and recovery is satisfactory, further investigation is indicated. Surgical correction of extracranial vascular lesions in patients who have suffered a stroke seems to protect them significantly against a recurrent attack.

When the symptoms of a patient are attributed to vertebrobasilar insufficiency, the diagnosis and the therapeutic strategy ought to be based on the angiogram. Noninvasive techniques are inadequate for the evaluation of the posterior circulation, and the flow patterns may be quite complex. In cases of combined disease of the carotid and the posterior circulation with an intact circle of Willis, carotid surgery alone will probably eliminate the symptoms of vertebral insufficiency. If the carotid arteries are normal or if the posterior communicating arteries are inadequate, direct vertebral revascularization may be needed. In cases of *subclavian steal,* simple *ligation* of the vertebral artery or subclavian *bypass* will successfully eliminate the steal.

Surgical Procedures

The treatment of extracranial vascular disease is basically surgical. Various antiplatelet agents have been employed in the treatment of this disease and may be beneficial in certain patients. However, the proven preventive value of carotid surgery cannot be matched by any kind of medical treatment.

The majority of symptomatic patients have combined disease involving either both carotid arteries or the carotid as well as the vertebral system. More than one operation may be occasionally necessary. Appropriate patient selection and timing of the proposed surgical procedures are essential. The most often performed procedure is a carotid endarterectomy. Ligation or revascularization of the vertebral arteries may be occasionally needed. Endarterectomy or bypass procedures to the subclavian arteries are indicated in a small number of patients.

Carotid Endarterectomy. A carotid endarterectomy is indicated in the treatment of symptomatic arteriosclerotic lesions of the distal common carotid artery and its bifurcation. It is a durable procedure with excellent results and a low mortality rate of 1 to 2 percent. The incidence of temporary and permanent neurologic deficits is in the range of 2 to 5 percent. Unlike other surgical procedures, a carotid endarterectomy demands meticulous and precise operative technique. It should be performed by experienced surgeons *only* so that mortality and morbidity will remain low.

Most of the controversy in carotid surgery involves the use of an intraluminal shunt. Several authors have reported their experiences with the use of a shunt. Some routinely use shunts, but some never use them. It seems that a selective approach is the proper one. Patients with single compensated lesions and excellent backbleeding from the internal carotid artery can be safely operated without a shunt. This makes the endarterectomy procedure much easier and eliminates problems associated with the use of a shunt such as debris embolization and intimal disruption. However, if the contralateral carotid artery is occluded, the lesion is poorly compensated, and the backbleeding is poor to fair, an intraluminal shunt will protect the patient from critical cerebral ischemia. Various techniques have been used in an attempt to detect the patient who needs shunting: (1) continuous *EEG* monitoring, (2) measurement of the carotid *stump pressure,* and (3) surgery under *local anesthesia.* These procedures have been advocated by some and challenged by others. This means that none of these controversies can significantly alter a successful outcome. It is the clinical judgment and the operative technique that count.

Operative Technique.   General anesthesia is preferred. After induction, the head is extended and rotated laterally, away from the operative side. The exposed sterile field extends from the ear lobe to the clavicle. A skin incision is made alongside the anterior border of the sternocleidomastoid muscle. The uppermost part of the incision should be placed right on the muscle edge and should be advanced at this plane. This eliminates the risk of injury to the marginal madibular branch of the facial nerve that loops around the angle of the mandible. The dissection is advanced through the platysma until the internal jugular vein is encountered. All of the branches of the jugular vein that cross medially are ligated and divided. The common carotid artery is so exposed in its location medially and posteriorly to the vein. The ansa hypoglossi that may be crossing the artery can be severed with impunity. The common carotid artery is dissected and looped with silastic tape. With care not to injure the vagus nerve that lies in a posterolateral position to the artery, the distal common carotid as well as the internal and external carotid arteries are dissected free. The *hypoglossal* nerve crosses over the internal carotid artery and is the upper limit of the dissection. Although not usually needed, additional exposure can be achieved inferiorly if the belly of the omohyoideus muscle is divided. The *carotid body* is injected with 0.5 ml 1 percent lidocaine solution by use of a hypodermic needle. The next steps are very important and should proceed in the following order:

1. Assure excellent exposure of the common, internal, and external carotid arteries.
2. Focus the light on the subject.
3. Verify the availability of all instruments that will be needed for vascular control, insertion of a shunt, and the endarterectomy procedure.
4. Fill the shunt with heparinized saline and clamp it in the middle.

5. Systemic heparinization.
6. Clamp the internal, common, and external carotid arteries in this order.
7. With a No. 11 blade, perform a vertical arteriotomy on the distal common carotid artery and extend it with fine scissors into the internal carotid artery, just past the stenotic lesion.
8. Wash out all luminal debris with saline irrigation.
9. Check backbleeding from the internal carotid artery and, if necessary, insert the distal limb of the shunt. Secure its intraluminal position with the special clamp and allow retrograde bleeding to flush and remove any air bubbles from cannula.
10. Insert the proximal wider tip of the shunt into the carotid artery and apply the appropriate clamp.
11. Establish flow through the shunt.

Under direct vision, an open endarterectomy is performed. The proper plane is through the layers of the media. Subintimal or subadventitial endarterectomies should be avoided. Dissection is advanced circumferentially in the common and internal carotid arteries to include the stenotic lesion. The proximal line of the endarterectomy is created sharply with scissors. Distally, the endarterectomy is terminated at the normal portion of the internal carotid artery. If necessary, the distal intimal flap may be tacked down with interrupted transverse mattress sutures of 6-0 prolene (Fig. 12-2). A limited endarterectomy of the proximal external carotid artery is performed, and a distal intimal separation line is created with gentle traction. The specimen is removed, and the endarterectomized area is inspected. Saline irrigation facilitates the detection of loose fibers that should be removed.

The closure of the arteriotomy is started with continuous suture of 6-0 prolene, advancing proximally. The last 1 to 1.5 cm of the arteriotomy is sutured quickly but precisely, under complete vascular control, after removal of the shunt. All clamps are removed, and flow is established in the external and internal carotid arteries. If the pulse in the distal internal carotid artery is not satisfactory, an intraoperative arteriogram is very helpful in demonstrating the nature and location of the problem. Hemostasis is secured. The wound is well irrigated and closed in layers. If any question exists, a small closed suction drain should be left in the wound for 24 hours. The use of skin sutures placed with a cutting needle is not recommended, as small wound hematomas occur frequently with this closure technique.

Complications. The surgeon's goal when performing a carotid endarterectomy is to make the patient asymptomatic and markedly reduce the chance of stroke. Unfortunately, an occasional patient undergoing this procedure will develop a neurologic deficit directly associated with the surgical procedure. This complication may be temporary or permanent and may present as acute

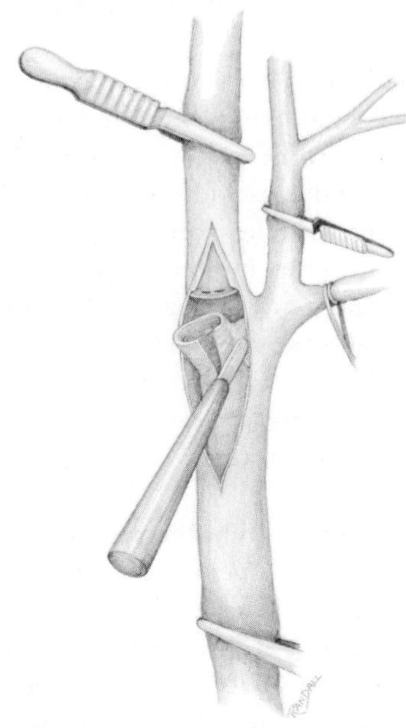

Figure 12-2. Carotid endarterectomy.

operative or delayed postoperative sequelae. *Acute operative* deficits are due either to (1) prolonged regional cerebral ischemia or to (2) debris or air embolization that may occur during dissection of the vessels, insertion of the shunt, or just after declamping. *Delayed* deficits occur in patients who are initially neurologically intact and develop a problem sometime in the postoperative period. This is usually associated with episodes of hypertension or hypotension and usually indicates the presence of an arterial *thrombosis* or *intracranial hemorrhage.* If a delayed deficit develops in association with signs of increased intracranial pressure, chances are that this patient had an intracranial hemorrhage, probably secondary to a hypertensive crisis. Computerized tomography of the brain will confirm the clinical diagnosis. Conservative management is indicated for this patient. If an ischemic hemispheric deficit develops, thrombosis of the carotid artery should be suspected. This patient should have prompt reexploration, thrombectomy, and correction of the problem that may have precipitated failure of the reconstruction.

For acute operative neurological complications, treatment should be conservative, followed by early rehabilitation. The overall incidence of neurologic complications is in the range of 2 to 5 percent, with many of these patients showing partial or complete recovery.

Unlike the complications associated with cerebral blood flow, neurological deficits may occur as a result of an injury to a cranial nerve (Fig. 12–3). Although the true incidence of iatrogenic injuries seems to be in the 15 percent range, only some of these patients will be symptomatic.

The marginal mandibular branch of the facial nerve, the hypoglossal, the vagus, and the recurrent and superior laryngeal nerves are occasionally injured. This may be due either to transection or more often to contusion of the nerve with resulting neuroapraxia and subsequent recovery of function. These complications may be avoided if the following is kept in mind: (1) The *mandibular branch* may be injured if the uppermost part of the incision is placed too medially instead of laterally, right on the anterior edge of the sternocleidomastoid muscle. (2) The *hypoglossal nerve* is routinely indentified and constantly kept in view. The nerve may be easily found if the ansa hypoglossi is dissected cephalad. (3) The *vagus nerve* should always be visualized whenever a clamp is applied on the arteries. This assures that it will not be accidentally cross-clamped.

Wound hematomas are occasionally seen following a carotid endarterectomy. They may be related to fluctuations of blood pressure but also to the surgical technique. If hemostasis is not satisfactory, the wound should never be closed. A soft closed-suction drain, placed away from the vessels, may have to be used oc-

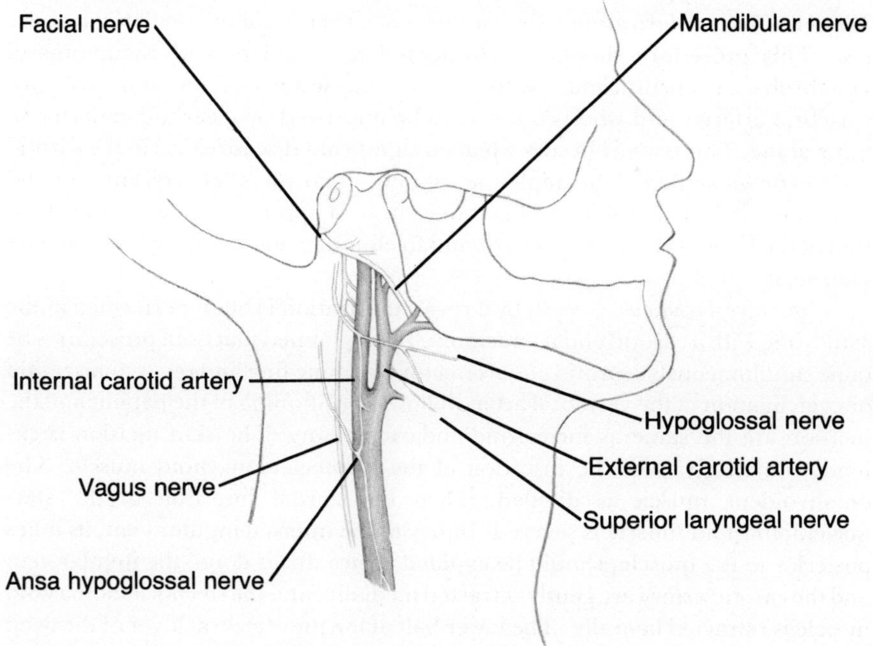

Figure 12-3. Cranial nerves.

casionally. Use of skin clips seems to lower the incidence of superficial wound hematomas. Once a hematoma is detected, it should be immediately drained by removing one or two clips and inserting a small Penrose drain. This may be done in the recovery room. If significant bleeding is encountered, the wound should be reexplored.

Infections are a rather rare complication of this neck wound. They have been seen mostly in association with wound hematomas.

After carotid endarterectomy, *hypertension* is occasionally seen in hypertensive or otherwise normotensive patients. It should be treated aggressively if the catastrophic complication of an intracranial hemorrhage is to be avoided. Titrated infusion of *nitroprusside sodium* solution is effective in promptly lowering the arterial pressure. However, it should be used only with continuous *monitoring* of the pressure through an arterial line. Even short periods of pharmacologic hypotension may produce severe cerebral or myocardial damage. For moderate hypertension, the combined use of loop diuretics and methyldopa intravenously is quite successful.

Cardiac arrest and *hypotension* are complications associated with stimulation of the carotid body either during dissection or with manipulation of the carotid bifurcation. Injecting the carotid body with lidocaine solution and limiting the dissection of the carotid bulb seem to offer adequate protection.

Vertebral Revascularization. Patients who need vertebral revascularization are few. This procedure should be considered in a patient with symptoms of vertebrobasilar insufficiency who has stenotic lesions of the subclavian or vertebral arteries and who is unlikely to be improved by a carotid endarterectomy alone. This usually occurs when no significant disease exists in the carotid arteries or when there is incomplete anastomotic pathways between anterior and posterior cerebral circulation. The same surgical approach allows simple ligation of the vertebral artery in an attempt to eliminate the symptoms of a subclavian steal.

Operative Technique. Vertebral revascularization is often performed at the same time with a carotid endarterectomy. If it is planned that both procedures be done simultaneously, carotid endarterectomy is done first and revascularization or even ligation of the vertebral artery follows. Positioning of the patient and the incision are the same as for carotid endarterectomy. The skin incision is extended inferiorly over the insertion of the sternocleidomastoid muscle. The omohyoideus muscle is divided. Then the sternal insertion of the sternocleidomastoid muscle is severed. Injury to the internal jugular vein, as it lies posterior to the muscle, should be avoided. Once this is done, the jugular vein and the carotid artery are gently retracted medially, and the sternocleidomastoid muscle is retracted laterally. The lower half of the prevertebral layer of the deep cervical fascia is now exposed and incised. The space between the scalenus anticus and the longus colli muscles is entered. On the left side of the neck, the thoracic duct overlying the arterial branches of the deeply situated subclavian artery is encountered. The inferior thyroid artery, a branch of the thyrocervical trunk, crosses over medially and supplies the ascending cervical branch. It may be divided for improved exposure. At a deeper plane, the vertebral vein and, behind it, the vertebral artery are seen. The vein is ligated and divided, and the vertebral artery is dissected for a 1.5- to 2-cm distance after systemic heparinization, and with a soft vascular clamp, the artery is divided as far proximally as possible and clamped as far distally as possible. The proximal stump is oversewn with continuous suture of 5–0 prolene. The cut end of the vertebral artery is then anastomosed to the proximal common carotid artery with continuous suture of 6–0 prolene (Fig. 12–4). This may be done with the use of a partial occlusion clamp applied on the common carotid artery. After completion of the anastomosis, the clamps are removed, and pulsatile flow in both carotid and vertebral arteries is verified. The wound is closed in layers. A soft drain may be left in the wound for 24 hours.

Complications. Injury to the internal jugular vein should be repaired. In-

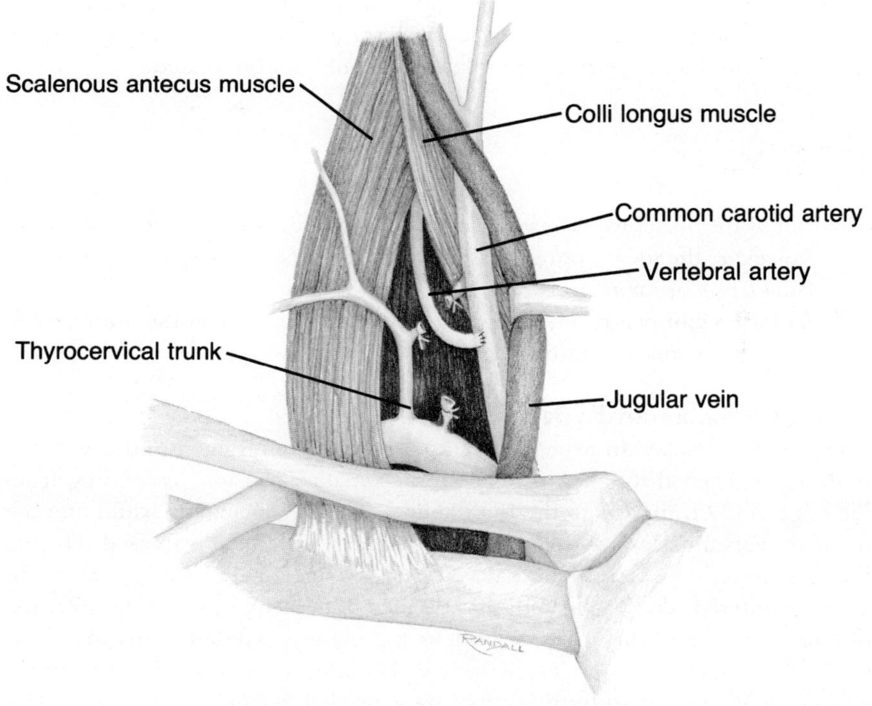

Figure 12–4. Carotid-vertebral bypass.

jury to the thoracic duct should be recognized, and the duct should be ligated. Injury to peripheral nerves is rather infrequent. The operating surgeon should be well familiar with the anatomy of this region. This will assure excellent results without undesirable sequelae.

Subclavian Steal Syndrome

DIAGNOSIS

In cases of high-degree stenosis or occlusion of the subclavian artery before the origin of the vertebral artery, blood flow to the upper extremity is maintained through various collaterals. The flow in the vertebral artery is reversed, and the cerebral circulation supplies the ipsilateral upper extremity. During exercise, the posterior cerebral circulation is depleted further, and symptoms of vertebrobasilar insufficiency appear. These are dizziness, *syncope,* vertigo, and bilateral visual blurring. Radiologic demonstrations of steal may be an incidental finding, and unless it is symptomatic, it should not be treated.

TREATMENT

Ligation of the vertebral artery has been successfully employed for this condition; however, the ideal approach is a bypass of the stenotic lesion, either as a *carotid-subclavian* or an *axillo-axillary* bypass.

Endarterectomy is rarely indicated, and as it requires a thoracotomy, it has higher mortality and morbidity rates.

Carotid-Subclavian Bypass

The stenotic subclavian artery and the ipsilateral common carotid artery are both approached through a simple supraclavicular incision, extending from the edge of the trapezius to the middle line. The sternocleidomastoid and the omohyoideus muscles are divided. The deep cervical fascia is incised. During this dissection, the external jugular vein and the suprascapular artery and vein are encountered, doubly ligated, and divided. The neurovascular bundle, the phrenic nerve, and the scalenus anticus muscle are exposed. This muscle is severed close to its insertion on the first rib. The subclavian artery is dissected for a distance of 2 cm. If additional exposure is needed, it can be accomplished by subperiosteal resection of the middle third of the clavicle. The proximal common carotid artery is dissected, and an 8-mm Dacron or PTFE graft is interposed. The common carotid artery can be safely clamped at this level without the need

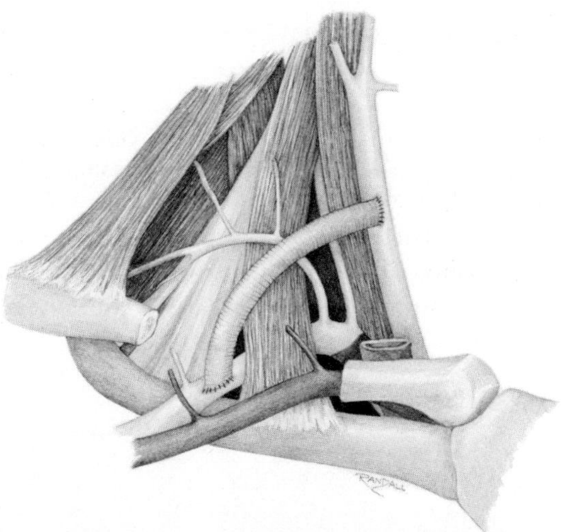

Figure 12-5. Carotid-subclavian bypass.

of an intraluminal shunt. The graft should lie behind the jugular vein (Fig. 12-5). The cut ends of the sternocleidomastoid muscle are approximated, and the wound is closed in layers.

Axilloaxillary Bypass

This bypass is indicated for the treatment of subclavian steal in patients with disease of the ipsilateral common carotid artery. However, some surgeons believe it is even preferable to carotid-subclavian bypass since it avoids manipulation of the carotid vessels. In such a case, the diseased as well as the donor contralateral axillary arteries are approached through bilateral infraclavicular incisions, as described for an axillofemoral bypass. An 8-mm graft is placed subcutaneously across the upper anterior chest wall (necklace graft; Fig. 12-6).

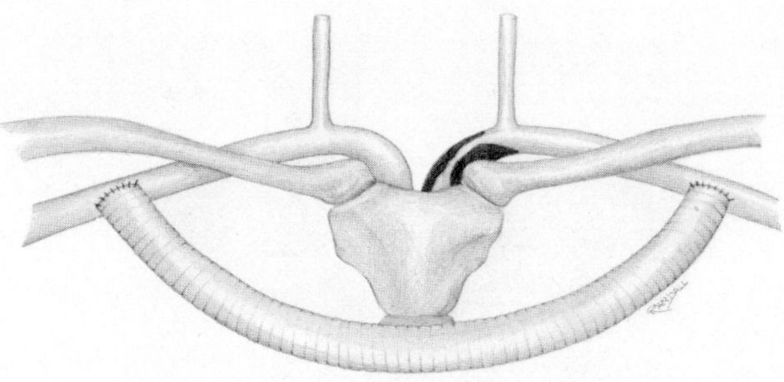

Figure 12-6. Axilloaxillary bypass.

Fibromuscular Dysplasia

Fibromuscular dysplasia (FMD) is predominantly seen in female patients. It is seen more often in the renal arteries, but recent reports have focused on the involvement of the carotid arteries.

The patient with FMD of the carotid artery presents with severe neurologic symptoms such as completed stroke, TIAs, amaurosis fugax, and various nonlocalizing neurologic symptoms. A usual complaint is constant ringing in the ip-

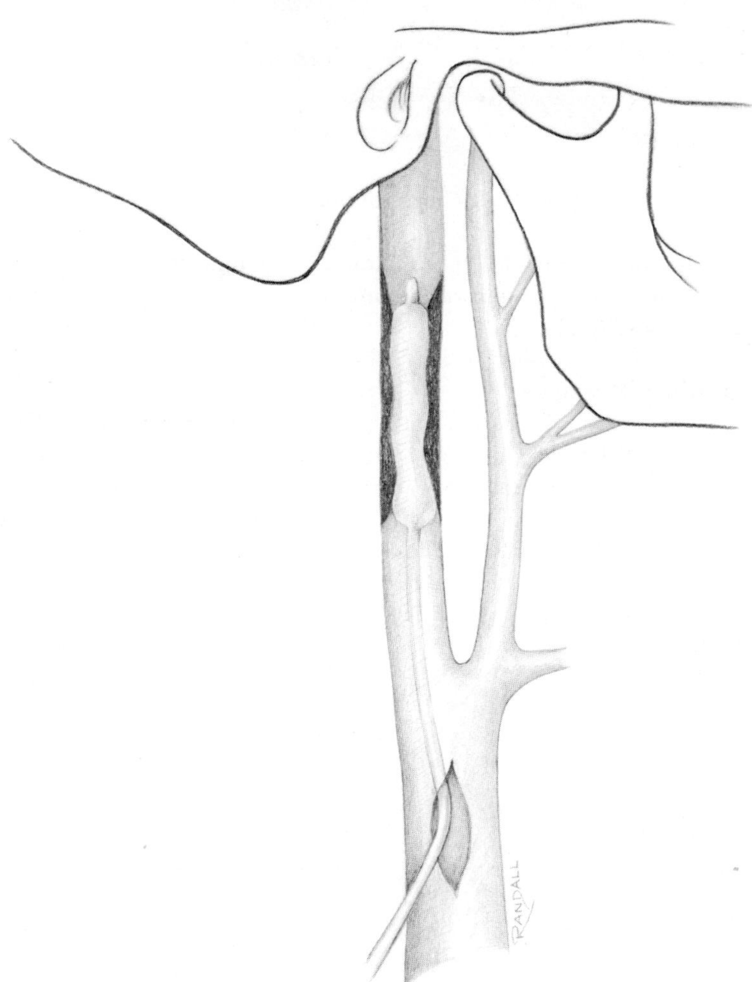

Figure 12-7. Fibromuscular dysplasia.

silateral ear. This represents the patient's perception of the flow turbulence in the involved internal carotid artery. Hypertension and other symptoms attributed to the presence of FMD in other vessels may be present. The common angiographic pattern of this disease is a "string of beads."

It is agreed that once carotid fibromuscular dysplasia becomes symptomatic, the patient should be treated in an attempt to prevent serious neurologic sequelae. The disease often extends quite distally into the internal carotid artery, well past the angle of the mandible. At this level, direct surgical reconstruction is impossible. For this reason, the favored treatment of FMD of the carotid artery is operative intraluminal dilatation with use of sized coronary dilators. Intraoperative, intraluminal balloon dilatation with Gruntzig catheters has also been successful (Fig. 12–7). This therapeutic approach has accomplished excellent long-term results with a low morbidity rate.

Spontaneous Dissection of the Internal Carotid Artery

Spontaneous, nontraumatic dissection of the internal carotid artery occurs usually in *young* individuals and presents with an acute neurologic deficit that may be transient or prolonged. Other unusual symptoms include ipsilateral headache, *neck pain,* and tenderness in the area of the angle of the mandible. On arteriography, these lesions present with tapered narrowing of the internal carotid artery that starts just beyond the carotid bulb and extends to the level of the bony foramen.

In general, these patients should be initially treated conservatively. It has been demonstrated that the luminal diameter will increase to near-normal caliber in most patients who are not operated. This may be due to absorption of the mural hematoma. Surgical intervention may be needed for repeated TIAs secondary to distal embolization. If the involved portion of the internal carotid artery is surgically accessible, resection with *vein graft interposition* is the appropriate treatment. However, when the lesion is too extensive, consideration should be given to simple ligation of the proximal internal carotid artery.

BIBLIOGRAPHY

Baker WH, Dorner DB, Barnes RW: Carotid endarterectomy: is an indwelling shunt necessary? *Surgery* 82:321, 1977.
Callow AD, Matsumoto G, et al: Protection of the high risk carotid endarterectomy patient by continuous electroencephalography. *J Cardiovasc Surg* 19:55, 1978.

Diethrich EB, Garrett HE, et al: Occlusive disease of the common carotid and subclavian arteries treated by carotid subclavian bypass. Analysis 125 cases. *Am J Surg* 114:800, 1967.

Effeney DJ, Ehrenfeld WK, Stoney RJ, et al: Why operate on carotid fibromuscular dysplasia? *Arch Surg* 115:1261, 1980.

Ehrenfeld WK, Wylie EJ: Spontaneous dissection of the internal carotid artery. *Arch Surg* 111:1294, 1976.

Fields WS, Lemak NA: Joint study of extracranial arterial occlusion. X. Internal carotid artery occlusion. *JAMA* 235:2734, 1976.

Hays RJ, Levinson SA, Wylie EJ: Intraoperative measurement of carotid back pressure as a guide to operative management for carotid endarterectomy. *Surgery* 72:953, 1972.

Hertzer NR, Feldman BJ, Beven EG, et al: A prospective study of the incidence of injury to the cranial nerves during carotid endarterectomy. *Surg Gynecol. Obstet* 151:781, 1980.

Kartchner MM, McRae LP, Morrison FD: Non-invasive detection and evaluation of carotid occlusive disease. *Arch Surg* 106:528, 1973.

Raines J: Controversies in the noninvasive evaluation of extracranial arterial disease, in Bernstein EF (ed) *Noninvasive Diagnositc Techniques in Vascular Disease.* St. Louis, Mosby, 1978, p 258.

Rich NM, Hobson RW: Carotid endarterectomy under regional anesthesia. *Am Surg* 41:253, 1975.

Rosenthal JJ, Gaspar Max R, Movius HJ: Intraoperative arteriography in carotid thromboendarterectomy. *Arch Surg* 106:806, 1973.

Thompson JE, Patman RD, Persson AV: Management of asymptomatic carotid bruits. *Am Surg* 42:77, 1976.

Thompson JE: Complications of carotid endarterectomy and their prevention. *World J Surg* 3:155, 1979.

Whitney DG, Kahn EM, Estes JW, et al: Carotid artery surgery without a temporary shunt. *Arch Surg* 115:1393, 1980.

CHAPTER THIRTEEN

Thoracic Outlet Syndrome

INTRODUCTION

Thoracic outlet syndrome is ascribed to compression of the brachial plexus and the subclavian vessels as they exit the thoracic cavity, crossing over the first rib. Various space-limiting factors have been associated with the development of this syndrome. These are cervical ribs, the scalenus anticus and medius muscles, anomalous ligaments and bands, and the subclavius and pectoralis minor muscles. The increased frequency of this syndrome among middle-aged, asthenic-type women suggests that weakness of the suspensory muscles of the shoulder girdle may be a contributing factor.

The diagnosis is made when the clinical symptoms are considered together with the findings of the physical examination and the information derived from various tests. Once the diagnosis is established, the patient should be treated in accordance with the severity of the symptoms and the degree of existing disability.

ANATOMY

Certain anatomic considerations are essential for the understanding of the etiologic mechanism and the proposed modes of treatment. The brachial plexus and the subclavian artery cross over the first rib through the space between the scalenus anticus and medius muscles. Just anterior to the scalenous anticus muscle, the subclavian vein exits the chest cavity. These structures pass under the clavicle, the costocoracoid ligament, and the insertion of the pectoralis minor muscles as they enter the axilla. Cervical ribs and abnormal bands may further restrict the narrow passage between the first rib and the scalenus muscles. *Neurovascular compression* at any point along their course generates the symptoms that are referred to as the thoracic outlet syndrome.

DIAGNOSIS

Symptoms

The most frequent complaints are generally attributed to compression of the brachial plexus and are (1) pain, (2) numbness, and (3) tingling. Fatigue, coldness, swelling, and discoloration are seen when the vascular structures are involved. The pain is in the shoulder and subscapular area and extends down to the entire upper extremity. It may occur at night and is often associated with paresthesias of *ulnar nerve distribution.* These symptoms ought to be differentiated from cervical radiculitis, disc syndromes, angina, and carpal tunnel syndrome, which may manifest a similar pain pattern.

Physical Examination

Vascular evaluation is essential. Bilateral determination of blood pressure may reveal differences attributed to arterial compression. Auscultation over the distal subclavicular area may reveal the presence of a bruit, indicating an arterial stenosis or even aneurysmal dilatation. If significant venous compression exists, edema and skin discoloration may be noted.

In thoracic outlet syndrome, vascular involvement is not present in all cases. It is the compression of the brachial plexus that is responsible for most symptoms. Neurological examination may reveal ulnar anesthesia, atrophy of the hypothenar, and weakness of the intrinsic muscles of the hand. A *Tinel test* may be positive, as carpal tunnel syndrome is sometimes seen in association with the thoracic outlet syndrome.

Various maneuvers have been described in an attempt to develop a reliable test for evaluation of the thoracic outlet syndrome. The military position testing and the *Adson maneuver* are designed to reproduce the symptoms by further limiting the space of the thoracic outlet. In the stress test, which seems to be reliable, symptoms are reproduced when the patient has the affected side abducted and external rotation at shoulder, 90° flexion at elbow, and then opens and closes for 30 seconds.

Investigative Tests

A treadmill electrocardiogram is essential to rule out angina as the cause of the shoulder pain. X-rays of the neck may reveal cervical ribs or other bony abnormalities. Tonometry and nerve conduction studies offer objective evidence of muscle group atrophies and conduction deficits. Plethysmographic studies are necessary if vascular compression seems to be part of the syndrome. Arteriography is only indicated in certain cases where vascular complications occur and reconstruction is planned. It should be realized that thoracic outlet syndrome is largely a diagnosis by exclusion and that there is not a single test that is diagnostic.

TREATMENT

Once the diagnosis of thoracic outlet syndrome is established, the patient should be treated according to the degree of disability. Conservative management consists of exercises that increase the tone of the suspensory muscles of the shoulder girdle. This exercise program should be closely supervised by a competent physical therapist. Approximately 50 percent of patients will respond favorably to this mode of treatment. The rest of the patients either show no improvement or may even get worse. It is this group of patients that are considered for surgical decompression.

Although various anatomic structures may contribute to the development of thoracic outlet syndrome, *removal of the first rib* has proved to offer adequate relief in the majority of patients. The approaches that have been successfully employed in the treatment of this condition are (1) the supraclavicular, (2) the posterior, (3) anterior, and (4) the transaxillary. Transaxillary resection of the first rib is the most popular procedure and offers a good to excellent result in over 90 percent of patients.

Operative Technique

Positioning of the patient is of paramount importance. The patient is placed in a 90-degree posterolateral position with a sandbag placed under the spine. The entire upper extremity is prepped and draped with a sterile stockinette so that an assistant can manipulate it for adequate exposure. The chest is also prepped and draped appropriately, as for an axillary thoracotomy. A 3- to 4-inch transverse skin incision is made below the inferior border of the hair stubble, extending from the border of the latissimus dorsi to the pectoralis major muscle (Fig. 13–1). This incision is advanced directly to the rib cage in order to avoid the axillary lymph nodes and vessels. A plane is then created in the areolar tissue overlying the rib cage and is advanced superiorly until the first rib is encountered. The intercostobrachial nerve is seen as it exits the second intercostal space. This sensory nerve may be sacrificed if so needed. The assistant should now raise the arm and the shoulder in a vertical position. This maneuver opens the axillary tunnel and exposes the important structures. From time to time, this traction is released to prevent postoperative discomfort from undue and prolonged tension of the brachial plexus. The exposure may be further im-

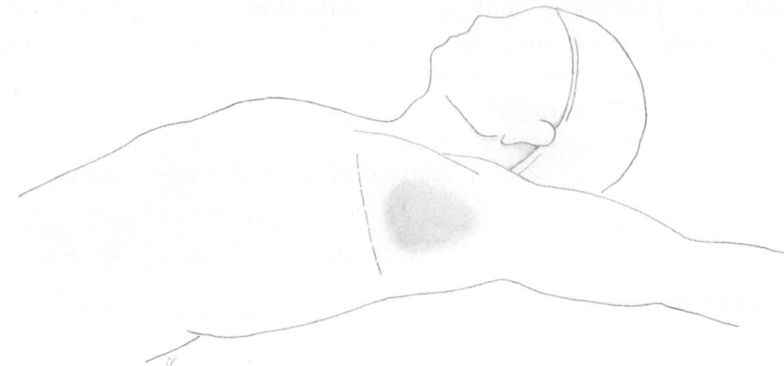

Figure 13-1. Transaxillary approach.

proved with retraction of the pectoralis major and latissimus dorsi muscles. The scalenus anticus and medius are severed at their tendinous insertions on the first rib, which is easily recognized by its flat shape (Fig. 13-2). This is followed by a subperiostal resection of the first rib from the costal cartilage, anteriorly to the transverse process of the vertebra, posteriorly (Fig. 13-3). During this procedure, the subclavian vein and artery and the brachial plexus are kept in view, avoiding any injury to these structures. Any cervical bands should be resected. If a cervical rib is present, it is separated from the first rib and resected with its periosteum back to its transverse process. The bone edges are rongeured to smooth. The pleura is inspected by irrigation during inflation of the lung. Bubbling during this procedure indicates the presence of a pleural tear.

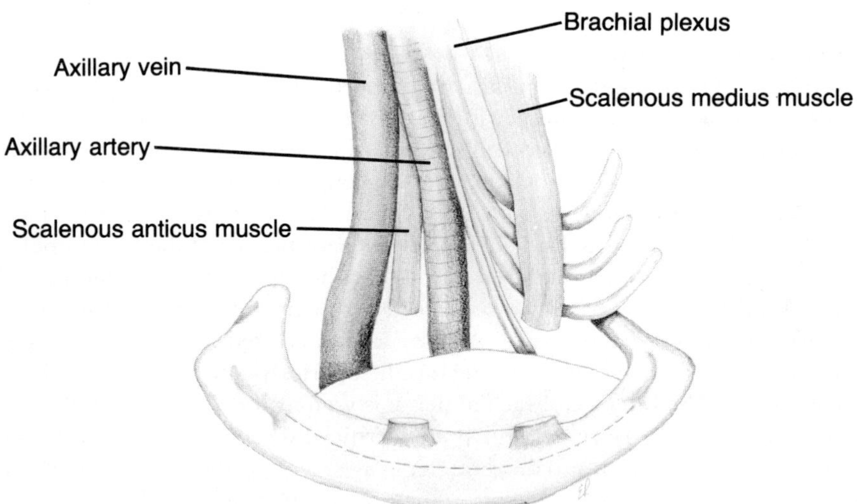

Figure 13-2. Exposure of the first rib.

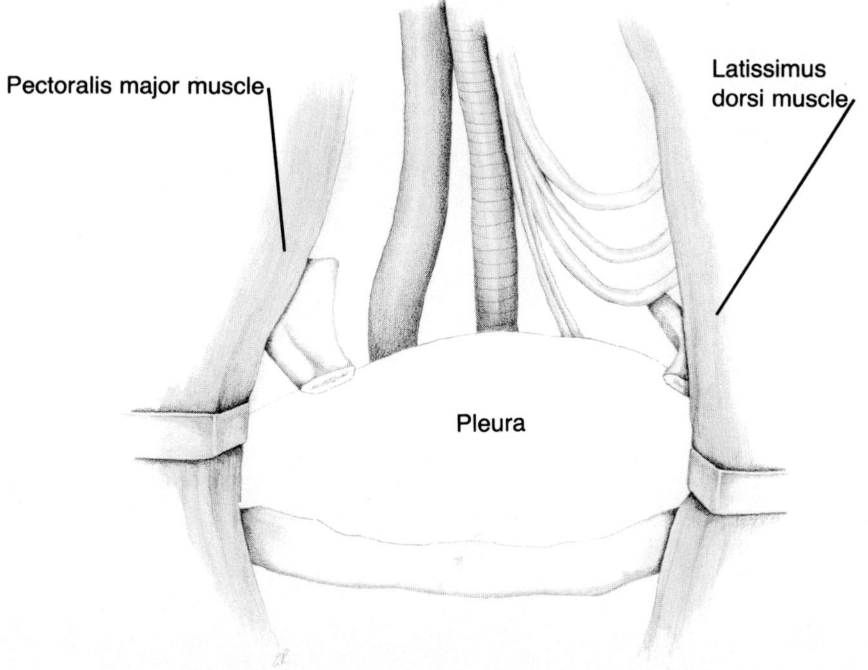

Figure 13-3. Resection of the first rib.

The subcutaneous tissue and the skin are closed in layers. With this approach, there are no muscles to suture, and if the maneuvering of the arm is done with caution, no significant postoperative discomfort is encountered.

BIBLIOGRAPHY

Blank R, Conner RG: Arterial complications associated with thoracic outlet compression syndrome. *Ann Thorac Surg* 17:315, 1974.
Calgett OT: Presidential address: research and prosearch. *J Thorac Cardiovasc Surg* 44:153, 1962.
Martinez MS: Posterior first rib resection for total thoracic outlet syndrome decompression. *Contemp Surg* 15:13, 1979.
Peet RM, Henriske JE, et al: Thoracic outlet syndrome. *Mayo Clin Proc* 31:281, 1956.
Roos DB: Transaxillary approach for first rib resection to relieve thoracic outlet syndrome. *Ann Surg* 163:354, 1966.
Roos, DB: Experience with first rib resection for thoracic outlet syndrome. *Ann Surg* 173:429, 1971.
Thomas GI, Jones TW, Stavery LS, Manhas DR: Thoracic outlet syndrome. *Am Surg* 44:483, 1978.

CHAPTER FOURTEEN

Angioaccess

INTRODUCTION

The survival of most patients with chronic renal failure depends on maintenance hemodialysis. Even patients who have had successful transplantation are usually placed on dialysis for a certain period of time. Angioaccess surgery has been developed in order to offer to these patients the necessary routes for hemodialysis. These vascular procedures, both temporary and permanent, often fail. The surgeon has the responsibility of maintaining a patent route at all times. Thrombectomies, revisions, and new procedures are frequently necessary to keep this patient alive. Angioaccess surgery challenges the ingenuity and creativity of the surgeon. Precise knowledge of the various anatomic structures and meticulous surgical technique are essential for success.

ANATOMIC EXPOSURES

All angioaccess procedures in the forearm require a broad operative field extending from the proximal palm to the upper arm. Surgeons involved in these procedures should be familiar with the anatomic exposures of the vessels at all different levels. Local anesthesia is preferred, but axillary block or general

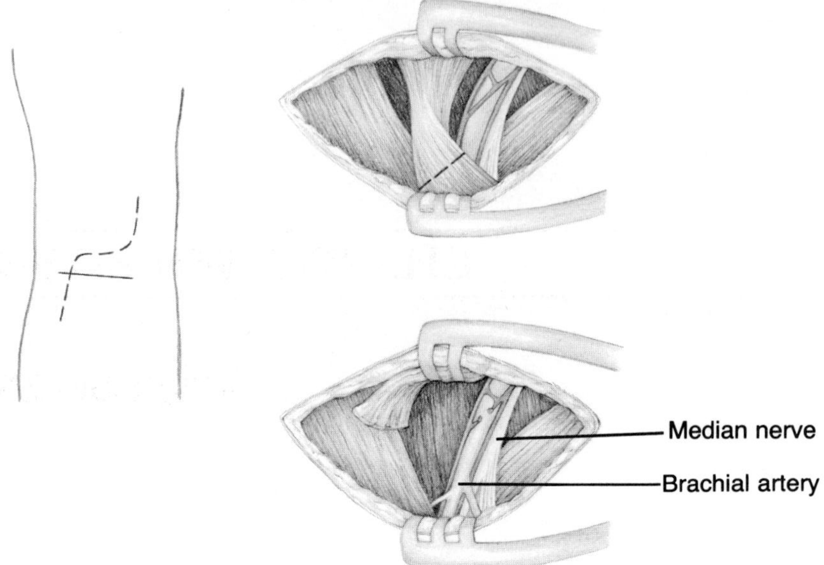

Figure 14–1. The distal brachial artery.

anesthesia may be used, depending on the nature of the procedure and acceptance by the patient.

Brachial Artery

The brachial artery is used for construction of a proximal end-to-side arteriovenous fistula and for placement of looped grafts in the forearm. It enters the forearm in a slightly oblique direction, accompanied medially by the median nerve. It is approached through a transverse or an S-shaped skin incision. The fascia is incised, and the bicipital aponeurosis is sectioned, exposing the distal brachial artery and its bifurcation (Fig. 14–1).

Ulnar Artery

The ulnar artery may not be widely used in angioaccess surgery, as it is the dominant vessel to the palmar arch and its interruption may result in significant hand ischemia. The Allen test is helpful in determining the adequacy of arterial inflow to the hand. This vessel takes off at a 30-degree angle from the brachial artery, passes under the medial nerve and the pronator muscle, and meets the ulnar nerve. They both descend distally, lying posteriorly and in between the flexor carpi radialis and flexor carpi ulnaris muscles. The distal two-thirds of the artery are accessible through incision on a line from the medial epicondyle to the area of ulnar pulsation at the wrist. Exposure requires incision of the fascia and retraction of the tendons of the flexor carpi ulnaris and the flexor digitorum superficialis muscles.

Radial Artery

The radial artery is the arterial component for most arteriovenous shunts and fistulas. This vessel is the direct continuation of the brachial artery, overlies the pronator teres muscle, and anteriorly and laterally is covered by the brachioradialis muscle. Exposure of the proximal third of the radial artery requires incision on a line from the distal brachial to the distal radial pulsation. After incision of the overlying fascia, the brachioradialis muscle is laterally retracted, exposing the proximal portion of the vessel (Fig. 14-2).

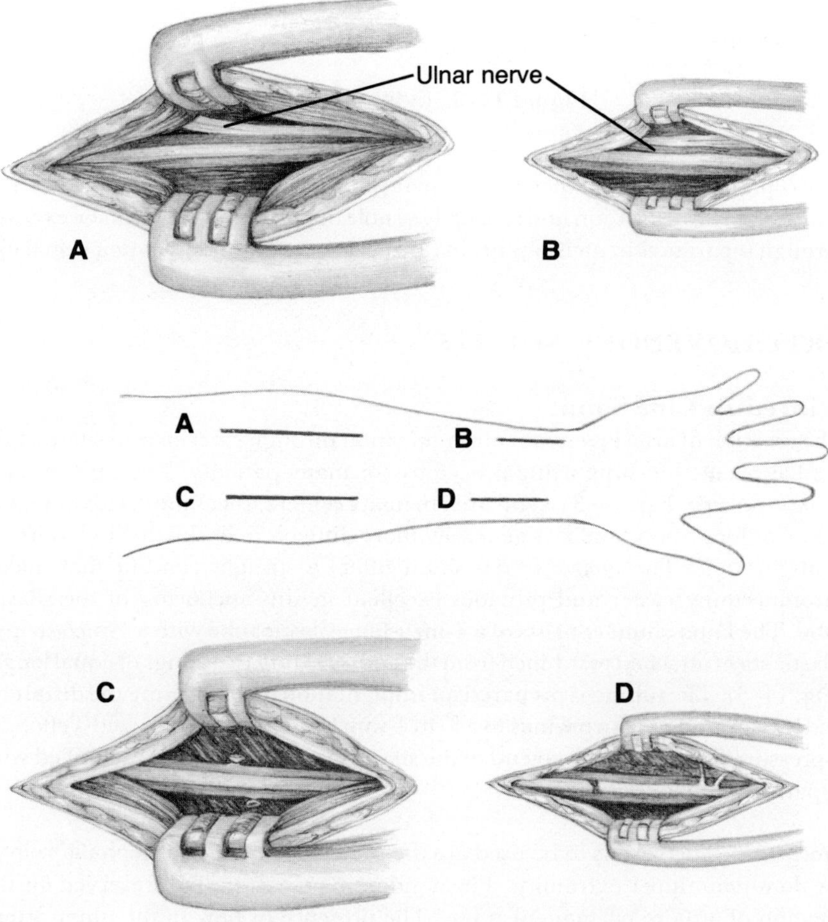

Figure 14-2. Ulnar and radial arteries.

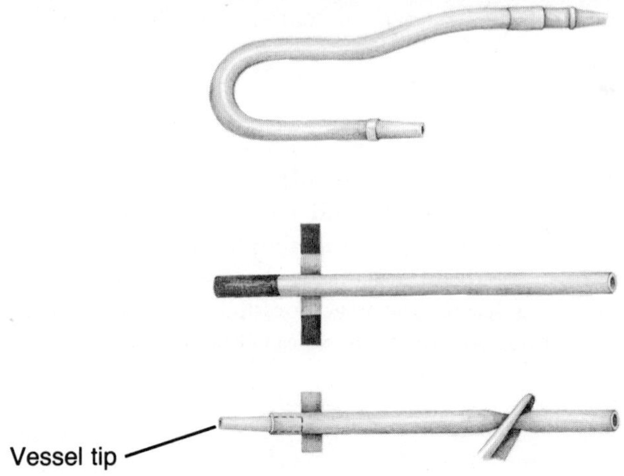

Figure 14-3. External shunts.

Veins

The cephalic, basilic, medial basilic, or any other prominent vein of the forearm is in a superficial location and is usually visible or palpable. They can be exposed through separate skin incisions or, in rare occasions, by undermining skin flaps.

ARTERIOVENOUS SHUNTS

Winged-In Line Shunt

The creation of arteriovenous communication through exteriorized silastic tubing has been a life-supporting procedure for many patients. The conventional *Quinton cannula* (Fig. 14–3) is still used in many centers. It has the disadvantage of easy clot formation, and it is generally more difficult to declot due to its curved configuration. The *winged-in line* shunt offers a straight conduit that makes thrombectomy easier and provides excellent in situ anchoring of the silastic tube. The latter shunt consists of a 7-inch-long silastic tube with a 1-inch strip of silastic sheet attached to it 1 inch from the end, creating two wings of equal length (Fig. 14–3). The tubing is prepared for implantation by shortening the distal end and by trimming the two wings to a 3- to 4-mm length. A proper-sized Teflon tip is pressure fitted to the distal end of the silastic cannula, which is then filled with heparinized saline solution.

Procedure. The vessels to be used are the radial artery and the cephalic vein of the dominant upper extremity. The nondominant extremity is reserved for the creation of a more permanent route. The presence of flow in the ulnar artery should be verified either by palpation or by a Doppler flow detector. Two separate skin incisions are made directly overlying the distal portion of the artery and the vein. We favor this approach over the single midway incision because it does not require undermining of the flaps, which may become necrotic. It also facilitates surgical removal of the cannulas through the same incisions. The vein is exposed in its subcutaneous location, and its patency is confirmed. Then the artery is exposed in a subfacial plane. Both vessels are cannulated with an appropriate-sized Teflon tip, and a ligature of 3–0 silk is tied around the vessel containing the tip. The artery and the vein are both ligated distally, and the wings are anchored to the fascia with 3–0 chronic sutures. This protects against axial dislodgement of the tubing and rotational movements of the Teflon tip. The silastic tubes are passed in a deeply located subcutaneous tunnel and are exteriorized through a snag cutaneous opening placed 2 cm distal to the incisions. The exteriorized tubes are shortened to appropriate length and are connected with a straight Teflon connector, establishing arteriovenous flow (Fig. 14–4). The wounds are closed in two layers. A sterile gauze dressing is applied without pressure, and the tubes are covered and protected. The shunt can be used immediately for hemodialysis.

Problems. Cannula failure is the result of infection, repeated clotting episodes, necrosis of the overlying skin, and hematoma. In general, arterial cannulae last longer than venous ones. The survival rates vary in different reports from an average of 7.6 to 24.5 months for the arterial cannula and from an average of 5.2 to 13.6 months for the venous one. Every attempt should be made to save the shunt. When clotted, both arterial and venous sides are thrombectomized at the bedside with a short No. 3 Fogarty catheter. If conversion to an arteriovenous fistula is planned, it should be done before cannula failure occurs. Severe hemorrhage from dislodgement of the tubes or disconnection during dialysis are rare but potentially lethal problems. The patient and the nursing staff should be instructed on how to react to such an event. Although the presence of a shunt limits

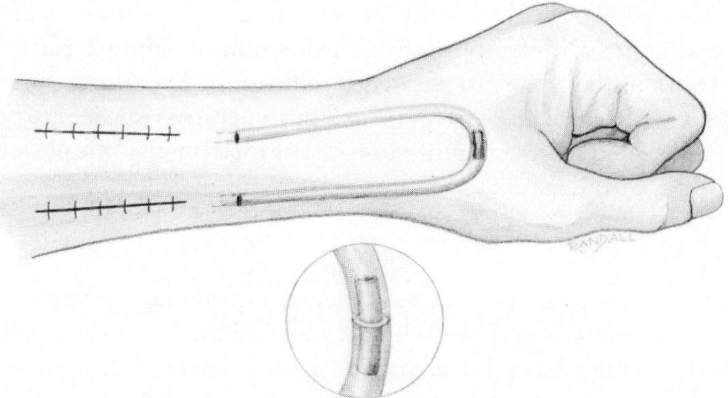

Figure 14–4. The winged-in line shunt.

use of the hand, it is generally well tolerated by inpatients and well accepted by outpatients.

Allen-Brown Shunt

The limb of an Allen-Brown shunt consists of silastic tubing with a Dacron cuff attached to it. This allows the placement of an external shunt without interruption of the distal arterial flow. It involves an end-to-side anastomosis between the artery and the Dacron cuff. The venous limb of the shunt can be constructed either by anastomosing an Allen-Brown shunt to the recipient vein or by inserting a conventional Teflon-tip cannula. This shunt may be removed simply by dividing the Dacron cuff close to the artery and closing the stump with a continuous prolene suture.

Thomas Shunt

The Thomas shunt is designed to be used for large-lumen vessels, usually the femoral artery and the saphenous vein. The artery and the vein are anastomosed to the Dacron cuff that is attached to the silastic tubing of the Thomas shunt. The cannulas are exteriorized. The use of this shunt is limited because of (1) the higher possibility of a groin prosthesis infection and (2) the possibility of interference with the arterial flow to the lower limb. It may be used in children.

DISTAL ARTERIOVENOUS FISTULA

Since its original description by Brescia, the distal forearm arteriovenous fistula has been the most effective route for long-term hemodialysis. It can be constructed as a side-to-side, end-to-side, and end-to-end anastomosis between the radial artery and the largest neighboring vein, usually the cephalic. This surgically created arteriovenous fistula delivers a flow volume of 250 to 300 ml/minute without significantly altering cardiac output. The arterial flow in the venous network initiates the process of arterialization. The fistula should not be used for hemodialysis during the first 2 to 3 postoperative weeks. Early failures have been associated with venopunctures performed during this period, which were necessary for the fistula to mature.

Procedure

The presence of adequate flow in the ulnar artery should be confirmed. The whole upper extremity is prepped with betadine solution and surgically draped from the wrist to the elbow. Local anesthesia of 1 percent lidocaine is used. A 5-cm-long skin incision is made midway between the radial artery and the vein

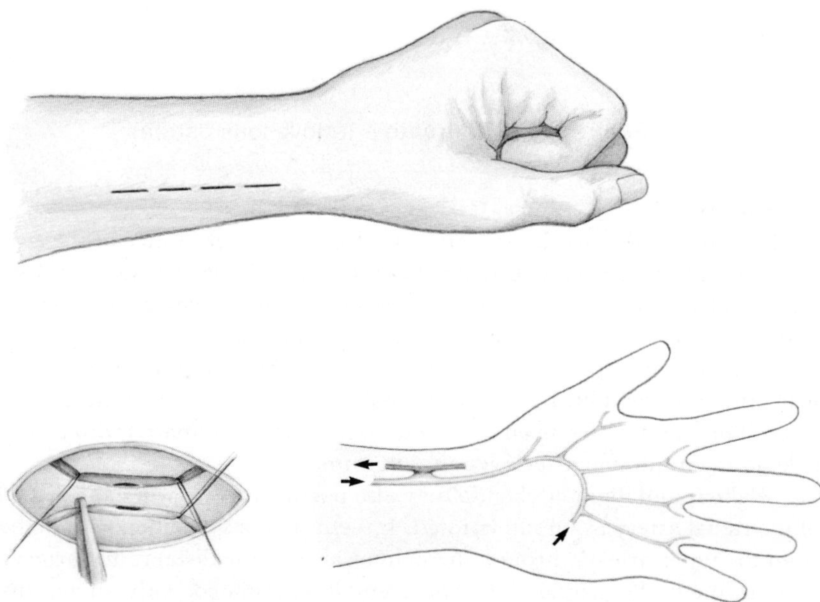

Figure 14–5. Distal arteriovenous fistula.

that is selected to accept the arterial flow. A medial and a lateral skin flap are undermined, and both vessels are identified and dissected free for a 3- to 4-cm length. Arterial and venous branches that are encountered are doubly ligated and divided. Regional installation of heparinized saline (5000 units in 250 ml normal saline) is used for anticoagulation. For a side-to-side anastomosis, proximal and distal control is accomplished with fine silastic vessel loops held under moderate tension in opposing directions so that the artery faces the vein (Fig. 14–5). A small vascular clamp is used for complete proximal control of the arterial flow.

A lateral arteriotomy and a venotomy are started with a fine blade and are enlarged with fine scissors for a total length of 8 to 10 mm. We prefer the use of 6–0 or 7–0 prolene for the anastomosis. Meticulous technique with accurate and precise suturing of the proximal corner are requirements for success. The use of magnifying loops is optional. A trill and a good pulse on the proximal part of the vein should be present at the completion of the anastomosis. The lack of these findings, even if a pulse is present on the distal portion of the vein, indicates a technical error and demands a revision at this time.

For an end-to-side and an end-to-end distal arteriovenous fistula (Fig. 14-6), the above steps are followed, and the anastomosis is appropriately constructed. The wound is closed in two layers, and a light dressing is applied.

Figure 14–6. Alternate arteriovenous fistulas.

Problems

Early failure of the fistula presents with lack of disappearance of the trill, the bruit, and the pulse in the proximal vein. It is due either to technical error or to inadequate venous outflow with high resistance. The former is a technical error, and the latter is the result of faulty operative judgment.

Venous incompetence occurs occasionally, resulting in edema, increased warmth, and even bluish discoloration of the hand. It is due to the presence of arterial pressure in the distal limb of the vein and is eliminated with an end-to-side or an end-to-end arteriovenous anastomosis.

Palmar and digital ischemia may also pose a problem when the distal limb of the radial artery is not interrupted. It seems that a steal phenomenon occurs from the ulnar artery, through the palmar arch to the distal radial artery, and then through the fistula. This problem is eliminated with an end-to-end anastomosis. Despite the above disadvantages of a side-to-side fistula, it is the one that most surgeons know how to do well, and it is an operation that works well. We prefer the side-to-side fistula with ligation of both the artery and vein distally so it is functionally and end-to-end fistula.

PROXIMAL ARTERIOVENOUS FISTULA

Creation of a distal arteriovenous fistula provides an excellent route for dialysis without significantly affecting cardiac output. Arteriovenous fistulas constructed closer to the heart (Fig. 14–7) tend to have high flows and may present serious hemodynamic problems. The conventional side-to-side arteriovenous fistula in the antecubital fossa may deliver 500 to 800 ml/minute, which could alter the cardiovascular dynamics. It also has a preferential antegrade flow in the proximal venous limb so that the distal venous system of the forearm fails to distend and arterialize. These two major problems are eliminated with a distal end-to-side arteriovenous anastomosis.

Procedure

Axillary block or general anesthesia is used. A transverse or S-shaped incision is made as for exposure of distal brachial artery. The basilic or the medial basilic vein is dissected free. The bicipital aponeurosis is severed, and the bifurcation of the brachial artery is exposed. The distal brachial artery is dissected, and proximal and distal control of the vessel is achieved. A 4- to 5-mm arteriotomy is

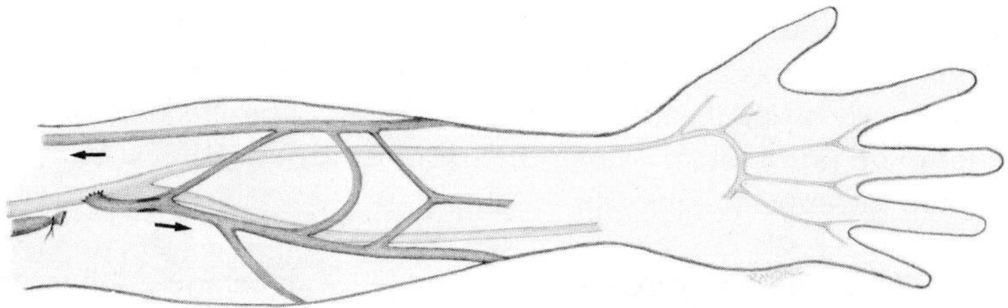

Figure 14–7. Proximal arteriovenous fistula.

made, and the previously dissected vein is proximally ligated and distally transected. A No. 3F dilator is inserted in the vein until a valve is encountered. This valve is destroyed to allow for retrograde flow. An end-to-side venoarterial anastomosis is done with 6–0 prolene sutures. The wound is closed in layers.

Problems

Early failure can occur either as a result of poor venous runoff or because of inability of the arterial pressure to induce retrograde flow in the veins of the forearm, usually associated with the presence of a *competent valve* in the proximity of the anastomosis. This can be prevented with destruction of the valve by introduction of a probe or a small vein dilator in the lumen of the transected vein. The process of retrograde arterialization leads to relative venous incompetence and to possible development of slight edema of the forearm.

GRAFTS IN THE FOREARM

An arteriovenous fistula is considered the primary procedure for long-term hemodialysis in the majority of patients. But there is the occasional patient with hypoplastic or thrombosed superficial veins who is not a good candidate for a primary procedure. There is also a larger group of patients who have been on dialysis for some time with shunts and fistulas that have failed. Both these groups of patients need a vascular conduit for their survival and present a challenge to the surgeon who is in charge of their care.

In angioaccess surgery, there is a great demand for vessels, and one should try to utilize the most distal portion of any available vessel. Use of various vascular grafts allows the surgeon to establish a vascular route in the forearm or the upper arm. The grafts used are autogenous saphenous vein, bovine heterografts, and prosthetic tubes made with Dacron or *PTFE. Polytetrofluoroethylene* has gained wide acceptance for this use. They are placed subcutaneously in a straight or a looped configuration. They may deliver flow volumes ranging from *300 to 800 ml/minute.*

Straight Grafts

Most shunts and fistulas fail because of inadequate venous runoff. In these instances, the arteries are still patent distally, and they can be effectively utilized in the absence of an infection. We favor the use of the distal radial artery and the basilic vein in the antecubital fossa.

Procedure.   The whole upper extremity is prepped with betadine solution, and adequate exposure of the forearm is achieved. Local anesthesia is usually sufficient. The distal radial artery is approached as previously described. The basilic or medial basilic vein is exposed through a transverse skin incision placed medially in the antecubital fossa. A straight subcutaneous tunnel is created between the exposed vessels by use of a tunneling forceps or a pair of dissecting scissors. An appropriate-sized graft is selected and prepared for the anastomosis. Regional heparinization is sufficient (5000 units heparin in 250 cc normal saline). Under adequate vascular control, a longitudinal venotomy is performed, and the graft is sutured in place with 6–0 prolene continuous suture. The graft is then passed through the tunnel, shortened, and tailored for anastomosis with the radial artery. With the arterial flow controlled, an arteriotomy is made, and the graft is sutured to the artery with the same material. Before completion of the anastomosis, the graft is unclamped and allowed to fill with venous blood. Also, the artery is temporarily unclamped to allow flushing of the vessel. Then the last one or two sutures are placed, and arteriovenous flow is established through the graft (Fig. 14–8). The wounds are closed in two layers.

Looped Grafts

Whenever the status of the distal artery is unsuitable for placement of a graft, a more proximal artery has to be used. Many surgeons consider the creation of an arteriovenous communication with use of a looped graft the ''secondary'' procedure of choice. It allows use of the longer graft technique and it also preserves adequate flow in the distal upper extremity.

Procedure.   With the whole upper limb prepped and draped, anesthesia is achieved with skin infiltration of 1 percent lidocaine. A 5-cm-long skin incision is made 1 cm distal to the antecubital crease. The distal brachial artery and the basilic vein are exposed for a 3-cm length, as previously described. A 6- or 8-mm prosthetic graft is selected and appropriately prepared according to its nature. After regional heparinization and flow control with small vascular clamps or silastic loops, a 1-cm anterolateral arteriotomy is performed. The placement of the arteriotomy and a 45- to 60-degree beveling of the graft are essential in order to avoid angulation or torsion of the graft and the artery (Fig. 14–9). The anastomosis is performed with 5–0 prolene suture. The subcutaneous route of the graft is then marked with a sterile marking pen on the skin. The area to be

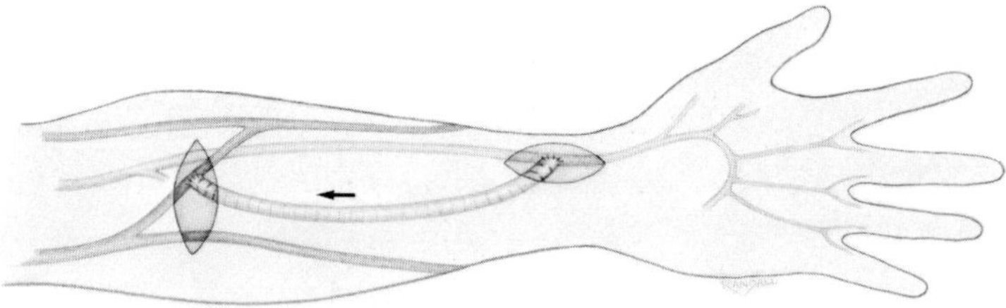

Figure 14-8. Straight graft in the forearm.

tunneled as well as the area for the 2-cm-long incision at the apex of the loop are anesthetized. The tunnel is created with tissue scissors or tunneling forceps. The graft is marked alongside its anterior surface in order to secure proper orientation during the two-step subcutaneous placement. Once the graft is in the subcutaneous position, it is trimmed and beveled at the distal end and sutured end to side with 6-0 prolene sutures to the basilic vein. The clamps are removed, and flow is established. Both the transverse and the vertical incisions are closed in two layers. The looped configuration allows insertion of a 30 to 40 cm graft, which offers sufficient length for multiple punctures. The graft can be used in 2 weeks or even sooner if absolutely necessary.

Problems

Thrombosis of the graft is not infrequent and should be managed by thrombectomy and possibly revision of the graft. Proper puncture of these grafts in alternate sites and avoidance of excessive pressure at the end of a dialysis session are essential in order to prolong the life of the graft. A thrombosed but not infected graft may remain in place. However, an infected prosthetic graft should be removed, and the patient should be protected with appropriate antibiotics.

GRAFTS IN THE UPPER ARM

Prosthetic grafts may be placed in the upper arm, between the axillary artery and the basilic or cephalic vein (Fig. 14-10). The subcutaneous placement of the

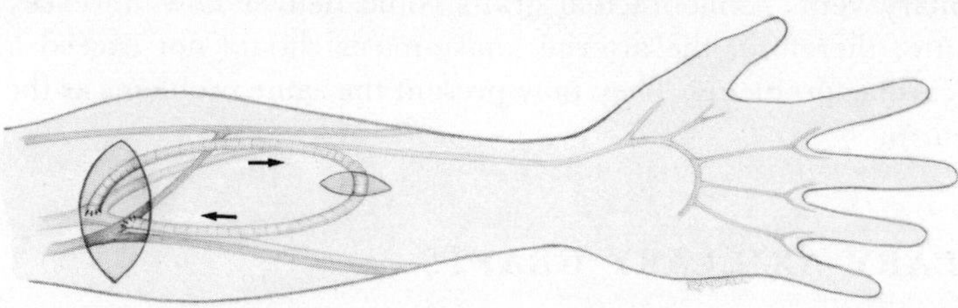

Figure 14-9. Looped graft in the forearm.

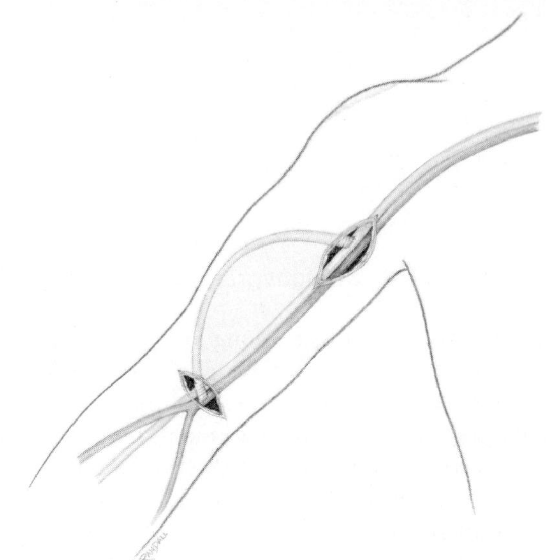

Figure 14–10. Axillobrachial graft.

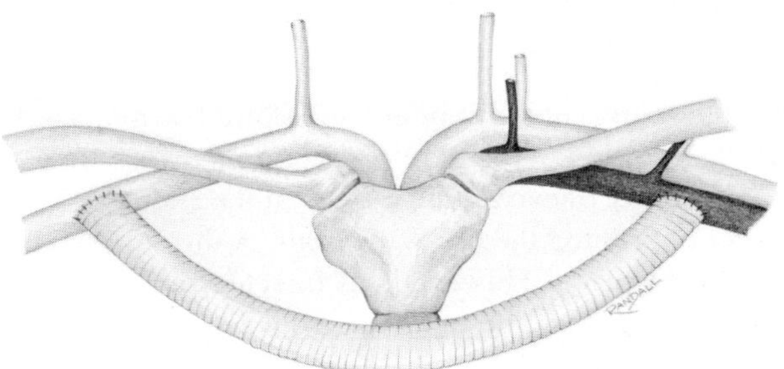

Figure 14–11. Axilloaxillary graft.

graft allows easy access for hemodialysis. The technique involves dissection of the distal axillary artery through a longitudinal incision and dissection of the basilic vein through a small transverse incision. We prefer to use brachial artery and axillary vein. Axillobrachial grafts could deliver flows in excess of 600 ml/minute; therefore, the arterial anastomosis should not exceed 5 mm to reduce cardiac problems. They may present the same problems as the graft in the forearm.

AXILLARY–AXILLARY GRAFTS

The axillary artery and the controlateral axillary vein may be connected through a subcutaneously placed, necklace-shaped, prosthetic graft (Fig. 14–11). We prefer the use of an 8-mm PTFE graft. Each vessel is exposed through a separate subclavicular skin incision after separation of the fibers of the pectoralis major muscles. Flow through these grafts is excellent.

BIBLIOGRAPHY

Brescia MJ, Camino JE, Appel K., et al: Chronic hemodialysis using venipuncture and a surgically created arteriovenous fistula. *New Engl J. Med.* 275:1089, 1966.

Burdick FJ, Scott W, Cosmi B: Experience with Dacron graft arteriovenous fistulas for dialysis access. *Ann Surg* 187:262, 1978.

Butler GH, Baker DL, Johnson MJ: Vascular access for chronic hemodialysis: PTFE versus bovine heterografts. *Am J Surg* 134:791–793, 1977.

Ehrenfeld KW, Grausz H, Wylie JE: Subcutaneous arteriovenous fistula for hemodialysis. *Am J Surg* 124:200–206, 1972.

Haimov M, Burrows L, et al: Alternatives for vascular access for hemodialysis experience with autogenous vein-saphenous vein autografts and bovine heterografts. *Surgery* 75:447, 1974.

Haimov M, Baez A, et al: Complications of arteriovenous fistulas for hemodialysis. *Arch Surg* 110:708, 1975.

Kaplan SM, Mirahmadis K, et al: Comparison of PTFE and bovine grafts for blood access in dialysis patients. *Trans Am Soc Artif Intern Organs* 22:388, 1976.

Lefrak AE, Noon PG: Surgical technique for creation of an arteriovenous fistula using a looped bovine graft. *Ann Surg* 182:782, 1975.

May J, Tiller D, et al: Saphenous vein arteriovenous fistula in regular dialysis treatment. *New Eng J Med* 280:770, 1969.

Mohaideen AH, Avram MM, Mainzer AR: Polyterrafluoroethylene grafts for arteriovenous fistula—preliminary report. *N Y State J Med* 76:2152, 1976.

Quinton WE, Dillard DE, Cole JJ, et al: Eight months' experience with silastic-teflon bypass cannulas. *Trans Am Soc Artif Intern Organs* 8:236, 1962.

Paruk S, Koenig M, et al: Arteriovenous fistulas for hemodialysis in 100 consecutive patients. *Am J Surg,* 131:552, 1976.

Ramirez O, Swartz C, et al: The winged in line shunt. *Trans Am Soc Artif Intern Organs* 12:220–221, 1966.

Rosenthal JJ, Spigelman A, et al: Problems with bovine heterografts for hemodialysis-recognition, correction, and prevention. *Am J Surg* 130:182, 1975.

Salomon J, Vidne F, et al: Our experience with the use of A–V fistula in chronic dialysis: modified surgical technique. *Surgery* 63:899–902, 1968.

Schwartz AB, DeClement FA, et al: Conversion of external A–V hemodialysis shunt to internal fistula. *JAMA* 239:1782, 1978.

Shimizu A, Triedi H, et al: Straight A–V shunt for long term hemodialysis. *JAMA* 216:645, 1971.

CHAPTER FIFTEEN

Surgery In Portal Hypertension

INTRODUCTION

Portal hypertension is usually the result of increased resistance to blood flow as it passes through the portal venous system. In most patients, it is caused by cirrhosis of the liver. The increased pressure stimulates the development of various collateral pathways that drain portal venous blood directly into the systemic venous circulation. Of these collateral beds, the most significant one is located at the esophagogastric junction. The submucosal gastroesophageal varices often rupture spontaneously, resulting in massive and often fatal hemorrhage. The surgeon's task is (1) to surgically control bleeding from gastroesophageal varices when all conservative measures have failed and (2) to decompress selectively the portal circulation in patients who have already suffered one or more episodes of variceal bleeding.

DIAGNOSIS

The presence of esophageal varices should be suspected in all cirrhotic patients who develop upper gastrointestinal bleeding. Hepatomegaly, jaundice, spleno-megaly, ascites, and vascular spiders are all findings frequently encountered in patients with chronic liver disease. The laboratory investigation may reveal compromised hepatic function, anemia, and coagulation deficits.

The specific diagnosis of bleeding esophageal varices can be reached with the following diagnostic techniques:

Endoscopy

Fiberoptic gastroesophagoscopy, when performed by a competent endoscopist, will accurately diagnose the presence of bleeding varices and rule out other causes of hemorrhage. This procedure should be carried out first in the work-up for upper gastrointestinal bleeding.

Selective Angiography

Recent improvements in angiographic techniques to evaluate the splanchnic vasculature represent a major advance in the management of patients with portal hypertension. The availability of retrograde femoral mesenteric angiography has almost completely eliminated the need for preoperative splenoportography. Mesenteric angiography provides considerable information that is helpful in evaluating the patient and planning for an appropriate operation. It has also been of therapeutic value in stopping esophageal variceal bleeding by a pitressin infusion into the superior mesenteric artery. The typical tortuosity of intrahepatic arteries supports the diagnosis of cirrhosis. An aberrant hepatic artery can be visualized. Essential information regarding the patency of the portal, superior mesenteric, and splenic veins can be obtained. Esophageal varices can be visualized. However, visualization of the bleeding site from the esophageal varix by visceral arteriography is very rare.

Splenoportography

Splenoportography was the conventional diagnostic procedure before the availability of retrograde femoral mesenteric angiography. Splenoportography, however, has several advantages: (1) it can measure the splenic *pulp pressure* to document the presence of portal hypertension; (2) it can give more accurate information relevant to the diameter of the splenic and portal veins; and (3) it can visualize esophagogastric varices better than any other diagnostic procedure. However, it is associated with the risk of bleeding and is usually done immediately before scheduled surgery.

Upper Gastrointestinal Series

An upper gastrointestinal series, including esophagogram, gives only information as to whether or not esophageal varices and any other lesions are present. It cannot demonstrate the bleeding site. We no longer use it in the diagnosis of acute gastrointestinal bleeding.

Sengstaken-Blakemore Tube

Since its initial introduction in 1945, this double-balloon tube has been extensively employed in the management of variceal hemorrhage. This tube is effective in temporarily ceasing bleeding from the esophageal varices of the majority of patients. Therefore, it is of diagnostic as well as therapeutic value. The complications associated with the use of this tube include: (1) *aspiration* of blood and nasopharyngeal secretions that may accumulate above the balloon; (2) erosion, laceration, or *rupture* of the esophagus from the pressure of the inflated balloon; and (3) *asphyxiation* from the gastric balloon's being drawn up by external weights to the level of the larynx.

TREATMENT

Decision Making

The patient who is diagnosed to be actively bleeding from esophageal varices should be initially treated *conservatively*. Control of the acute hemorrhage may be obtained with: (1) a Sengstaken-Blakemore tube and (2) intravenous infusion of pitressin or, preferably, intra-arterial infusion through a catheter with the tip placed in the superior mesenteric artery. Occasionally, both of the above therapeutic maneuvers are necessary in order to cease the bleeding. The goal of this conservative management is to allow enough time for optimal preparation of the patient before a definite elective procedure of portal decompression.

Although the majority of patients with active variceal bleeding will favorably respond to the above treatment, an occasional patient may develop multiple repeated episodes of bleeding within a short period of time or may suffer bleeding that is resistant to all conservative measures. In this last small group of patients, *an emergency procedure to control the bleeding is necessary*. The procedures that are available for the surgical control of acute variceal bleeding are (1) *direct shunting* procedures and (2) *nonshunting* procedures that directly attack the bleeding site. If shunting is elected, the surgeon should attempt to achieve definite portal decompression with an operation that can be performed within a reasonably short period of time.

The end-to-side portocaval shunt or the H-graft mesocaval shunt seem to meet the above relative criteria. If a nonshunting procedure is elected for immediate control of the bleeding, it should be realized that it does not offer adequate protection from a recurrent episode of variceal bleeding.

Preoperative Care and Evaluation

Once an acute episode of variceal bleeding is under control, the patient should be considered for portal decompression. Intensive medical treatment and proper nutritional support are essential in order to decrease the degree of ascites and to improve the nitrogen balance.

The preoperative evaluation of a patient scheduled for surgery may include:

1. *Percutaneous liver biopsy.* If there is evidence of tissue necrosis or acute alcoholic hepatitis, surgery should be postponed.
2. *Arteriography.* Splenic and superior mesenteric arteriography with venous phase are necessary in order to define the degree of portal perfusion and visualize the anatomy of the portal system (Fig. 15–1).
3. *Venography.* This will demonstrate the hepatic veins and allow measurement of the hepatic *wedge pressure.* If selective distal splenorenal shunt is considered, a *left renal* venogram with or without pressure measurement is essential in order to locate the renal vein in relation to the splenic vein.
4. *Electroencephalogram (EEG).* Patients who demonstrate slowing on EEG are considered subclinically encephalopathic and are in high risk of developing postoperative encephalopathy.

The day before surgery, the patient should undergo mechanical bowel preparation. Prophylactic antibiotics and cimetidine are started 6 hours prior to surgery.

Operative Procedures

Shunting Procedures. *Portocaval Shunt.*   Transportal decompression successfully decompresses gastroesophageal varices and protects against recurrent variceal bleeding. For this reason, it is considered the procedure of choice in emergency situations and, by some, in elective cases, too. As pharmacologic control of encephalopathy is now visible in most patients, this procedure is much appreciated because it offers long-term, excellent portal decompression.

There are three types of portocaval shunts, depending on the tailoring of the anastomosis between the portal vein and the inferior vena cava: (1) an *end-to-side* portocaval shunt with ligation of the distal portal vein assures portal decompression and effectively prevents recurrence of variceal bleeding. (2) A *side-to-side* portocaval shunt effectively relieves portal hypertension. Its disadvantages are (a) a technical problem in freeing the vessel for a long enough segment to allow construction of a shunt and (b) the shunt's permission of retrograde flow away from the liver through the distal portal vein, which may accelerate the development of hepatic failure and higher incidence of encephalopathy. (3) An *H-graft* interposition shunt between the portal vein and the inferior vena cava functions as a side-to-side shunt. In certain patients, it may be technically easier to perform than the other procedures, but it carries with it an increased risk of thrombosis.

Operative Technique.   The patient is placed in the left lateral position. The abdomen is entered through an extended right subcostal incision. The liver is retracted cephalad, exposing the hilum. The duodenum is mobilized with a Kocher maneuver. The portal vein is situated posteriorly to the common bile duct and the hepatic artery (Fig. 15–2). With gentle medial and forward retrac-

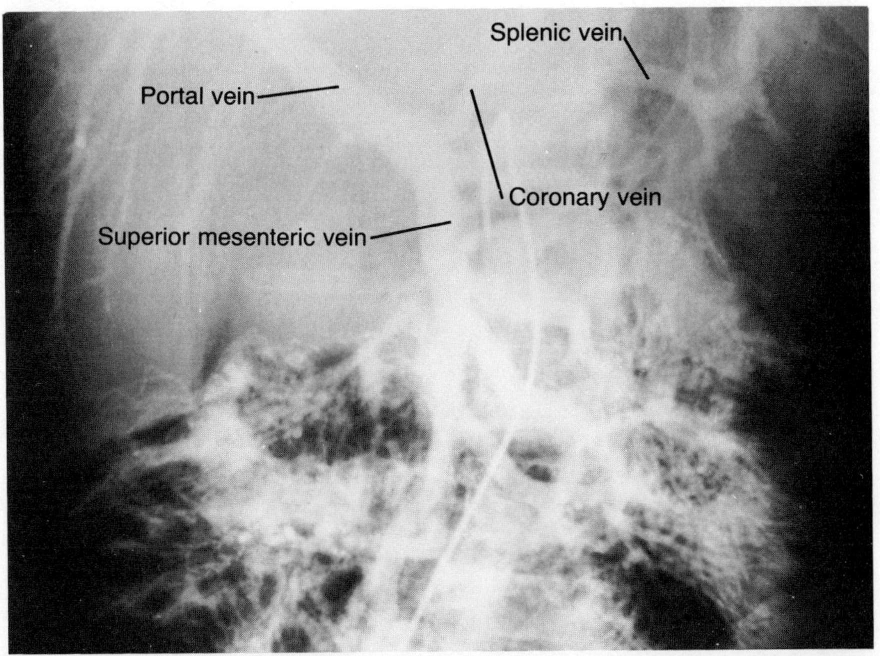

Figure 15-1. Portal circulation.

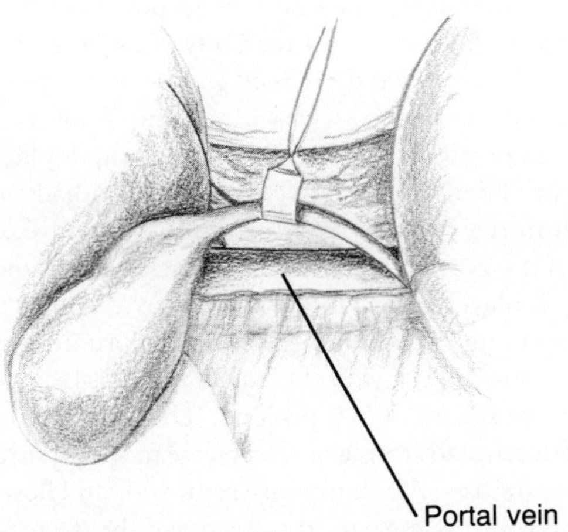

Figure 15-2. The portal vein.

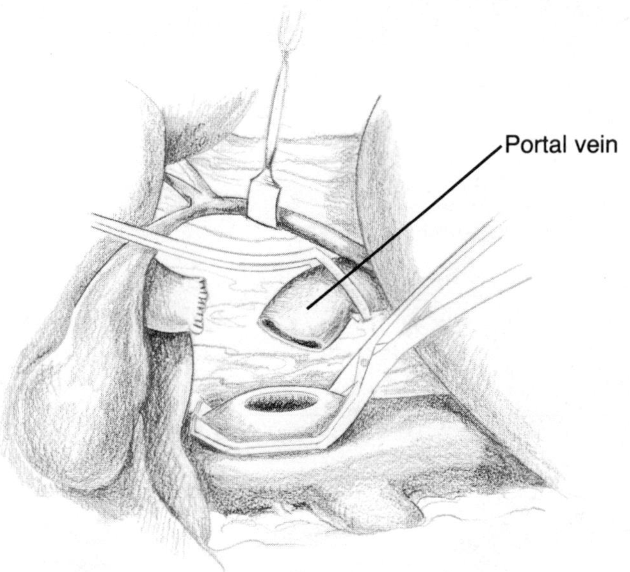

Figure 15–3. End-to-side portocaval shunt.

tion of the hilar structures and the gall bladder, the peritoneum that covers the portal vein is incised, and the portal vein is dissected free with combined blunt and sharp dissection. Silastic vessel loops are placed around it. The *portal pressure* is now measured through a No. 19 needle. Then the inferior vena cava is exposed through an incision over the retroperitoneum. The pressure in the vena cava should also be measured. The suprarenal portion of the inferior vena cava is dissected anteriorly, laterally, and medially. For an end-to-side anastomosis, the surgeon should assure that there is *adequate length* for portal vein mobilization in order to reach the vena cava. A vascular clamp is placed on the portal vein as close to the liver as possible. Another vascular clamp is placed close to the origin of the portal vein. Then the portal vein is divided adjacent to the distal clamp, and the distal stump is oversewn with continuous suture of 5–0 prolene. Once this distal end of the portal vein is closed, the clamp is removed. Then a partial occlusion clamp is placed on the inferior vena cava, and an anterior venotomy is performed, long enough to accommodate the cut proximal end of the portal vein (Fig. 15–3). The posterior row of the anastomosis is best done with continuous transverse mattress suture of 5–0 prolene. The anterior row is completed with continuous or interrupted simple or transverse mattress sutures, assuring an unconstricting anastomosis. All clamps are removed, and flow through the shunt is established. The result is measured in terms of the decrease of portal pressure

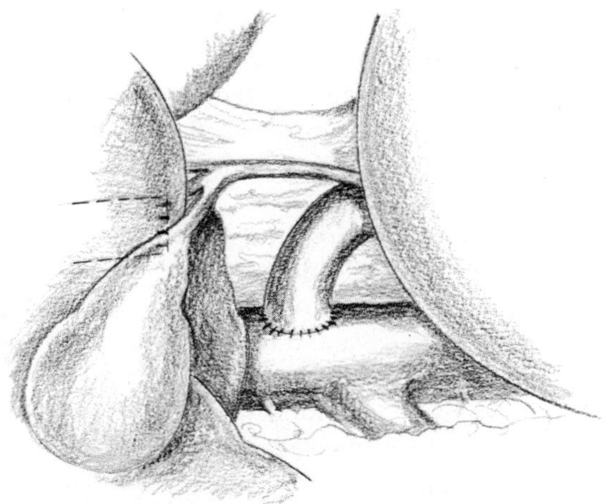

Figure 15-4. Portocaval shunt.

that is accomplished before and at the end of the end-to-side portocaval shunt (Fig. 15–4).

For a side-to-side shunt, the two vessels should be close to each other so that the anastomosis can be done without tension. Otherwise, an H-graft (Dacron or PTFE, 14 to 16 mm) may be interposed between the IVC and the portal vein (Fig. 15–5). A large caudate lobe can be partially resected with electrocauterization.

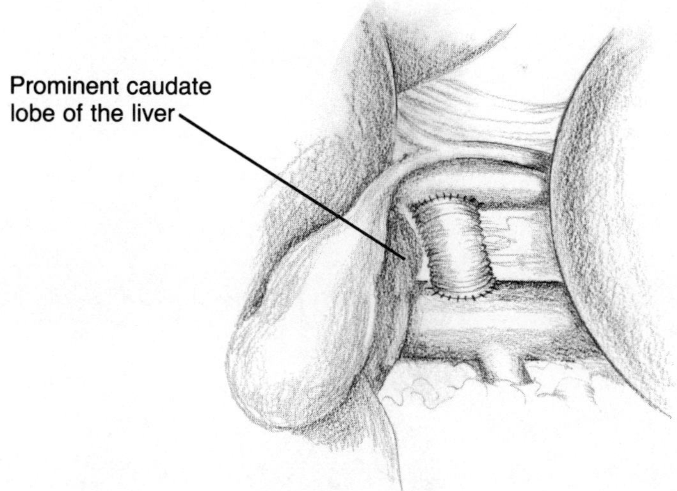

Figure 15-5. Portocaval shunt with an H-graft.

Mesocaval Shunt. The mesocaval shunt was originally introduced for relief of portal hypertension in pediatric patients with portal vein thrombosis. The vena cava is divided at the confluence of the common iliac veins. The distal stump is oversewn with continuous suture of 5–0 prolene, and the proximal end of the inferior vena cava is anastomosed end to side to the superior mesenteric artery (Fig. 15–6).

This original concept has been recently modified and applied in the treatment of portal hypertension with bleeding esophageal varices in the adult. It is now performed with the interposition of a prosthetic graft or a piece of jugular vein between the inferior vena cava and the superior mesenteric vein. For this reason, it is known as an *H-graft interposition shunt.* This procedure is a rather easy one to perform and effectively decompresses the portal circulation. The incidence of encephalopathy with a mesocaval interposition shunt is lower than it is with a portocaval shunt. A mesocaval interposition shunt is not contraindicated in the patient with a small amount of ascites. The main disadvantage of a mesocaval interposition shunt is that the graft may eventually thrombose in 15 to 20 percent of patients.

Operative Technique. The abdomen is entered through a long midline incision. The transverse mesocolon is retracted superiorly, exposing the root of the small bowel mesentery. The superior mesenteric vein is located on the patient's right in relationship to the artery. Another landmark for the identification of the

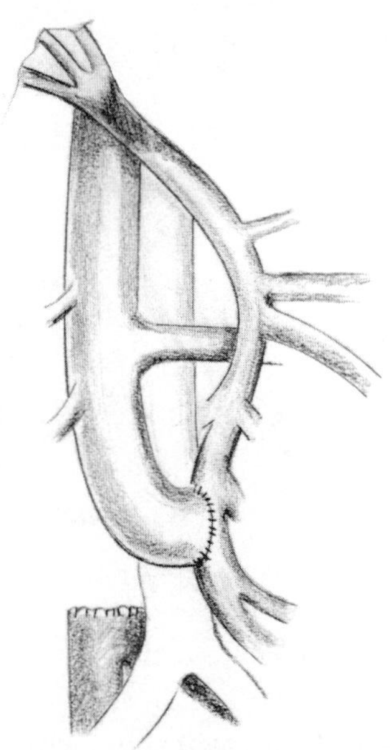

Figure 15–6. Mesocaval shunt.

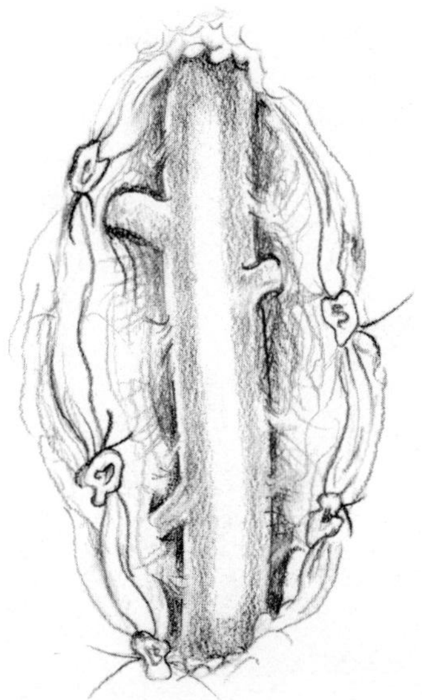

Figure 15–7. Superior mesenteric vein.

location of the vein is to follow the middle colic vein that crosses in the groove that is formed by the transverse mesocolon and the small bowel mesentery. The peritoneum is incised along the proposed course of the superior mesenteric vein, and the vein is dissected from the surrounding tissue. As there are multiple minute venous and lymphatic channels in the mesenteric fatty tissue, we recommend the technique of clamping, dividing, and ligating small amounts of tissue on top of the mesenteric vein (Fig. 15–7). This will assure a dry field and prevent the development of postoperative ascites. Once the superior mesenteric vein has been exposed for a distance of 3 to 4 cm, the portal pressure is directly measured. The next step is to expose the inferior vena cava. This is easily done through the transverse mesocolon by dissection close to the transverse portion of the duodenum. The anterior, lateral, and medial walls of the inferior vena cava are well dissected for a distance of 4 to 5 cm. A partial occlusion clamp is applied, and an elliptical incision is made on the anterior caval wall, properly sized in order to accommodate the prosthetic graft that will be interposed. A size 16- to 20-mm Dacron or PTFE graft is used. The graft-to-cava anastomosis is performed with continuous suture of 5–0 prolene (Fig. 15–8). It is now passed through a tunnel in the mesentery and is properly tailored for the anastomosis with a superior mesenteric vein. It should be confirmed that the graft will be neither redundant nor under tension. The superior mesenteric vein is clamped both proximally and distally with soft vascular clamps. A medially placed venotomy is performed, and the graft is sutured to the vein with continuous suture of 5–0 prolene (Fig.

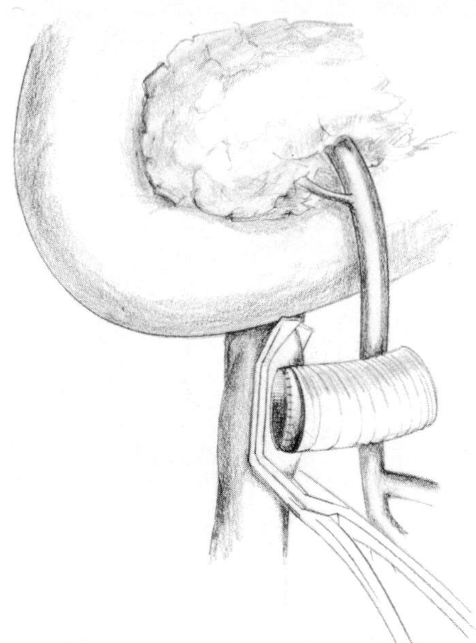

Figure 15-8. Mesocaval shunt.

15-9). The posterior row is best sutured with a *transverse mattress* technique. This will prevent an occasional inversion of the posterior anastomosis that renders the procedure thrombogenic. The anterior row is completed with continuous over-and-over sutures. Once the graft is in place, the portal pressure and the pressure across the graft are measured. If the portal pressure is not significantly reduced, a technical problem should be suspected and corrected at this time. The mesentery is reperitonealized, and the wound is closed in layers. The principles of this procedure are (1) dissection of the superior mesenteric vein first, (2) performance of the caval anastomosis first, and (3) provision for adequate length, usually 4 to 5 cm, and proper alignment of the graft.

Distal Splenorenal Shunt.   The distal splenorenal shunt is designed to selectively decompress gastroesophageal varices. It consists of (1) an end-to-side anastomosis between the distal splenic vein and the renal vein, (2) ligation of the *coronary vein* where it joins the portal vein, and (3) extensive *gastric devascularization* along the greater curvature of the stomach except for short gastric veins.

This shunt has proven to be effective in preventing recurrent variceal bleeding. It has additional advantages in that it does not decrease the nutritional flow to the liver and does not increase the incidence of postshunt encephalopathy. It is indicated as an elective procedure for variceal decompression in cirrhotic patients who have controllable ascites and no history of previous splenectomy. In the presence of slight or moderate ascites, a distal splenorenal shunt can be safely performed with subsequent placement of a peritoneal-jugular shunt. The mortality rate of this operation is in the range of 5 to 7 percent, which is comparable to that of other portal decompression procedures. The results of this procedure have been reported to be favorable for the majority of patients.

Operative Technique. The patient is positioned supine with the left flank and lower chest elevated. A bilateral subcostal incision with an extension to the left flank is performed, or a long midline incision is used. Once the abdomen is entered, an exploration is performed. The presence of small or moderate amounts of *ascitic fluid* should not be considered as a contraindication to the performance of a distal splenorenal shunt. The *falciform ligament* is ligated and divided. This will eliminate a collateral pathway to the umbilical vein. The next step is division of the *gastrocolic omentum* that extends from the pylorus to the short gastric vessels. This may be done close to the stomach, interrupting the gastroepiploic vessels. The stomach is retracted cephalad, and the lesser sac is entered. The posterior parietal peritoneum is divided alongside the inferior border of the pancreas. This will allow upward mobilization of the entire pancreas. The splenic vein that lies on the posterior surface of the pancreas can now be seen and palpated. The adventitial tissue is incised, and the posterior surface of the vein is dissected. Following this, the anterior surface of the vein is dissected as far medially as the junction of the superior mesenteric and splenic veins. If the inferior mesenteric vein joins the splenic vein, it is doubly ligated and divided

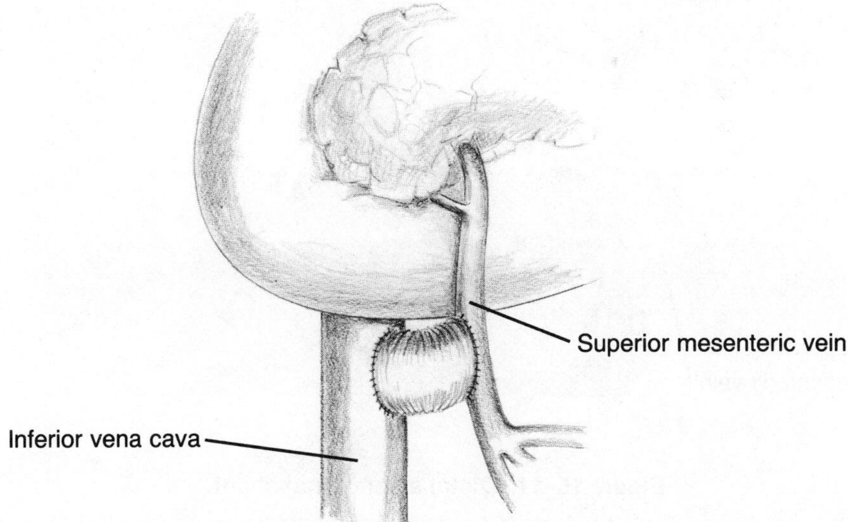

Figure 15–9. Mesocaval shunt.

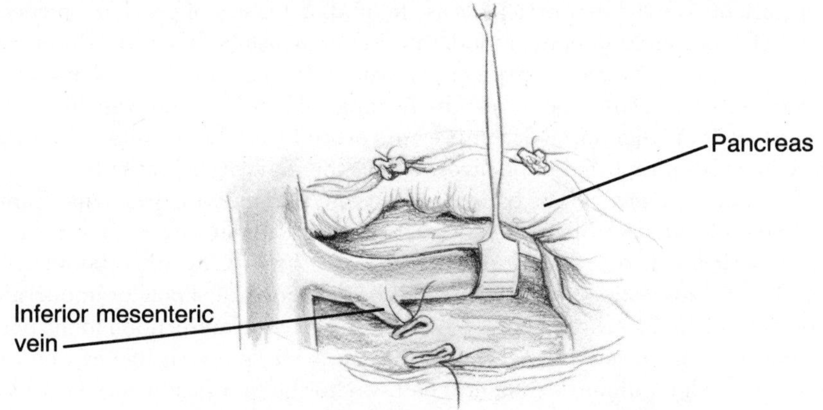

Figure 15–10. Distal splenorenal shunt.

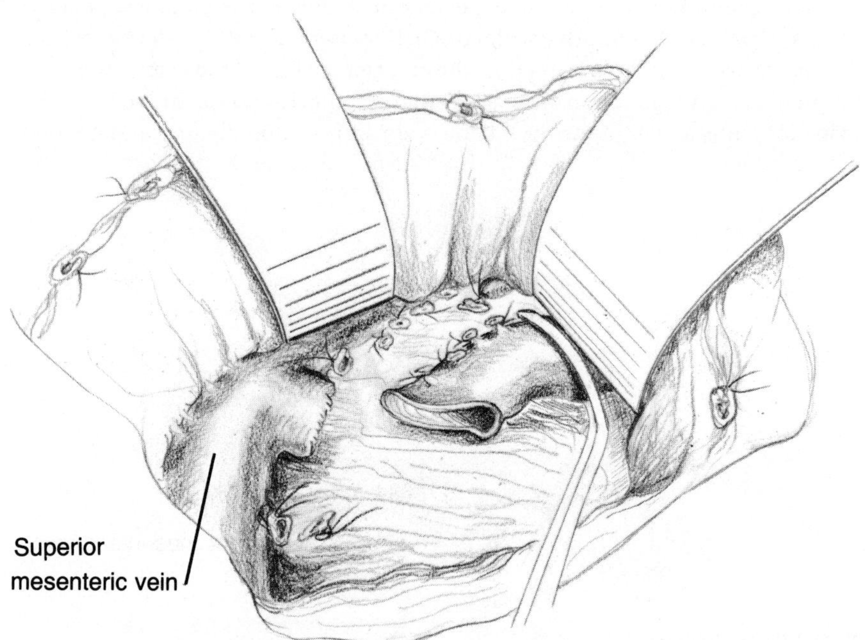

Figure 15–11. Distal splenorenal shunt.

(Fig. 15–10). The splenic vein is then divided between two vascular clamps right at its junction with the superior mesenteric and portal veins. The medial end is oversewn with continuous suture of 5–0 prolene (Fig. 15–11). The divided vein is now mobilized laterally. On the superior border of the vein, there are multiple venous tributaries to the pancreas. All of these branches are securely ligated and divided so that a 4 to 5 cm segment of the vein will be free. With the small bowel mesentery retracted medially in order to protect the superior mesenteric artery, a retroperitoneal dissection proceeds in a caudal direction until the left renal vein is encountered. The adrenal vein is divided between ligatures, but the gonadal vein is left intact (Fig. 15–12). This will allow complete mobilization of the left renal vein anteriorly as well as posteriorly. A portion of the left renal vein is now selected for the anastomosis. This is done in such a way that acute angulation of the splenic vein will be avoided. An anterior-superior venotomy, equal in length with the diameter of the divided splenic vein, is performed. The posterior side of the splenorenal anastomosis is done with continuous transverse mattress suture of 5–0 prolene. Interrupted simple or mattress sutures or continuous sutures are used for the anterior side of the anastomosis. All clamps are removed, and flow is established through the shunt. The coronary vein is now isolated in its suprapancreatic retroperitoneal location. The vein is ligated twice. Any other prominent varices that are seen in the gastrohepatic ligaments are also ligated. The wound is closed in layers.

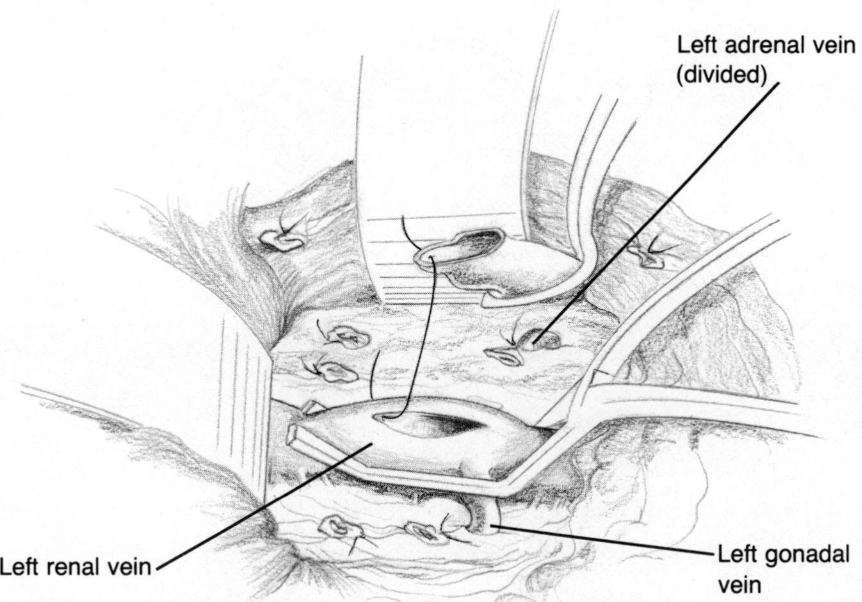

Figure 15–12. Distal splenorenal shunt.

Central Splenorenal Shunt. This is performed by an anastomosis between splenic end of splenic vein to left renal vein. It is an alternative to mesocaval shunt especially when splenectomy is indicated since the spleen is removed in this procedure. It is inferior to portacaval shunt as far as protection against recurrent bleeding and has a higher incidence of thrombosis.

Operative Technique. The spleen is first removed, then the splenic and renal veins are dissected as previously described. Anastomosis is performed between the splenic end of the splenic vein and the side of the renal vein.

Nonshunting Procedures. *Injection Sclerotherapy.* This procedure is used for control of acute variceal bleeding as well as for permanent obliteration of gastroesophageal varices. Under general anesthesia and through the rigid esophagoscope, 3 to 4 ml of sclerosing agent such as ethalolamine oleate are injected into each varix. Pressure is applied for a few minutes. This procedure is repeated every 4 to 6 weeks until all varices are obliterated.

Sugiura Procedure. This procedure aims to disconnect permanently the por-

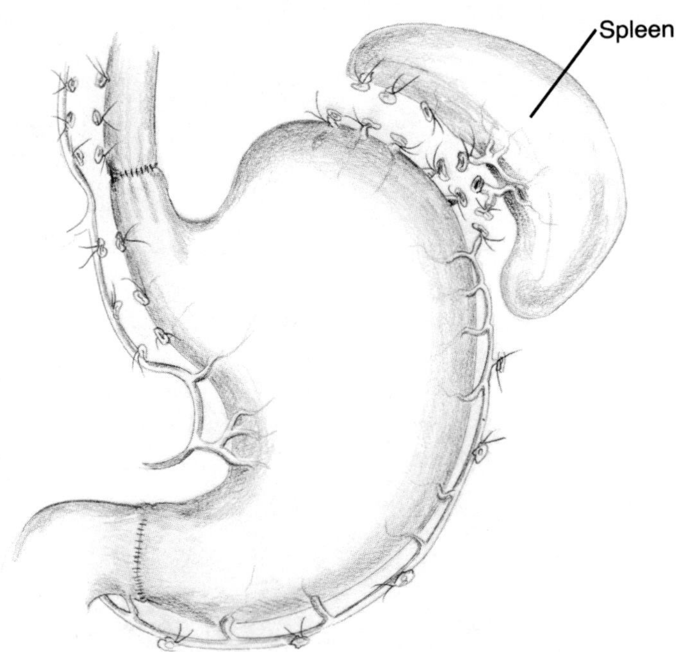

Figure 15–13. Sugiura procedure.

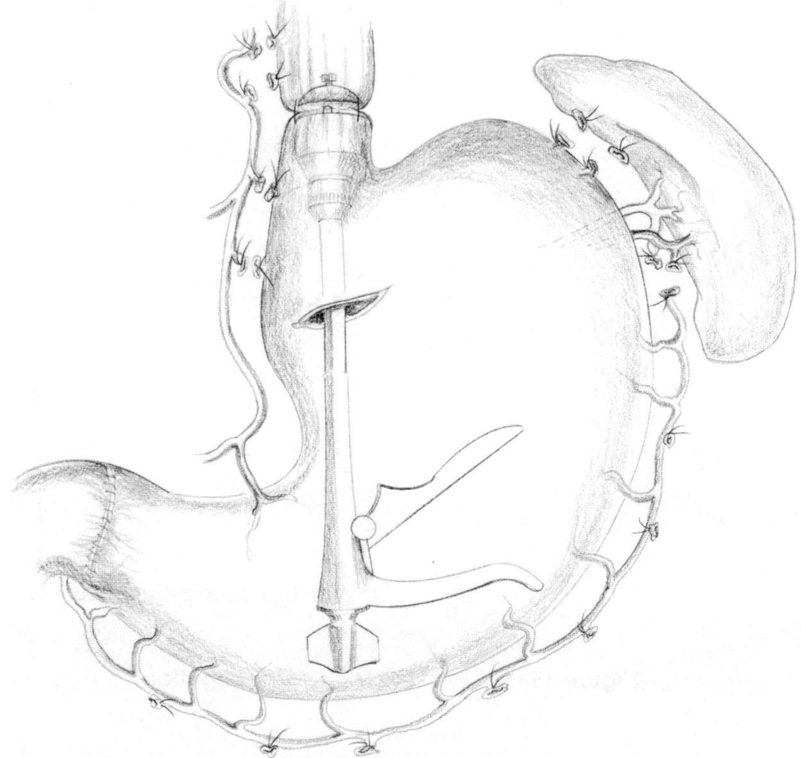

Figure 15–14. Stapling of the E-G junction.

tal system from the azygous system by eliminating the varices. It consists of complete devascularization of the esophagogastric junction, transection of the distal esophagus, and reanastomosis (Fig. 15–13). This may be accomplished either with a hand-sewn anastomosis or with use of the EEA stapler (Fig. 15–14). However, in our experience, manipulation of this instrument in the esophagogastric junction is quite difficult.

Splenectomy, Devascularization, and Intragastric Ligation of Varices (Matsumoto). This procedure is mainly indicated as a semiemergency procedure for control of acutely bleeding gastroesophageal varices resistant to all conservative measures in patients with poor hepatic function. The three major steps of this nonshunting procedure are (Fig. 15–15): (1) *splenectomy* and *devascularization of the greater curvature.* The gastrocolic ligament is divided outside the gastroepiploic arcade. All short gastric vessels are severed; (2) *division of the gastrohepatic ligament* and *ligation of the coronary vein* as it lies above the upper margin of the pancreas

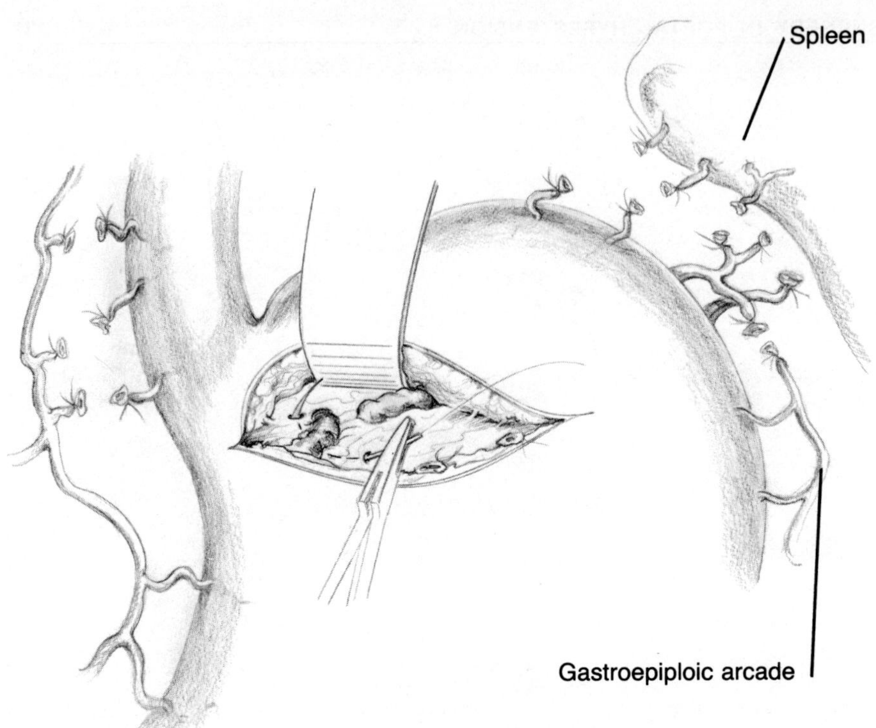

Figure 15–15. Intragastric variceal ligation.

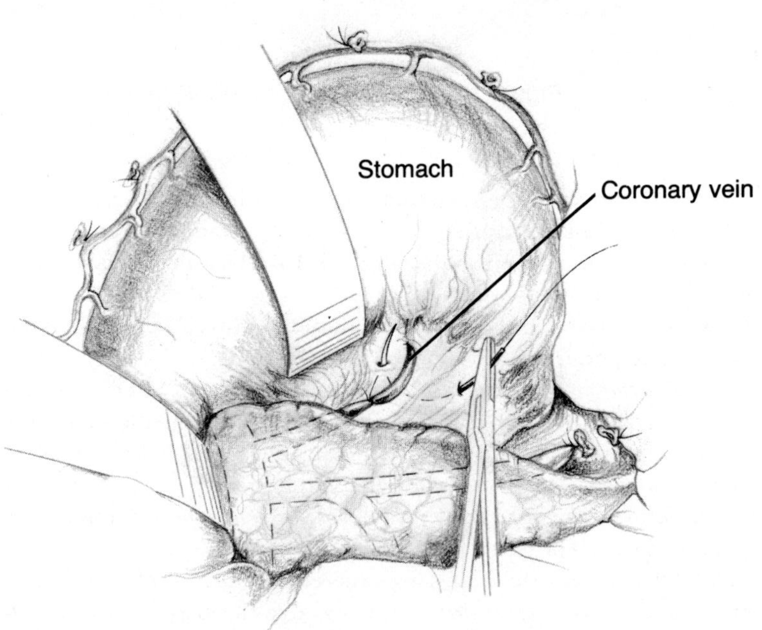

Figure 15–16. Ligation of the coronary vein.

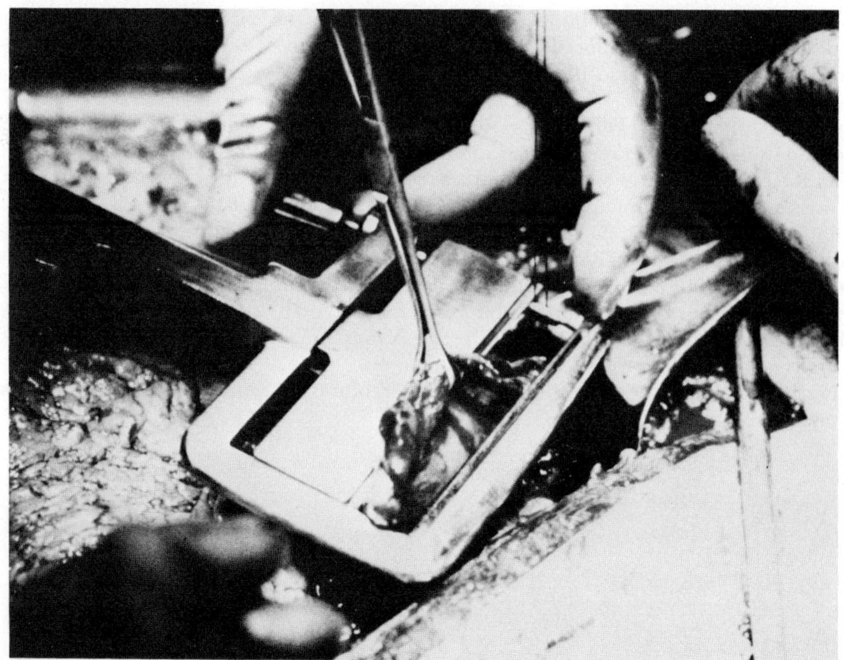

Figure 15-17. Closure of the gastrotomy.

(Fig. 15-16). The left gastric artery, the right gastric vein, and any visible retroperitoneal varices are suture ligated; and (3) *intragastric ligation of submucosal varices*. A high transverse anterior gastrotomy is performed, and all visible gastric and esophageal varices are suture ligated. The gastrotomy is closed with the TA90 stapler (Fig. 15-17).

The above procedure effectively disconnects and decompresses the submucosal esophagogastric venous plexus. Other procedures have also been described, eg, Tanner's gastric transection, Crile's transesophageal ligation of varices, etc., all of which aim at disconnecting the portal venous system from the azygos venous system.

BIBLIOGRAPHY

Blakemore AH: Portocaval shunting for portal hypertension *Surg Gynecol Obstet* 941:443, 1952.

Clatworthy AW, Wall T, Watman RN: A new type of portal to systemic venous shunt for portal hypertension. *Arch Surg* 71:588, 1955.

Cooperman AM, Hermann RG: Ligation procedures in the management of portal hypertension. *Surgery* 81:382, 1977.

DelGuercio LRM, et al: A shunt equation for estimating the splenic component of portal hypertension. *Am J Surg* 135:70, 1978.

Drapanas T: Interposition mesocaval shunt for treatment of portal hypertension. *Ann Surg* 176:435, 1972.

Jackson FC, Perrin EB, Felix WR, et al: A clinical investigation of portocaval shunt. Survival analysis of the therapeutic operation. *Ann Surg* 174:72, 1971.

Malt RA, Abbott WM, et al: Randomized trial of emergency mesocaval and portocaval shunts for bleeding esophageal varices. *Am J Surg* 135:584, 1978.

Orloff MJ, Duguay LR, Kosta LD: Criteria for selection of patients for emergency portocaval shunt. *Am J Surg* 134:146, 1977.

Reichle FA, Fahmy WF, Golsorkhi M: Prospective comparative clinical trial with distal splenorenal and mesocaval shunts. *Am J Surg* 137:13, 1979.

Rikkers LF, Rudman D, Galambos JT, et al: A randomized controlled trial of the distal splenorenal shunt. *Ann Surg* 188:271, 1978.

Sones PJ, Rude JC, Berg DO, et al: Evaluation of the left renal vein in candidates for splenorenal shunts. *Radiology* 127:357, 1978.

CHAPTER SIXTEEN

Syndromes of Intestinal Ischemia

INTRODUCTION

The blood supply of the alimentary tract is derived from the celiac axis, the superior and inferior mesenteric arteries, and the two hypogastric arteries. These vascular beds communicate with each other through numerous collateral vessels (Fig. 16–1). Arteriosclerotic disease of the visceral arteries may present either as occlusive or as aneurysmal disease. Stenosis or even occlusion of the visceral arteries is usually well compensated through various interconnecting intestinal vascular arcades. However, chronic uncompensated occlusive disease of the superior mesentery and celiac arteries results in symptomatic intestinal ischemia and requires prompt surgical treatment before the catastrophic event of fatal mesenteric infarction. The various syndromes of acute as well as chronic visceral ischemia will be individually discussed.

ACUTE OCCLUSION OF THE SUPERIOR MESENTERIC ARTERY

Mesenteric Embolism

Emboli to the superior mesenteric artery usually originate from *mural thrombi* associated with atrial fibrillation or myocardial infarction. They may also occur

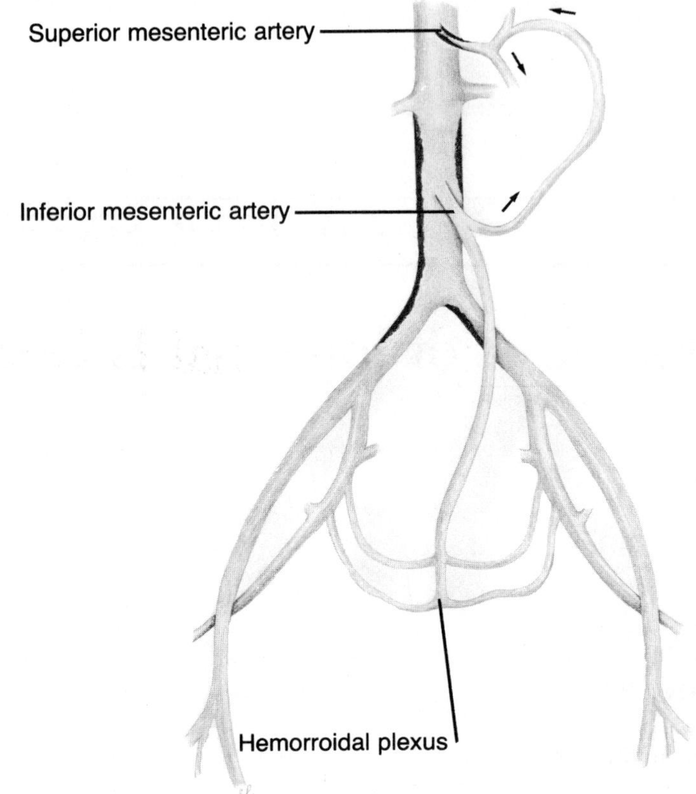

Figure 16-1. Marginal artery of Drummond.

in patients with valvular prostheses, ventricular aneurysms, and atrial myxomas.

The main symptom is cramping upper abdominal pain of *abrupt* onset. The pain soon becomes generalized. The resulting acute intestinal ischemia generates an intense muscular spasm of the bowel wall that is manifested with explosive upper and lower gastrointestinal evacuation. Various laboratory tests will reveal some rather nonspecific changes. The finding that is of great importance is the presence of significant metabolic acidosis, which should be corrected. Radiologic examination of the abdomen may demonstrate thickening of the bowel wall and the presence of gas in the intestinal wall or in the portal venous system. However, the preoperative diagnosis cannot be accurately established without arteriography. This should be done simultaneously with preparation for surgery.

The patient should be operated upon as soon as possible because prolonged ischemia is associated with irreversible tissue damage. At laparotomy, three clinical syndromes can be recognized: (1) *segmental infarction* of a portion of the small intestine. This should be managed with segmental intestinal resection and primary anastomosis, provided that the remaining intestine is of adequate length to maintain nutrition of the patient; (2) *extensive infarction* of the distal jejunum, the ileum, and right colon. In this situation, it is the length of the viable proximal jejunum that will determine the approach. If more than 2 feet of small bowel are viable, a small bowel resection and right hemicolectomy may be performed. However, if the demarcation line is very close to the ligament of Treitz, an embolectomy should be attempted, followed by a second-look operation within 24 to 48 hours; (3) *ischemia of the entire small bowel* and right colon. Any type of resection is not compatible with life. For this reason, an embolectomy followed by a second-look operation within 24 to 48 hours is the proper operative approach.

The colon is reflected cephalad, and the mesenteric root is exposed as it crosses over the duodenum. Through a transverse arteriotomy, a distal and proximal *embolectomy* is performed with use of a No. 3 Fogarty catheter (Fig. 16–2). Brisk backbleeding and satisfactory proximal flushing are usually associated with rewarding results. If no improvement is noted during the second-look operation, the only alternative in view of death is total intestinal resection and life long parenteral nutrition. Postoperative anti-coagulation should be considered in the patient who is apt to reembolize. If an extensive

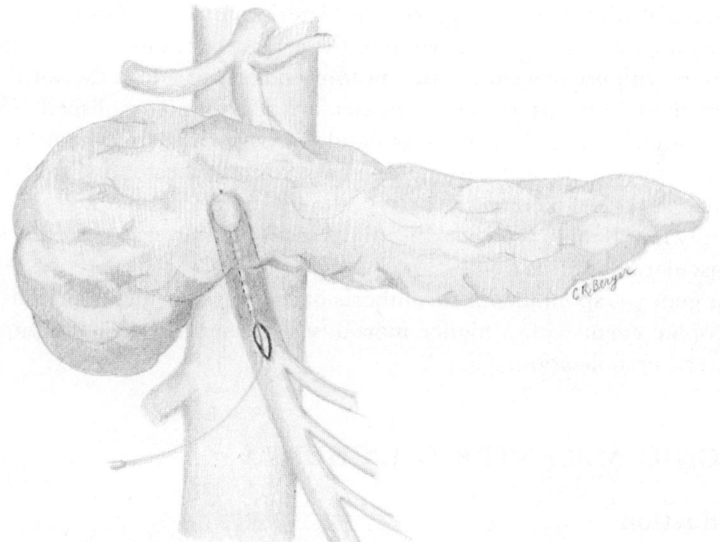

Figure 16–2. Thromboembolectomy of the superior mesenteric artery.

intestinal resection is performed, the patient should be covered with an H$_2$ blocker and antacids.

Thrombosis of the Superior Mesenteric Artery

Thrombosis of the superior mesenteric artery occurs at the site of an ulcerated arteriosclerotic lesion of this vessel. The patient often gives a history of previous gastrointestinal complaints associated with weight loss and symptoms consistent with chronic mesenteric ischemia. Thrombosis presents with continuous abdominal pain of insidious onset. The pain becomes gradually worse and may be associated with bloody diarrhea secondary to ischemic necrosis of the intestinal mucosa. Radiologic examination of the abdomen usually reveals nonspecific generalized bowel distention. *Arteriography* is essential in the diagnosis. *The occlusion of the superior mesenteric artery due to thrombosis is generally more proximal than it is with mesenteric embolism. The vessel also appears to taper at the level of the thrombosis.*

Because of the insidious onset of this process, diagnosis and treatment are usually delayed. At laparotomy, the extent of intestinal gangrene depends on the patency of the celiac axis and the inferior mesenteric artery. Unfortunately, in most cases, the degree of existing intestinal necrosis necessitates an extensive resection that is incompatible with life. Direct revascularization of the superior mesenteric artery is usually unsuccessful. However, it should be attempted in patients who are unlikely to survive an extensive intestinal resection. The proximal superior mesenteric artery is exposed at the root of the mesentery. The arteriosclerotic vessel can usually be palpated even in the absence of arterial pulsations. With the vessel exposed, an arteriotomy is performed. If there is backbleeding from the distal portion of the artery, revascularization should be performed with use of a vein graft anastomosed end to side to the aorta and the superior mesenteric artery. Once revascularization is accomplished, a second-look operation within 24 to 48 hours should be performed in order to determine accurately the extent of the residual necrosis. Thrombectomy of the occluded proximal superior mesenteric artery should not be attempted, for it will uniformly fail. If there is no backbleeding through the arteriotomy, any attempt to revascularize is futile.

In general, spontaneous thrombosis of the superior mesenteric artery is a catastrophic event with a higher mortality rate and a poorer prognosis than mesenteric embolization.

CHRONIC MESENTERIC ISCHEMIA

Introduction

Chronic occlusive disease of the celiac, superior, and inferior mesenteric arteries may become symptomatic despite the excellent collateral network of the mesenteric circulation. In the majority of patients, the cause is arteriosclerosis at the takeoff and proximal portion of the superior mesenteric artery. The celiac axis is also frequently involved. Occlusion of the inferior mesenteric artery may become symptomatic if it is associated with disease of the superior mesenteric or hypogastric arteries.

Diagnosis

The characteristic symptoms of chronic mesenteric ischemia are: (1) *postprandial* epigastric and middle abdominal *pain.* This typically occurs 20 to 60 minutes after eating; (2) significant *weight loss,* which is suggestive of malignancy. This is due to malabsorption, anorexia, and reluctance to eat induced by the fear of pain associated with food intake.

The physical examination is generally unrevealing with the exception of an epigastric bruit that is often detected. Other signs of generalized arteriosclerosis are usually present. In the absence of remarkable physical findings, various tests are usually performed. Upper and lower gastrointestinal series, abdominal sonography, and computerized tomography are seldom rewarding. Malabsorption testing may reveal an excess of fecal fat and decreased xylose absorption.

Examinations that are diagnostic are aortography and *selective angiography* of the celiac trunk and the superior mesenteric artery. The anterior projection will demonstrate the collateral circulation of the mesenteric vascular arch with the marginal artery of Drummond. However, the stenotic lesions can be clearly and accurately visualized in the *lateral projection.* Once the extent of the disease is well appreciated, the proper surgical procedure can be designed.

Treatment

Symptomatic occlusive disease of the visceral arteries is beyond the limits of any form of conservative approach. Acute thrombosis at the site of a stenotic lesion is a real threat with disastrous sequelae. Vascular reconstruction is the only realistic choice.

Revascularization of the Superior Mesenteric Artery. *Thromboendarterectomy with or without Patch Angioplasty* has been successfully employed in the treatment of mesenteric ischemia. The diseased proximal portion of the superior mesenteric artery is easily approached retroperitoneally by dissection on top of the aorta, just proximal to the left renal vein. The inferior mesenteric vein may have to be divided to allow liberal mobilization of the mesenteric root. Isolation of the vessel is sometimes difficult and necessitates interruption of multiple lymphatic channels and sympathetic fibers (Fig. 16–3). Aortic clamping is done proximal to the renal arteries and results in temporary ischemia of the kidneys. Because of the above disadvantages, this method of reconstruction is not widely used.

Bypass grafting is the preferred technique of revascularization of the superior mesenteric artery. This procedure is done through a midline incision. The transverse colon is retracted cephalad, exposing the mesenteric root. The

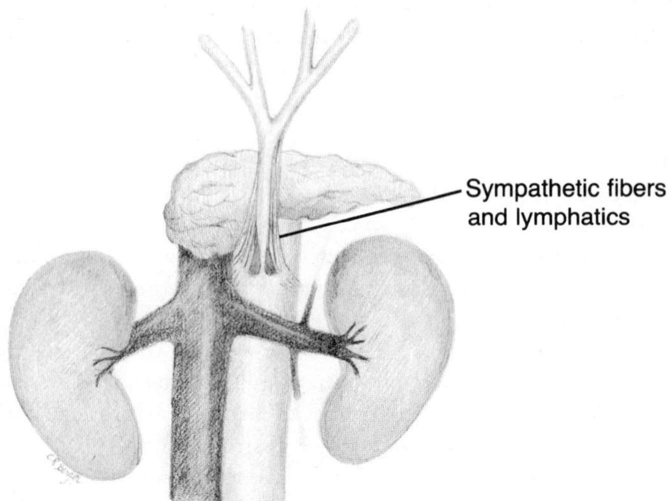

Figure 16–3. Exposure of the superior mesenteric artery.

arteriosclerotic superior mesenteric artery, which is deep-seated and considerably large in diameter, is detected by palpation. The overlying tissues are dissected, and the artery is exposed for a length of 3 cm. Silastic vessel loops are placed around it. A second team may harvest the saphenous vein. Then the infrarenal aorta is exposed as for an aortoiliac reconstruction. A tunnel is created through the mesentery. After systemic heparinization, the aorta is clamped with a partial occlusion clamp, and an aortotomy is performed. The reversed piece of the saphenous vein is sutured in place with continuous suture of 5–0 prolene. The graft is clamped next to the anastomosis with a soft Edward's clip, and the partial occlusion clamp is removed. The graft is passed through the tunnel and is anastomosed without tension to a soft portion of the superior mesenteric artery. The arteriotomy is best done on the medial aspect of the artery. All clamps are then removed, and flow through the graft is verified. This approach is technically easy and can be done with minimal time of warm intestinal ischemia. The peritoneum is approximated, and the wound is closed in layers.

Revascularization of the Celiac Axis. The celiac artery may be successfully revascularized by endarterectomy or by bypass grafting. In order to expose the artery, the lesser omentum is divided. The stomach is retracted inferiorly, and the liver is gently retracted upward. The peritoneum is incised proximal to the pancreas, and the muscular fibers of the diaphragmatic crus are severed with electrocautery. This exposes the *supraceliac* aorta and the celiac trunk (Fig. 16–4). For an isolated lesion of this vessel, a vein graft is used, anastomosed to the infrarenal aorta, and tunneled posteriorly to the pancreas. For combined revascu-

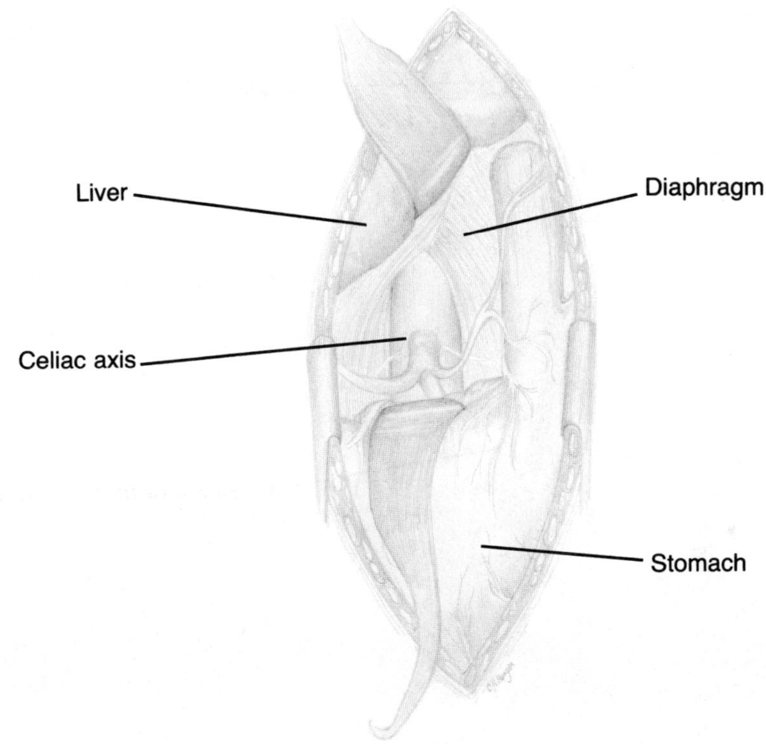

Figure 16-4. Exposure of the celiac axis and the supraceliac aorta.

larization of the superior mesenteric and celiac arteries, a 12- to 6-mm bifurcating Dacron graft is preferred (Fig. 16–5). In general, bypass of the aorta to one of the three branches of the celiac artery achieves the objectives of the surgeon.

ANEURYSMS OF THE SPLACHNIC ARTERIES

Aneurysm of the Splenic Artery

Aneurysms of the splenic artery are the most common aneurysms of the visceral arteries. The majority of patients are females in *their third* or *seventh decade of life.* Various contributing factors have been implicated in the pathogenesis of splenic artery aneurysms. The most common cause seems to be *medial degeneration* of the arterial wall. It is postulated that multiparity is a contributing factor to the development of medial degeneration of the visceral arteries. The second most common cause of splenic artery aneurysms is arteriosclerosis. Congenital and

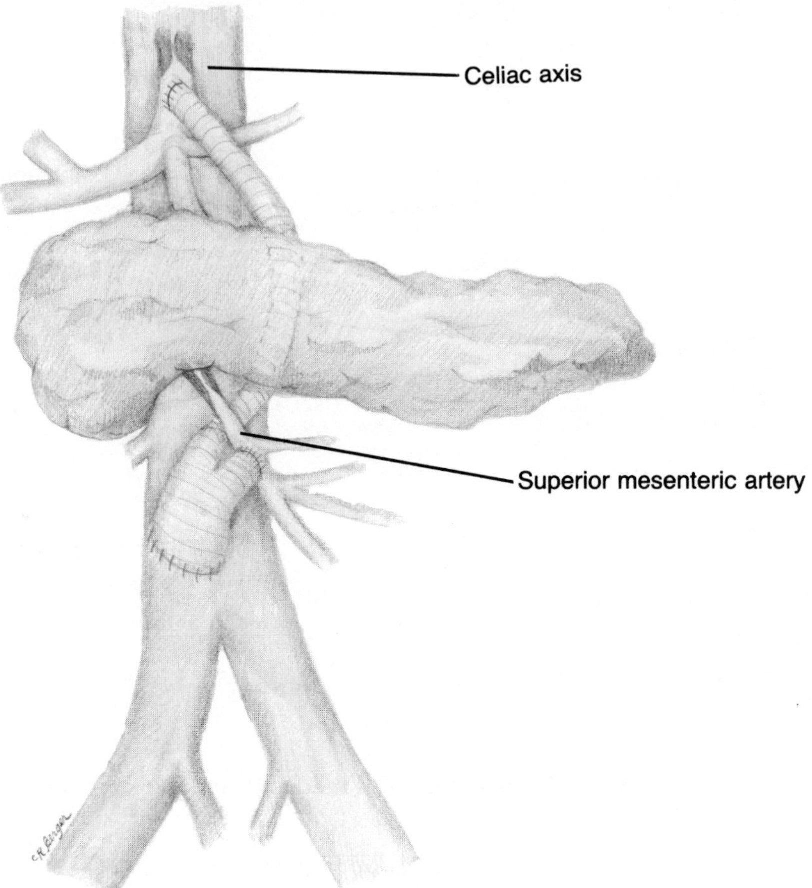

Figure 16-5. Combined revascularization of the superior mesenteric and celiac arteries.

mycotic aneurysms associated with an arterial injury or arteriopathy are seen infrequently.

The majority of patients with aneurysms of the splenic artery are asymptomatic. A few patients will complain of vague discomfort in the left upper quadrant. These lesions are usually detected incidentally during a radiologic examination. They may present as *calcifications* of the left upper quadrant. An arteriogram is necessary for a definite diagnosis of a splenic artery aneurysm. However, a bruit may be occasionally heard over the left upper quadrant. Unlike abdominal aortic aneurysms, which are palpable, aneurysms of the splenic artery are not usually detected on physical examination.

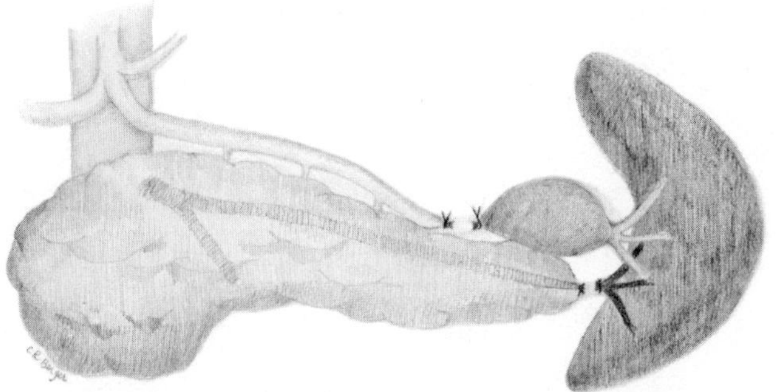

Figure 16-6. Distal splenic artery aneurysm.

Seven to 9 percent of these aneurysms will eventually rupture. The incidence of the rupture is much higher during pregnancy. The mortality rate associated with a rupture is over 25 percent. It may occur either as a free rupture, initially in the lesser sac and then extending into the free peritoneal cavity, or as a rupture in an adjacent viscus such as the stomach. Because of the considerable risk of rupture, all aneurysms of the splenic artery should be surgically treated with the exception of those in an elderly patient with multiple medical problems. An aneurysm of the distal splenic artery is best treated with *resection* and splenectomy (Fig. 16-6). When the aneurysm involves the proximal artery, proximal and distal ligation with preservation of the spleen is sufficient (Fig. 16-7). The results of surgical treatment of splenic artery aneurysms are excellent, and the operative risk is low.

Aneurysm of the Superior Mesenteric Artery

The majority of aneurysms of the superior mesenteric artery are *mycotic*. They should be suspected in a bacterial endocarditis patient who develops epigastric pain or an expanding tender abdominal mass. A few arteriosclerotic and traumatic aneurysms are occasionally seen. These may be either asymptomatic or present with symptoms of intestinal ischemia. They are prone to rupture; for this reason, they should be treated surgically. The preferred surgical procedure is ligation and resection of the aneurysms with distal revascularization with use of a reversed piece of autogenous vein.

Aneurysm of the Celiac Artery

Aneurysms of the celiac artery occur rather infrequently, and they are mostly associated with arteriosclerosis. A few mycotic, traumatic, and congenital aneurysms have also been reported.

The most frequent manifestations of these lesions are vague abdominal discomfort, occasional gastrointestinal complaint, or findings such as obstructive

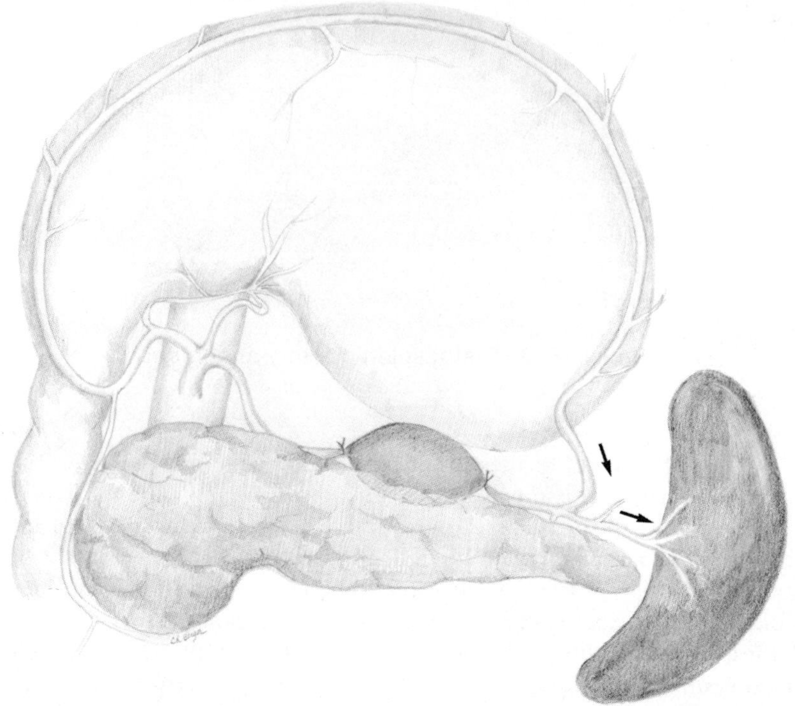

Figure 16–7. Proximal splenic artery aneurysm.

jaundice or gastrointestinal bleeding referred to adjacent organs. Occasionally, they may be associated with symptoms of intestinal ischemia.

The tendency to rupture justifies surgical approach to these lesions. The aneurysms may be either excised or excluded. Distal revascularization is accomplished with either a prosthetic or autogenous vein graft.

Aneurysm of the Hepatic Artery

The hepatic artery is *the second most common site of aneurysmal disease of the visceral arteries*. These aneurysms may be associated with (1) arteriosclerosis, (2) medial degeneration, and (3) trauma. They may be mycotic in origin.

The majority of these lesions are asymptomatic and are discovered incidentally during a laparotomy. In the symptomatic group of patients, the most frequent complaint is epigastric and right upper quadrant pain. The symptoms may mimic the pain of chronic cholecystitis. Aneurysms of the hepatic artery may present with various patterns of biliary symptomatology due either to obstruction or intrabiliary rupture. On x-rays, they may demonstrate calcification or displacement of adjacent structures. Arteriography is confirmatory. They are surgically treated by excision or obliteration.

RENAL ARTERY HYPERTENSION

Surgical importance of renal artery occlusive disease was considered by Goldblatt in 1938. Experimental renal artery hypertension in animals could be divided into two categories:

Two Kidney Hypertension

Two kidney hypertension is developed by clamping one renal artery while leaving the contralateral renal artery intact. In this animal, increased renin content and secretion in the clamped kidney with increased aldosterone secretions are observed. Sodium and water are retained initially, but these will be excreted by the opposite kidney due to increased blood pressure and glomerular filteration rate. Thus, sodium and water balance will be returned to normal.

Removal of the clamp on the renal artery cures two kidney hypertension, and this represents so-called unilateral renal artery stenosis and is considered to be renin dependent.

One Kidney Hypertension

One kidney hypertension is produced by clamping one renal artery following nephrectomy of the opposite side. In this situation, renin production from the clamped kidney increases and stimulates aldosterone production from the adrenal cortex. Excess sodium and water caused by the increased amount of aldosterone cannot be excreted since the opposite kidney does not exist. Therefore, volume-dependent hypertension develops that reduces the plasma-renin-angiotensin activity to normal. This type of hypertension is considered to be similar to bilateral renal artery stenosis and responds to the restriction of dietary salt and water.

It is also interesting to know that in the case of Goldblatt's experiment, the blood pressure elevation did not persist for more than 6 weeks after arterial constriction in the dog unless the contralateral renal artery was also constricted or the contralateral kidney was also removed, while in rats, sheep, and rabbits, constriction of one main renal artery alone usually caused persistent hypertension.

The common cause of renal artery stenosis is considered to be atherosclerosis, which usually obstructs the blood flow at the main renal artery, partially or completely. In contrast, another cause of renal artery stenosis or occlusion is fibromuscular dysplasia, which usually causes multiple areas of stenosis along the renal artery as a "chain of lakes" style. In addition, it is noteworthy to remember that following renal trauma, often renal ischemia may produce the same situation. Renal artery occlusive disease leading to renal ischemia may cause renal vascular hypertension, renal failure, or both.

Renin presumably acts on the substrate synthetized by the liver to produce decapeptide, angiotensin No. 1, which is eventually split by the enzyme in the blood to an octapeptide, angiotensin No. 2, which is the most important active pressor agent. (Vasoconstriction is due to constriction of the smooth muscle in the arteriolar wall and indirectly by increasing aldosterone production, which causes retention of sodium and water with expansion of extracellular fluid volume.)

DIAGNOSTIC APPROACHES

There are various tests available for detecting renal hypertension including radioisotope roentgenogram, angiotensin infusion, rapid sequence intravenous pyelogram, and pyelogram urea washout test, etc. The most common studies would be an arteriogram combined with split function study or renal vein renin study.

The split function study is based on the fact that the ischemic kidney reabsorbs more sodium and water. Excessive absorption of creatine, insulin, and pallor aminohippurate are also noted in addition to these chemical changes. Initially, this study (Howard test) was considered as positive when the urine volume from the affected kidney is reduced by 50 percent and the urinary sodium concentration is reduced by 15 percent or more compared to a patient with a well-hydrated and normal salt diet.

The most important test, however, is the renal vein renin determination. Care should be taken prior to renal vein renin study to assure adequate sodium depletion in the patient by maintaining a strict low sodium diet, using diuretics, etc. All antihypertensive medications must be discontinued at least 2 weeks prior to plasma renin determination. Should it be impossible, at least specific renin blocking substances including propranolol, α-methyldopa, etc., should be stopped. Guanethidine, which is the antihypertensive agent, may be of choice during this particular period since it does not block the renin. Administration of hydralazine before determining the level of plasma renin may stimulate the production of renin from the ischemic kidney. Positive renal vein renin ratio that exceeds 1.5 establishes the diagnosis of renal vascular hypertension, and prognosis is better with a higher ratio. It is important to know that the renin ratio may be lower than 1.4 in some patients with renal artery stenosis. It is also helpful to investigate the urinary catecholamine level and the urinary aldosterone level and, in addition, a rapid-sequence intravenous urogram. In intravenous pyelogram, discrepancy in renal length, calyceal appearance, time, and concentration of contrast medium on delayed film are three essential factors to assess renal artery stenosis.

Renal arteriography with oblique view is quite important with selected catheterization of each renal artery for evaluation and selection of corrective method.

TREATMENT

Decision Making

The objective of surgical procedure for the renal artery stenosis is to restore the normal circulatory flow through the renal artery of the affected kidney. However, renal vascular hypertension is usually an indication for such an operation. Accordingly, it is essential to consider that renal vascular hypertension and severe renal decompensation may both be indication for surgical repair of the renal artery stenosis.

Differentiation from other surgically correctable causes of hypertension such as pheochromocytoma, coarctation of the aorta, renal artery stenosis, Cushing's disease, and hyperaldosteronism should be done.

Surgical treatment is advised for all patients shown to have significant renal artery disease. The patients with the diagnosis of nonvascular hypertension should not be operated on but followed closely. Renal revascularization should be attempted only if renal function deteriorates in order to prevent further deterioration even though hypertension may not be improved. The best surgical treatment at this time is considered to be aortorenal bypass with autogenous saphenous vein. Autogenous artery such as the splenic artery in nonarteriosclerotic patients may be considered as an alternative, but the performance of such a procedure may prolong the surgical procedure and may not be necessary or recommendable. Because of the progressive nature of this disease, careful postoperative follow-up is essential. These patients should be followed monthly and then annually, and renal arteriography should be done if graft occlusion is suspected.

Surgical Approach

Aortorenal Bypass. This could be easily done by using a reverse saphenous vein. If the diameter of the autogenous saphenous vein is less than 5 mm, PTFE (polytetrafluoroethylene) graft may be in order (Fig. 16–8). The right renal artery is located behind the vena cava, so care should be taken in dissection and retraction in that area.

Endarterectomy. The second method of renal artery reconstruction that is not as popular as bypass would be endarterectomy. In this situation, however, it is important to make the incision beyond the junction of the renal artery and the aorta and to extend the incision to the aortic side in order to remove the entire atheromatic material. In addition, it is often necessary to secure the distal portion if the intima with a 6.0 prolene in order to avoid flapping when the flow is established. Finally, patch angioplasty is often required in order to minimize unnecessary narrowing of the renal artery (Fig. 16–9). It is considered, however, that aortorenal bypass may be the superior procedure over endarterectomy.

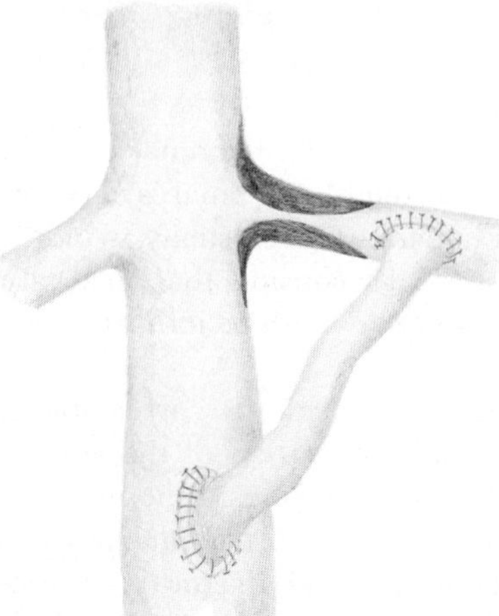

Figure 16–8. Aortorenal bypass.

Another important factor is to minimize the period of time that the renal blood supply is occluded. It is generally accepted under normal thermic conditions that the renal artery may be clamped within a 45-min duration without further difficulty. If such renal anoxia is prolonged, postoperative renal shutdown may develop. In such a situation, local hypothermia with saline or hypothermic perfusion could be used.

The result of surgical treatment in such patients is excellent. Approximately more than half are completely cured. Forty percent are significantly improved, and only 10 percent were ineffective. It is also interesting to know that treatment of renal vascular hypertension in children is quite promising not only in the results of the high cure rate of renal hypertension but also in preventing the deterioration of renal function.

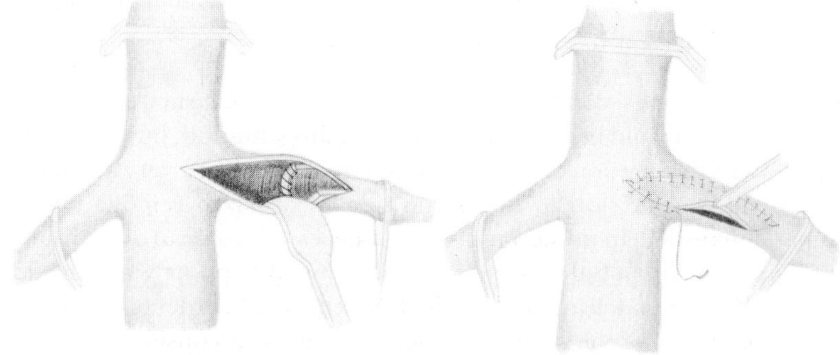

Figure 16–9. Endarterectomy of renal artery.

Percutaneous Transluminal Angioplasty of the Renal Artery. Another procedure is percutaneous transluminal dilatation of the renal artery. This procedure, known as Grantzig procedure, is gaining popularity; however, longterm results await to be seen.

Ex Vivo Renal Artery Reconstruction. This procedure is so-called benchwork surgery. In this procedure, the kidney with the renal artery is removed from the body and subjected to careful reconstruction and then reimplanted. This procedure is not desirable because of the ischemia that occurs during the repair.

BIBLIOGRAPHY

Bergan JJ: Recognition and treatment of intestinal ischemia. *Surg Clin North Am* 47:109, 1967.

Harper DR, Buist TAS: Selective angiography in acute mid-gut ischemia. *Gut* 19:132, 1978.

Jones EL, Finney GG: Splenic artery aneurysms: a reappraisal. *Arch Surg* 97:640, 1968.

Kraft RO, Fry WJ: Aneurysms of the celiac artery. *Surg Gynecol Obstet* 117:563, 1963.

Lord RSA, Stoney RJ, Wylie EJ: Coeliac-axis compression. *Lancet* 2:795, 1968.

Ottinger LW: The surgical management of acute occlusion of the superior mesenteric artery. *Ann Surg* 188:721, 1978.

Pierce GE: Brockenbrough ED: The spectrum of mesenteric infarction. *Am J Surg* 119:233, 1970.

Reul GJ Jr., Wukasch DC, Sandiford FM, et al: Surgical treatment of intestinal angina. Report of 25 patients. *Surgery* 75:682, 1974.

Rob D: Surgical diseases of the celiac and mesenteric arteries. *Arch Surg* 93:21, 1966.

Stanley JC, Thompson NW, Fry WJ: Splanchnic artery aneurysms. *Arch Surg* 101:689, 1970.

Stoney RJ, et at: Revascularization methods in chronic visceral ischemia caused by atherosclerosis. *Ann Surg* 186:468, 1977.

Weaver DH, Fleming RJ, Barnes WA: Aneurysm of the hepatic artery. Value of arteriography in the surgical management. *Surgery* 64:891, 1968.

Westcott JL, Ziter FMH: Aneurysms of the splenic artery. *Surg Gynecol Obstet* 136:541, 1973.

CHAPTER SEVENTEEN

Inferior Vena Cava Interruption

Pulmonary embolism is the most common cause of hospital deaths. This is secondary to thrombus formation in the deep veins of the calf or pelvis.

Most patients with venous thromboembolism can be treated successfully by anticoagulation; however, certain patients will require surgical interruption of the vena cava to prevent pulmonary embolism.

INDICATIONS

1. Pulmonary embolism in spite of adequate anticoagulation.
2. Presence of a contraindication to anticoagulation, eg, bleeding, recent cerebrovascular accident or after neurosurgery.
3. Recurrent embolism.
4. Septic embolism.
5. Less common causes include core pulmonale believed to be due to recurrent embolism, and prophylactically when a large thrombus is identified in a proximal vein.

METHODS

Vena caval interruption can be achieved by two main techniques:

1. Direct surgery on the inferior vena cava.
2. Percutaneous transjugular interruption.

Direct Surgery on the Inferior Vena Cava

This is achieved by an operation that requires general anesthesia and stopping of anticoagulation. After the inferior vena cava is exposed by a retroperitoneal approach, it can be ligated, plicated or clipped with a serrated clip.

Ligation is associated with an incidence of leg swelling and a rate of venous insufficiency complications higher than with the other techniques. It is also associated with a higher incidence of hemodynamic disturbances such as temporary hypotension. On the other hand, it provides complete occlusion of the inferior vena cava, which is necessary for septic embolism.

Both plication and clipping allow for some flow through the inferior vena cava, and although eventually the vena cava at that point will completely occlude, sufficient collaterals might develop and therefore reduce the incidence of leg swelling and sequela of venous insufficiency.

All these procedures should be done at a level just below the renal veins to avoid a cul-de-sac formation and to exclude the right gonadal vein. If the procedure is done by a transperitoneal approach as recommended by some surgeons, the left ovarian vein should be ligated in females. The procedures just described are still associated with about 7.6 percent recurrent embolism. This has been attributed to large collaterals entering the inferior vena cava above the interruption site and to the presence of a thrombus at a higher level (for example, in the renal vein or the right atrium). The mortality from direct surgery on the inferior vena cava has been reported in the range of from 6 to 40 percent, although it should be remembered that the underlying disease in these very sick patients contributes significantly to this mortality.

Percutaneous Transjugular Procedures

In the last decade two new devices have been introduced: the Mobin-Udin umbrella and the Hunter-Session occluder. Both can be inserted under local anesthesia and under fluoroscopic control, a distinct advantage over other procedures since general anesthesia and more traumatic surgery are avoided in this usually very sick population of patients.

The Mobin-Udin umbrella is available in two sizes, 23 mm or 28 mm. The appropriate size should be used to avoid dislodgement of the umbrella. Its separation from the stylet should be assured prior to insertion. The umbrella is usually released just below the renal vein, usually between L3 and 4 (Fig. 17–1). Although it is made of thrombogenic material, its perforations remain open for

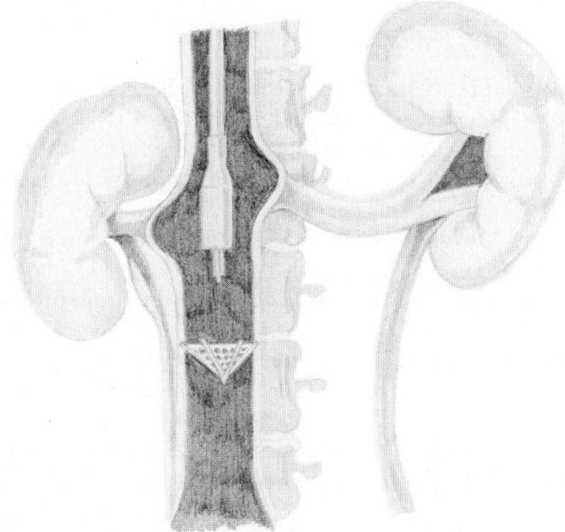

Figure 17–1. Mobin-Udin umbrella.

long periods of time. Because of the sharp needle points of this umbrella that help fix it in position to the walls of the inferior vena cava, complications due to perforation and hematomas have been reported. The reported mortality rate for insertion of the Mobin-Udin umbrella is 4 to 16 percent.

The Hunter-Session detachable balloon occluder (Fig. 17–2) can be inserted while the patient is still on anticoagulants, since it has no sharp edges. It also has a built-in capability for venography to permit precise placement and, in addition, it fits any size vena cava. The balloon deflates slowly over 12 to 14 months, but it also incites fibrous reaction where it contacts the venous wall to cause the vena cava to scar and encapsulate the balloon remnant. Although it completely occludes the vena cava, the incidence of leg swelling is about 13 percent in the patients who remain on heparin and about three times that number if the patients are off heparin. The reported mortality rate with this procedure is 14 percent and is due to the original disease.

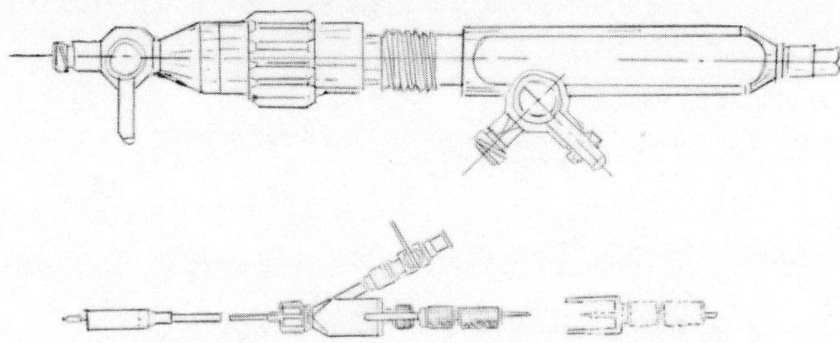

Figure 17–2. Hunter-Session occluder.

BIBLIOGRAPHY

Hunter JA, Dye WS, Javid H, Najafi H, Goldin MD, Serry C: Permanent transvenous balloon occlusion of the inferior vena cava. *Ann Surg* 186:491, 1977.

Donaldson MC, Wirthlin LS, Donaldson GA: Thirty-year experience with surgical interruption of the inferior vena cava for prevention of pulmonary embolism. *Ann Surg* 191:367, 1980.

Adams JT, Feingold BE, DeWeese JA: Comparative evaluation of ligation and partial interruption of the inferior vena cava. *Arch Surg* 103:272, 1971.

Couch NP, Baldwin SS, Crane C: Mortality and morbidity rates after inferior vena cava clipping. *Surg* 77:106, 1975.

Mobin-Udin K, Utley JR, Bryant LR: The inferior vena cava umbrella filter. In Sasahara AA, Sonnenblock EH, Lesch M (eds.): *Pulmonary Emboli,* New York, Grune & Stratton, 1975, pp 163–171.

Pollack EW, Sparks FG, Barker WF: Inferior vena cava interruption: Indications and results with caval ligation, clips and intra caval devices in 110 cases. *J. Cardiovasc Surg.* 15:69, 1974.

Wingrel M, Bernhard VM, Madisson F, et al: Comparison of caval filters in the management of venous thromboembolism. *Arch Surg* 113:1264, 1978.